RECLAIM YOUR HEALTH

Learn how to overcome the most common chronic illnesses

MEN'S HEALTH

By Award Winning Author

Dr. Harris Phillip

BSc, MSc, MBBS, FRCOG, FACOG, LLM

Table of Contents

Foreword

By Professor Ali Nakash

While continuing with his 30+ years of experience in clinical practice, Harris has decided to sum up much of what he has gained from seeing and treating thousands, maybe millions, of patients with many medical problems over the years. In his summary, compiled into a series of twelve chunk-sized books, the reader is provided with usable tools presented in a simple, readily digestible format to allow everyone to benefit. From the least medically inclined among us to the nursing student, the pharmacy student, the nurse, the pharmacist, the midwifery student, the midwife, the medical student, and the trained doctor, whether junior or senior. In essence, there are useful nuggets of easy-to-follow guidance for all. In the first book in the series, he starts with a disease we all dread. Many, including my wife, call it that disease.... You certainly know the disease to which I refer; it is cancer. Reading through the pages of the first book in this series, I was immediately impressed with the presentation. Such a complex condition was condensed into such simple and easy-to-follow guidance. Not only has he addressed cancer from its cellular level, but he has also extended the discussion to allow you, the reader, to appreciate plausible causative agents for this condition once it is initiated. He gives some Reclaim Your Health-Cancer, he gives some insight into how the disease process flourishes, and towards the end of the book, he addresses how we can make ourselves cancer-proof. Making ourselves cancer-proof, I find, is particularly interesting since it allows both medical and non-medical personnel to explore avenues through which they can empower both themselves and their patients as together we fight this dreaded disease. In the other books of this series, which are being completed, the approach is the same, whether it is addressing Alzheimer's disease, cardiovascular disease, diabetes, or the other chronic health challenges of our time. I am particularly impressed with the presentation, the relative simplicity, and the inherent usefulness of this series, which doubtlessly will empower and serve as a useful companion handbook on our journey to reclaiming our health. Mr Phillip is an award-winning author for his book STOP! It's Not Too Late: Adding Years to Your Life and Life to Your Years Using the BMS Model, a book which I call an encyclopaedic guide to healthy living. But in this book series, I think he has outdone himself as he seeks to provide the tools that we all need to reclaim our health. He has most definitely put his years of training and experience in capsule form through the various books in this series. Mr Phillip is a trained senior consultant obstetrician and gynaecologist. He has displayed his abundance of knowledge through the ease with which he addresses the various chronic health challenges of our times. This series, for me, represents an interesting and empowering piece of medical science which has been presented in a digestible format for even the non-medical personnel among us. I am therefore moved to make this bold prediction that once you start reading these books, you will find it difficult to stop because of the timeliness and appropriateness of their contents.

A Note from the author

In a world where healthcare often feels impersonal, reactive, and fragmented, Reclaim Your Health offers a bold and compassionate alternative. This twelve-book series was born from a simple yet powerful conviction: that patients deserve not only access to care, but ownership of it.

As a clinician, innovator, and educator, I have witnessed first-hand the transformative impact of knowledge—when patients understand their bodies, their conditions, and their options, they become active participants in their healing. This series is designed to bridge the gap between clinical expertise and everyday experience, translating complex medical concepts into clear, actionable guidance.

Ten volumes have already been published, this is the eleventh, each tackling a vital dimension of conservative care—with clarity, empathy, and scientific rigor. The remaining volume is in an advanced stage of preparation, and I will complete the series by the end of March.

Reclaim Your Health is more than a collection of books. It is a movement toward autonomy, dignity, and informed decision-making. It complements our broader mission—through medical device innovation and workforce development—to reshape healthcare from the ground up.

Whether you are a patient seeking answers, a clinician striving to educate, or a policymaker looking to support sustainable care models, this series is for you. May it inspire confidence, spark dialogue, and above all, help you reclaim what matters most: your health.

Harris Phillip

Founder, Philburn Academy

Healthcare Entrepreneur & Innovator

United Kingdom

Introduction

Several years ago, I was employed as a teacher, which incidentally was my first professional job. While entering the classroom to deliver a biology lecture to a group of students at Saint Andrews High School, who were preparing to write the General Certificate of Education examination (GCE or GCSE as referred to in the UK), a young man who claimed he had no interest in biology collected his books and was leaving the classroom to go to the library. The lecture was designed to highlight the characteristics of living things and to help distinguish the living from the dead. I commenced the lecture with the statement, 'Once one starts living, he/she starts dying'. Inherent in that statement is that both living and dying are processes. Even deeper is the realisation that what we refer to as life is simply a grant. You see, we are given two dates and a dash. The dash is our life, the period between our date of birth and our date of death. Upon hearing this introduction, the young man made an about-turn and asked permission to attend my lecture. I did not convert him into a biologist, but he left the class much better informed. Today, this young man is a politician. The dash is the focus of this book: how can we extend the dash to delay our date of death? I prefer to look at the whole scenario as a rubber band that can be stretched between two points, the two points being the date of birth and the date of death. We can do nothing about our date of birth; that date is beyond our control, but if my analogy of a rubber band is fully understood and since our date of birth cannot be seriously influenced by our action or inaction, the rubber band concept to hold, it means that the dash can be extended and thus we can delay our date of death. My paternal grandmother, for instance, lived to a ripe old age of 115. She lived a fully independent life, still being able to cook and care for herself in her 115th year. This is not widespread, I hear you say, and my response is: why not? Do we have any skills, knowledge, or abilities in the current era to approach this lifespan and make it more of the expected norm as opposed to an occasional event? It is with this burning desire that I have used my medical knowledge gleaned in the field, as well as my extensive research, the skills of which I learned as a university student in organic and biochemistry at a top 10 USA university, as I pursued a PhD degree in Biochemistry. This training not only provided me with the skills and tools which I needed to pursue the more inquisitive aspect of my person but also alerted me to the value of research. Thus, when faced with a challenging question, I revert to research to help me determine the answer. In observing the lifestyle of my paternal grandmother, my 30+ years of medical practice, drawing on the knowledge gleaned through my research and from my study in organic chemistry, leading to my master's degree and my sojourn through the biochemistry classroom, I believe that we have an opportunity to delay the second date, the date of death, by stretching in rubber band style the duration of the dash. This is the purpose of this book series: providing tools, suggestions, and basic information that will hopefully allow you to prolong your dash and live a more dynamic and healthier lifestyle, thus adding years to your life and life to your years. I will aim to provide books on each of the nine chronic ailments, suggesting how best one can delay the insult on our bodies, hence allowing us to live a more complete, fun-filled life, a guide to which has been developed in one of my earlier books, using the BMS approach, an award-winning book. In this book series, we will look at cancer, Alzheimer's, dementia and diseases of the brain, heart disease and strokes, diabetes, arthritis, obesity, chronic lung disease, and chronic kidney diseases, hoping that this serves as a useful handbook – guide, if you will – in understanding and defeating the most common chronic ailments affecting human beings on planet earth. I know that you may be stunned: why have a trained obstetrician and gynaecologist got involved in the writing of books addressing various aspects of health, some of which may be remote from obstetrics (care of pregnant ladies during their pregnancy and childbirth) and gynaecology (the branch of medicine which deals with the functions and diseases specific to women and girls, specifically those related to the reproductive system)? This discipline is the only medical discipline which allows one to practise all the facets of medicine. It, therefore, means that any good obstetrician or gynaecologist, because of the demands on his scope of practice, needs to be above average in his knowledge of internal medicine, surgery, paediatrics, social and preventive medicine, care of the elderly, and neonatology. Hence, my familiarity with these various disciplines and the related physiology has empowered me in the provision of this book series, which I am hopeful will be an empowering tool to help many understand elements of their health while simultaneously allowing them to know when things are wrong and therefore the need to seek medical advice. Hopefully, the message is that the earlier a disease process is found, the more options will be available for management, and the more likely a full cure will be realised.

Chapter 1
Male Health from Birth to Middle Age: A Lifespan Overview

Infancy and Early Childhood (0–5 years) Infancy (Birth–2 years)

Biological & Physical Development

- **Sex differentiation** occurs prenatally under the influence of testosterone and dihydrotestosterone (DHT).
  - At birth:
  - Testes may not fully descend (cryptorchidism); most descend by 6 months.
  - Penis size varies; micropenis is rare and usually hormonal.
- **"Mini-puberty"** (first 3–6 months):
  - Temporary surge in testosterone.
  - Important for brain masculinization, penile growth, and testicular development.

Immune & General Health

- Immune system is immature → higher infection risk.
- Circumcision (if performed) slightly lowers future UTI and STI risk.
- Higher risk than females for:

- Sudden Infant Death Syndrome (SIDS)
- Respiratory distress
- Congenital anomalies

Neurodevelopment

- Male brains mature slightly slower than female brains, hence the abused belief that females mature earlier than males.
- Early motor skills often develop faster, language skills slightly later on average.
- Growth is rapid, with significant development of the brain, immune system, and motor skills.
- Boys tend to be slightly heavier at birth and may experience more earlier-life respiratory infections due to narrower airways.
- Nutrition, vaccinations, and safe physical exploration play major roles in long-term health.
- Early bonding and emotional security support healthy stress responses later in life.

Childhood (6–12 years)

Growth & Hormones

Physical Development

- Growth remains linear.

- Body composition: slightly more lean muscle mass than females.
- Testes and penis remain small until puberty.

Cognitive & Emotional Health

- Logical reasoning improves.
- Emotional expression often socially discouraged → early emotional suppression patterns may begin.
- Boys may be less likely to report pain or distress.

Health Patterns

- Obesity risk may begin if diet/activity is poor.
- Dental issues common.
- Sports injuries increase.

Puberty & Adolescence (10–19 years)

Hormonal Changes

Physical Changes

- Growth spurt (typically 12–16 years).
- Increased muscle mass, bone density, and lung capacity.
- Testicular enlargement precedes penile growth.
- Spermatogenesis begins.

Brain Development

- Limbic system (emotion/reward) matures faster than prefrontal cortex (judgment).
- Increased impulsivity and risk-taking.
- Sleep cycle shifts later (circadian delay).

Mental Health

- Rising risk of:
  - Depression
  - Anxiety
  - Substance use
- Male suicide rates begin to exceed female rates in late adolescence.
- Body image concerns focus on muscularity rather than thinness.

Sexual & Reproductive Health

- Onset of sexual interest.
- Risk of STIs increases.
- Gynecomastia (temporary breast tissue growth) is common and usually resolves.
- Activation of the hypothalamic-pituitary-gonadal axis.
- Testosterone increases 20–30× from childhood levels.
- DHT drives:

  - Facial/body hair
  - Voice deepening
  - Genital maturation

Physical Changes

- Stable, low testosterone.
- Steady growth in height and weight.
- Genital growth is minimal.

Brain & Behaviour

- Increased physical activity and risk-taking tendencies.
- Higher incidence of:
  - ADHD
  - Autism spectrum disorders
- Emotional regulation still developing.

Health Risks

- Injuries (falls, burns, accidents) are a major cause of morbidity.
- Asthma more common in boys before puberty.

Preventive Focus

- Vaccinations
- Vision/hearing screening

- Early behavioural and developmental monitoring
- Steady physical growth continues, with boys often showing higher activity levels and greater muscle mass development.
- Common health concerns include asthma, allergies, and minor injuries due to active play.
- Cognitive and social development accelerates, making this a key period for building healthy habits around sleep, nutrition, and physical activity.
- Emotional regulation skills begin to solidify, influenced by family, school, and environment.

Adolescence (13–19 years)

- Puberty brings major hormonal changes, including increased testosterone, growth spurts, voice deepening, and reproductive maturation.
- Boys often experience rapid increases in muscle mass, height, and strength.
- Mental health becomes a critical focus: identity formation, peer pressure, and academic stress can influence emotional wellbeing.
- Risk-taking behaviours may increase due to brain development patterns, making guidance and supportive environments essential.

Early Adulthood (20–30 years)

Physical Peak

- **Peak testosterone**, muscle strength, reaction time, and fertility.

- Bone density peaks in late 20s.
- Cardiovascular system at maximal efficiency.

Health Risks

- Accidents remain the leading cause of death.
- High rates of:
- Alcohol use
- Risky behaviours
- STIs remain a concern.

Mental & Emotional Health

- Identity consolidation (career, relationships).
- Men are less likely to seek mental health care.
- Stress related to performance, finances, and masculinity norms.

Reproductive Health

- Fertility is high.
- Sperm quality optimal but sensitive to:
- Heat
- Smoking
- Obesity
- Anabolic steroid use

Pause for Thought

- For ease of convenience both in terms of reference and association, the male's life is sub-divided into convenient epochs.
- Infancy and early childhood refer to the period extending between birth and early childhood, a subject of that period, infancy extends between birth and two years.
- In males, sex differentiation occurs before birth and this is under the control of both testosterone and dihydrotestosterone (DHT).
- It is not unusual to find empty scrotal sacs in baby boys at the time of birth, the condition in which the testis does not fully descend is called cryptorchidism, however by six months of age the testis are usually fully descended into the scrotal sac.
- Within the first 3-6 months of life there is a temporary testosterone surge, referred to by some as a mini-puberty. This testosterone surge is important for brain masculinization, penile growth and testicular development.
- At this stage the immune system is immature, thus presenting a higher infection risk, there seems to be a higher risk for sudden infant death syndrome (SIDS), respiratory distress and congenital abnormality among young males than among females of similar ages.

- Male circumcision which is practiced in many cultures and in many religious groupings is thought to slightly lower the risk of a urinary tract infection as well as sexually transmitted diseases.
- There seems to be a higher risk for sudden infant death syndrome (SIDS), respiratory distress and congenital abnormality among young males than among females of similar ages.
- Male brains mature slightly slower than female brains, hence the belief that females mature earlier than males. Early motor skills tend to develop faster whilst language skills may lag.
- Boys tend to be heavier at birth and may experience more earlier life respiratory infections due to narrower airways.

Take home Nuggets

- In the age range 6-12 years, the period is dominated by physical development, linear growth and hormones, with a distinct difference in body's composition, with males slightly leaner and more muscular than females.
- Difference is also seen between boys and girls in the sphere of cognitive and emotional health. Logical reasoning improves during that time, because of the social discouragement of emotional expression, early emotional suppression patterns may begin and as a result boys may be less likely to report pain or distress.

- Health problems within this age group may be associated with obesity risk, if diet and activity levels are poor, dental issues and sports injuries.
- In the period between 10-19 years, hormonal changes induce physical changes which may include growth spurts between 12-and 16-year, increased muscle mass, bone density, and lung capacity. There may also be testicular enlargement which tends to precede penile growth. Spermatogenesis also begins.
- Brain development: the limbic system (emotion and reward) matures faster than the area of the brain (prefrontal cortex) which deals with judgement as a result there is an increased impulsivity and risk-taking activities. There is also evidence of circadian delay (that is a later shift in sleep cycles).
- There is also a rising risk of depression, anxiety, and substance use. Male suicide rates also begin to exceed female rates in late adolescent. There is a greater focus on masculinity rather than thinness and body image.
- In terms of sexual interest, it begins, so too is an increased risk of Sexually Transmitted Infections and temporary breast tissue growth or gynaecomastia. There is also an activation of the Hypothalamic-pituitary-gonad axis and an increase in testosterone level by 20 to 30 times over the childhood levels.

- The dihydrotestosterone drives facial/body hair, voice deepening, genital maturation and physical changes. There is also a steady growth in height and weight with minimal growth in the genitals.
- There is generally an increase in physical activity and risk taking tendencies with a higher incidence of Attention Deficit Hyperactivity Disorder, autism spectrum disorders, and emotional regulation is still being developed. Morbidity in this age group are mainly from falls, burns and accidents. Asthma is more common in males before puberty
- In early adulthood between 20-30 years, the male is at his physical peak, testosterone is at its peak, which ensures muscle strength, reaction time and fertility is at their peak. The cardio-vascular system is at its peak at this time whereas bone density peaks in the late 20's.

Chapter 2
Early midlife and Male/Female comparison

Early Midlife Transition (30–40 years)

Hormonal Shifts

- Testosterone declines ~1% per year after ~30.
- Changes are gradual, not abrupt like menopause.

Physical Changes

- Slower metabolism.
- Gradual increase in fat mass (especially visceral fat).
- Muscle mass declines if resistance training is absent.

Health Risks Begin to Rise

- Hypertension
- Dyslipidaemia
- Insulin resistance
- Sleep apnoea (especially with weight gain)

Mental Health

- Chronic stress accumulation.

- Increased risk of:
- Depression
- Burnout
- Emotional suppression may manifest as irritability or somatic symptoms.

Reproductive Considerations

- Fertility remains possible but sperm quality slowly declines.
- Increased genetic mutation risk in sperm with age.
- **7. Midlife (40–50 years)**

Endocrine Changes

- Testosterone decline may become clinically noticeable in some men:
- Fatigue
- Reduced libido
- Decreased muscle mass
- Mood changes
- Not all men experience symptoms.

Cardiovascular Health

- Heart disease risk rises sharply.
- Men develop coronary artery disease ~10 years earlier than women.
- Central obesity becomes a major risk factor.

Prostate & Urogenital Health

- Benign prostatic hyperplasia (BPH) may begin.
- Urinary symptoms can appear.
- Prostate cancer risk begins increasing (screening debates start here).

Mental & Cognitive Health

- Midlife reassessment ("midlife crisis" stereotype).
- Suicide risk peaks in middle-aged men in many countries.
- Cognitive speed may slow slightly; knowledge and expertise remain strong.

Cross-Cutting Themes in Male Health

- **1. Men Seek Less Preventive Care**
- Lower healthcare utilization.
- Higher likelihood of late diagnosis.
- **2. Socialization Effects**
- Emotional suppression
- Risk-taking encouraged
- Stoicism rewarded → delayed care

3. Key Modifiable Factors Across Life

- Physical activity

- Nutrition
- Sleep
- Stress management
- Social connection

Stage	Key Focus
• Birth–2	• Hormonal imprinting, immune vulnerability
• 2–10	• Brain development, injury prevention
• 10–19	• Puberty, mental health, risk behaviour
• 20–30	• Physical peak, identity formation
• 30–40	• Metabolic shift, stress accumulation
• 40–50	• Cardiovascular & hormonal health

Male vs Female Health Trajectories (Birth → Middle Age)

Early Life (Birth to ~10 years)

- **Similarities**
- Both sexes share broadly similar physiology before puberty, with only small differences in height and growth timing.
- **Differences**
- **Male infants**: Slightly higher vulnerability to respiratory infections and early mortality (supported by global health patterns).
- **Female infants**: Slightly stronger immune responses on average.

Adolescence (10–19 years)

- This is where sex-based health differences become clearly visible.

Males

- Testosterone drives rapid muscle growth, increased height, and higher physical risk-taking.
- Higher rates of injuries, road accidents, and early cardiovascular risk factors begin to appear.
- Mental health challenges often manifest as externalising behaviours (risk-taking, aggression).

Females

- Higher rates of non-fatal conditions begin to emerge, including headaches, musculoskeletal pain, and mood disorders.
- Hormonal cycles influence iron levels, mood, and metabolic patterns.
- Mental health challenges often manifest as internalising symptoms (anxiety, depression).
- **Young Adulthood (20–35 years)**

Males

- Peak physical performance but also higher rates of premature death from injuries, cardiovascular issues, and respiratory/liver diseases.
- Lifestyle factors (alcohol, smoking, occupational hazards) contribute significantly.

Females

- continue to experience higher rates of non-fatal illness and disability, including migraines, autoimmune conditions, and mental health disorders.
- Pregnancy and reproductive health add unique physiological demands.

Middle Age (36–50 years)

Males

- Cardiovascular risks accelerate hypertension, cholesterol imbalance, and heart disease become more common.
- Testosterone gradually declines, affecting energy, muscle mass, and mood.
- Higher mortality persists across most major disease categories.

Females

- Continue to live longer but with more years spent in ill-health due to chronic, non-fatal conditions.
- Musculoskeletal disorders, mental health conditions, and headaches remain more prevalent.
- Perimenopause begins for many, influencing mood, metabolism, and cardiovascular risk.

Why These Differences Occur

- Recent research shows that:
- Biology alone doesn't explain everything.
  A 2025 study found that while thousands of proteins differ between males and females, only a small fraction of these differences is genetically driven.

- Social and environmental factors—work, stress, education, lifestyle, and access to resources—play a major role in shaping health outcomes.
- Gender roles influence risk exposure, health-seeking behaviour, and stress patterns.

The Big Picture

Aspect	Males	Females
Life Expectancy	shorter	Longer
Illness burden	Low illness, higher death rates	Higher illness, lower death rates
Leading issues	Cardiovascular disease, injuries, liver and respiratory disease	Musculo-skeletal pain, mental health, headaches
Onset of differences	adolescence	adolescence
Midlife trajectory	Rising metabolic and cardiac risk	Rising chronic non-fatal conditions

Male health from birth to middle age is shaped by biology, environment, lifestyle, and emotional development. The most powerful protective factors across all stages include:

- Consistent physical activity
- Balanced nutrition
- Supportive relationships
- Healthy stress management
- Regular preventive health checks

Pause for Thought

- In early midlife from about age 30-40 years, there is a gradual decline in the male sex hormone by about 1% a year These changes though are gradual, unlike the relatively abrupt change seen in menopause.
- With the decline in the male sex hormone, comes physical changes, metabolism slows down and there is a gradual increase in fat and a decline muscle mass particularly if there is no effort in establishing a resistance training regime.
- Health challenges begin to rise, challenges like hypertension, dyslipidaemia, insulin resistance and sleep apnoea which is usually associated with weight gain.

- Mental health factors start having an effect which may be brought on by chronic stress, features such as depression and burnout, the effect of emotional suppression begins to manifest as irritability or somatic symptoms
- This decline also influences reproduction. Fertility is still possible, but the sperm quality slowly declines and with that there is an increased genetic mutation risk in sperm as one age.
- Between the ages of 40-50, the effect of endocrine changes mainly the decline in testosterone become clinically noticeable, this normally manifest as fatigue, reduced libido, and decreased muscle mass. This may be further accompanied by mood changes, though these changes may not be universal.
- These endocrine changes is also reflected in a sharp rise in heart disease. It is noted that men develop coronary artery disease about ten years earlier than women. Central obesity is a major risk marker.
- Issues with the prostate gland and urogenital system start to rise. Issues like benign prostatic hypertrophy may begin, urinary symptoms may appear and prostate cancer risk begins to rise.
- Mental and cognitive health typically takes a hit at this time and this is commonly referred to as midlife crisis, in this phase, suicide risks peaks, cognitive speed may slow slightly but knowledge and expertise remain strong.

- Unfortunately, men utilisation of health care services is less than females, as a result there is a higher likelihood of late diagnosis and socialisation may be also adversely affected with emotional suppression, risk taking behaviour and stoicism which may lead to delayed care.

Take home nuggets

- Though midlife presents the male with numerous potential adverse challenges, many of them are modifiable through physical activity, nutrition, sleep etiquette, proper stress management and improved social connectivity.
- Interestingly life for both males and females are virtually identical from birth to 10 years, that is both sexes share similar physiology with only small differences in height and growth timing.
- The slight differences noted between the sexes at this stage are male infants are more vulnerable to respiratory infections and early mortality as per findings found globally. In the female, there is a stronger immune system on average.
- During adolescence, the sex-based health differences become more clearly visible, testosterone, the dominant male sex hormone drives rapid muscle growth, increased height, and higher physical risk-taking, there are higher rates of injuries, road accidents, and

early cardiovascular risk factors appear, mental health challenges often manifest as risk taking behaviour and aggression.

- Females on the other hand have higher rates of non-fatal conditions such as headaches, musculoskeletal pains, and mood disorders. Their moods, metabolic patterns and iron levels are influenced by hormonal cycles. Here mental health challenges manifest as anxiety and depression, products of internalising symptoms.
- In young adulthood (age range 20-35), the differences between sexes continue to manifest. In males, there is peak physical performance but also a higher rate of premature death from injuries, cardiovascular issues and respiratory and liver disease, but lifestyle factors such as alcohol use, smoking, and exposure to environmental hazards contribute significantly.
- Females on the other hand, continue to experience higher rates of non-fatal illness and disability, including migraines, autoimmune conditions, and mental disorders with pregnancy and reproductive health adding unique physiological demands.
- In males age range 36-50, the period considered as middle age, cardiovascular risk accelerates secondary to hypertension, and cholesterol imbalance. Testosterone gradually declines, affecting energy, muscle mass, and mood. Sadly, higher mortality rates persist across most major disease categories.

- With females, though they live longer, more years are spent in ill health due to chronic, non-fatal conditions, musculoskeletal conditions, mental health conditions and headaches remain more prevalent. The effect of the perimenopause begins to show up, influencing mood, metabolism and cardiovascular risk.
- These differences can't be simply explained by biology; though there are thousands of different proteins between males and females, only a small fraction of these is genetically driven. Social and environmental factors seem to play a major role in shaping health outcomes. It must be noted though, that gender roles influence risk exposure, health seeking behaviour and stress patterns.

Chapter 3
Understanding Andropause

The Biological Changes in Men

As men approach andropause, they experience various biological changes that can significantly impact their overall health and well-being. Andropause, often referred to as male menopause, typically occurs in middle-aged men and is characterized by a gradual decline in testosterone levels. This hormonal shift can lead to a multitude of physiological changes, including weight gain, reduced muscle mass, and altered fat distribution. Understanding these biological changes is crucial for both men and their partners as they navigate this transitional phase in life.

One of the most notable changes during andropause is the decrease in testosterone production. Testosterone plays a vital role in maintaining muscle mass, energy levels, and metabolic rate. With lower testosterone levels, many men notice an increase in body fat, particularly around the abdomen. This redistribution of fat can lead to a more pronounced waistline, which is often linked to various health risks, including cardiovascular disease and diabetes. Recognizing this pattern can help men take proactive steps to manage their weight and overall health.

In addition to hormonal changes, andropause can also affect other biological systems. For instance, there is often a decline in the production of growth hormone and insulin-like growth factor, which are essential for muscle growth and maintenance. This decline contributes to the difficulty many men face in maintaining muscle mass as they age. As muscle mass decreases, metabolism slows down, making it easier to gain weight and harder to lose it. Addressing these changes through targeted exercise and nutrition can help mitigate some of the effects of andropause.

Psychological factors also play a role during this transitional phase, as men may experience mood swings, fatigue, and decreased motivation. These psychological changes can influence lifestyle choices, including diet and exercise habits. Men may find themselves less inclined to engage in physical activity or may turn to comfort foods, further exacerbating weight gain. It is essential for men and their partners to recognize these emotional and psychological changes as part of the andropause experience, fostering open communication and support to navigate these challenges together.

Ultimately, understanding the biological changes associated with andropause empowers men to take control of their health. By acknowledging the decline in testosterone and its effects on weight management, men can implement strategies that support their physical and emotional well-being. This might include regular exercise, a balanced diet rich in whole foods, and seeking guidance from healthcare practitioners. By addressing these changes proactively, men can navigate andropause more effectively, maintaining their strength and vitality during this life transition.

Symptoms and Emotional Impact

As men approach andropause, a variety of physiological and emotional symptoms may emerge, significantly impacting their daily lives and relationships. Common physical symptoms include fatigue, reduced libido, and changes in body composition, such as increased fat accumulation and decreased muscle mass. These changes are often accompanied by hormonal fluctuations, particularly a decline in testosterone levels, which can lead to further complications, including diminished energy levels and mood instability. Understanding these symptoms is crucial for both men experiencing andropause and their partners, as it fosters empathy and encourages open communication about the challenges faced during this transition.

Weight gain is a prevalent concern associated with andropause, often exacerbated by hormonal changes and a decrease in physical activity. Men may find it increasingly difficult to maintain their previous weight due to metabolic slowdowns and potential shifts in appetite regulation. This weight gain can lead to a cycle of frustration and discouragement, as men struggle with their body image and self-esteem. The physical changes can also prompt feelings of vulnerability, as societal expectations around masculinity and physical fitness weigh heavily on men during this period, further complicating their emotional landscape.

The emotional impact of andropause extends beyond individual experiences, affecting relationships with partners and families. Men may experience heightened irritability, anxiety, or sadness, which can strain communication and intimacy with their significant others. Partners may feel uncertain about how to provide support or may misinterpret these emotional shifts as personal grievances, leading to misunderstandings. Establishing an open dialogue about these changes is essential for maintaining healthy relationships, as it allows both partners to express their feelings and work together to navigate the complexities of this transitional phase.

Moreover, the psychological responses to andropause symptoms can lead to increased stress and even depression. Men who feel overwhelmed by their physical changes may withdraw from social interactions or activities they once enjoyed, compounding feelings of isolation and dissatisfaction. This emotional toll can create a vicious cycle where declining mental health further exacerbates physical symptoms, including weight gain. It is vital for men to recognize the importance of seeking professional help, whether through counselling, support groups, or discussing their feelings with healthcare practitioners, to address these emotional challenges effectively.

Ultimately, understanding the symptoms and emotional impact of andropause is crucial for men and their partners. By recognizing the interplay between physical changes and emotional well-being, individuals can adopt a proactive approach to manage their health during this transition. This awareness not only helps in mitigating the effects of weight gain but also promotes stronger relationships and fosters a supportive environment for both men and their partners as they navigate the complexities of andropause together.

The Connection Between Andropause and Weight Gain

Andropause, often referred to as male menopause, is a phase that many men experience as they age, typically around their late 40s to early 60s. This transitional period is marked by a gradual decline in testosterone levels, which can lead to a range of physical and emotional changes. One of the most significant issues associated with andropause is weight gain. Understanding the connection between andropause and weight management is crucial for men and their partners, as it allows for proactive strategies to address these changes and maintain overall health.

As testosterone levels decrease during andropause, men may notice an increase in body fat, particularly around the abdomen. This shift in body composition can be attributed to several factors, including hormonal changes that affect metabolism and fat distribution. Lower testosterone levels can lead to a decrease in muscle mass, which is vital for maintaining a healthy metabolic rate. With less muscle, the body burns fewer calories at rest, making it easier to gain weight. Recognizing this connection is the first step in addressing weight gain during this transition.

Additionally, andropause is often accompanied by changes in lifestyle and mental health. Many men may experience symptoms such as fatigue, depression, or decreased motivation, which can contribute to a more sedentary lifestyle. This reduction in physical activity can further exacerbate weight gain. Moreover, emotional challenges related to andropause, such as stress and anxiety, can lead to unhealthy eating habits as a coping mechanism. Understanding these interrelated factors can help men and their partners develop healthier lifestyle choices and strategies for managing weight.

Nutrition plays a critical role in managing weight during andropause. A balanced diet that includes adequate protein, healthy fats, and a variety of fruits and vegetables can support hormonal balance and overall well-being. Men should focus on nutrient-dense foods that promote muscle retention and fat loss. Additionally, being mindful of caloric intake and portion sizes is essential, as metabolism slows down during this transition. Encouraging partners to participate in meal planning and preparation can foster a supportive environment for making healthier choices together.

Physical activity is equally important in combating weight gain associated with andropause. Incorporating regular exercise into daily routines can help maintain muscle mass, boost metabolism, and improve mood. Resistance training, in particular, is beneficial for counteracting muscle loss and promoting fat loss. Engaging in activities that both partners enjoy can enhance motivation and adherence to a fitness regimen. By addressing the connection between andropause and weight gain, men and their partners can work collaboratively to navigate this transition with strength and resilience, fostering a healthier lifestyle together.

The Science of Weight Management

Metabolism and Aging

Metabolism plays a crucial role in how our bodies respond to various life stages, particularly during andropause. As men transition through this phase, they often experience significant shifts in hormonal levels, particularly testosterone. These hormonal changes can lead to a decrease in metabolic rate, making it more challenging for men to maintain a healthy weight. Understanding the relationship between metabolism and aging is vital for both men and their partners as they navigate these changes. By recognizing how metabolism evolves, individuals can adopt strategies that support weight management and overall health during andropause.

As men age, there is a natural decline in muscle mass, often referred to as sarcopenia. This loss of muscle tissue can significantly impact resting metabolic rate because muscle burns more calories than fat, even at rest. When muscle mass decreases, the body's ability to burn calories diminishes, leading to potential weight gain if caloric intake remains unchanged. It is essential for men facing andropause to engage in regular strength training exercises to counteract this muscle loss. By incorporating resistance training into their routine, they can help preserve muscle mass, boost metabolism, and improve body composition.

Hormonal fluctuations during andropause also influence fat distribution in the body. Many men find that they gain weight around the abdomen rather than in other areas, leading to an increase in visceral fat. This type of fat is particularly concerning as it is associated with higher risks of chronic diseases, including cardiovascular issues and diabetes. Partners can play a supportive role by encouraging healthier eating habits and exercise routines that focus on fat loss and overall well-being. Understanding these changes can foster a collaborative approach to weight management.

Dietary choices are pivotal in managing metabolism and weight during andropause. A balanced diet rich in lean proteins, healthy fats, and complex carbohydrates can help sustain energy levels and support metabolic function. Nutrient-dense foods, such as fruits, vegetables, and whole grains, provide essential vitamins and minerals that can enhance metabolic processes. Additionally, staying hydrated is important, as even mild dehydration can impair metabolism. Men and their partners should consider meal planning and healthy cooking together, making the journey toward weight management a shared experience.

In conclusion, addressing metabolism and its effects during andropause is crucial for maintaining a healthy weight and overall health. Men can take proactive steps by incorporating strength training, making informed dietary choices, and fostering a supportive environment with their partners. By understanding the metabolic changes that occur with aging, individuals can navigate this transition more effectively, ensuring they remain physically active and healthy. With the right strategies in place, men can manage their weight and thrive during andropause, leading to improved quality of life.

Hormonal Influences on Weight

Hormones play a crucial role in regulating various bodily functions, including metabolism, appetite, and fat distribution. As men approach andropause, which is often characterized by a gradual decline in testosterone levels, they may experience significant changes in their weight and body composition. Testosterone is essential for maintaining muscle mass, promoting fat loss, and supporting overall metabolic health. When levels of this hormone decrease, men may find it increasingly difficult to maintain their weight or even prevent weight gain, leading to a cycle that can be challenging to break.

One of the most notable effects of declining testosterone is the shift in body composition. Men often experience an increase in visceral fat, which is the fat stored around internal organs. This type of fat is associated with a higher risk of metabolic disorders, such as diabetes and cardiovascular disease. Research indicates that lower testosterone levels are linked to increased fat mass and reduced lean muscle mass. This change can further exacerbate weight gain, as muscle is more metabolically active than fat, meaning that having less muscle can lead to a slower metabolism and more difficulty in managing weight.

Additionally, hormonal fluctuations can also affect appetite and energy levels. Men facing andropause may experience changes in their hunger-regulating hormones, such as ghrelin and leptin. Ghrelin stimulates appetite, while leptin signals satiety. An imbalance in these hormones can lead to increased hunger and cravings, making it harder to adhere to a healthy diet. Furthermore, fatigue and reduced energy levels often reported during andropause can result in decreased physical activity, which can contribute to weight gain over time.

Stress is another factor that can influence hormonal balance and, consequently, weight management. As men approach andropause, they may face various life stressors, including career changes, relationship dynamics, and health concerns. Elevated levels of cortisol, the stress hormone, can lead to increased appetite and cravings for unhealthy foods. Chronic stress can also disrupt sleep patterns, further impacting hormonal regulation and contributing to weight gain. Understanding the interplay between stress and hormonal changes is vital for developing effective weight management strategies.

Addressing hormonal influences on weight during andropause requires a multifaceted approach. Encouraging healthy lifestyle changes, such as regular physical activity, strength training, and a balanced diet, can help counteract the effects of hormonal decline. It is also essential for men and their partners to communicate openly about these changes and seek professional guidance when necessary. Healthcare practitioners can provide valuable insights into hormone testing and management options, as well as support in implementing lifestyle interventions that promote healthy weight management during this transitional phase of life.

The Role of Muscle Mass

Muscle mass plays a critical role in the overall health and well-being of men, particularly as they approach andropause. During andropause, which is often characterized by a decline in testosterone levels, many men experience changes in body composition, including an increase in body fat and a decrease in muscle mass. This decline can lead to a variety of health issues, including decreased metabolism, increased risk of chronic diseases, and diminished quality of life. Understanding the importance of maintaining muscle mass during this transitional phase is essential for effective weight management and overall health.

One of the primary functions of muscle mass is its impact on metabolism. Muscle tissue is metabolically active, meaning it requires energy to maintain itself. As men lose muscle mass with age and hormonal changes, their resting metabolic rate declines, leading to weight gain if caloric intake remains the same. By preserving and even increasing muscle mass through resistance training and proper nutrition, men can counteract this metabolic slowdown. This not only helps in managing weight but also improves energy levels and overall physical performance.

Additionally, maintaining muscle mass is vital for hormonal balance. Testosterone is closely linked to muscle growth and maintenance. As testosterone levels drop during andropause, the ability to build and retain muscle diminishes. This creates a cycle where reduced muscle leads to further hormonal imbalances, exacerbating the symptoms of andropause. Engaging in regular strength-training exercises can help stimulate testosterone production, promoting not only muscle preservation but also enhancing mood and reducing feelings of fatigue often associated with andropause.

The psychological benefits of maintaining muscle mass should also not be overlooked. Engaging in strength training can boost self-esteem and confidence, which may be challenged during andropause. The physical changes that accompany this life stage can affect how men perceive themselves, leading to issues such as anxiety and depression. By focusing on building and maintaining muscle, men can foster a sense of accomplishment and control over their bodies, which can significantly improve mental health and emotional resilience.

Finally, muscle mass serves as a protective factor against chronic diseases. Research indicates that higher muscle mass is associated with a lower risk of conditions such as type 2 diabetes, cardiovascular disease, and osteoporosis. For men facing andropause, prioritizing muscle maintenance through targeted exercise and proper nutrition can lead to long-term health benefits. By taking proactive steps to preserve muscle mass, men not only improve their physical health but also enhance their quality of life during this transitional period and beyond.

Nutrition for Men in Transition

Essential Nutrients for Men

Understanding the essential nutrients for men, especially those approaching andropause, is crucial for maintaining overall health and managing weight effectively. As men age, hormonal changes can lead to an increase in body fat, decreased muscle mass, and various metabolic shifts. A well-balanced diet rich in essential nutrients can help counter these effects, promote optimal health, and support weight management during this transition.

Protein is one of the most critical nutrients for men experiencing andropause. It plays a vital role in preserving lean muscle mass, which tends to decline with age. Incorporating lean meats, poultry, fish, eggs, legumes, and dairy products into the diet can provide the necessary amino acids that support muscle repair and growth. Additionally, protein has a higher thermic effect than fats or carbohydrates, meaning it requires more energy to digest, which can aid in managing body weight.

Healthy fats are equally important for men in this stage of life. Omega-3 fatty acids, found in fatty fish, walnuts, flaxseeds, and chia seeds, are known for their anti-inflammatory properties and support heart health. They can also enhance mood and cognitive function, both of which may be impacted during andropause. Including monounsaturated fats like olive oil and avocados can further contribute to a balanced diet, promoting satiety and helping to regulate body weight.

Vitamins and minerals such as vitamin D, zinc, and magnesium are also essential for men facing andropause. Vitamin D is crucial for bone health and can influence testosterone levels, while zinc plays a significant role in hormone production and immune function. Magnesium supports muscle function and can help reduce the risk of metabolic syndrome, which is often associated with weight gain. Incorporating foods rich in these nutrients, such as leafy greens, nuts, seeds, and fortified products, can help maintain optimal health.

Lastly, hydration cannot be overlooked. As men approach andropause, the body's ability to regulate hydration may decline. Drinking adequate water is vital for metabolic processes, digestion, and overall bodily functions. Additionally, staying hydrated can help manage appetite, as thirst is sometimes mistaken for hunger. Encouraging consistent water intake and being mindful of hydration can significantly impact weight management and overall well-being during this transitional phase.

Creating a Balanced Diet

Creating a balanced diet is crucial for men approaching andropause, as it plays a significant role in managing weight and overall health. During this transitional phase, hormonal changes can lead to an increase in body fat, particularly around the abdomen. A well-structured diet can help mitigate these effects by providing essential nutrients, stabilizing energy levels, and supporting metabolic functions. Understanding the components of a balanced diet is the first step towards achieving and maintaining a healthy weight during andropause.

A balanced diet should include a variety of food groups to ensure adequate nutrient intake. This encompasses fruits, vegetables, whole grains, lean proteins, and healthy fats. Each of these food groups contributes unique vitamins and minerals that are vital for bodily functions. For instance, fruits and vegetables are rich in antioxidants, which can help combat oxidative stress associated with hormonal changes. Whole grains provide fibre, which aids in digestion and helps maintain a healthy weight by promoting satiety. Lean proteins, such as chicken, fish, and legumes, support muscle mass, which is essential for metabolism, while healthy fats from sources like avocados and nuts can improve heart health.

Portion control is another essential aspect of creating a balanced diet. As metabolism slows down during andropause, it becomes increasingly important to monitor caloric intake. Men should focus on understanding serving sizes and listening to their body's hunger cues to avoid overeating. Utilizing smaller plates and being mindful of food choices can help manage portions effectively. Additionally, planning meals ahead of time can prevent impulsive eating and ensure that healthier options are readily available.

Hydration is often overlooked but is a vital component of a balanced diet. Adequate water intake is necessary for various bodily functions, including digestion, nutrient absorption, and temperature regulation. Men experiencing andropause may find that dehydration can exacerbate feelings of fatigue and affect their overall well-being. It is recommended to aim for at least eight glasses of water per day, adjusting based on activity levels and personal needs. Incorporating hydrating foods, such as cucumbers, oranges, and soups, can also contribute to overall fluid intake.

Lastly, it is essential to recognize that dietary changes should be sustainable and enjoyable. A balanced diet does not require complete restriction of favourite foods or indulgences. Instead, it encourages moderation and the inclusion of a wide range of flavours and textures. Engaging partners in meal planning and preparation can enhance the experience and foster a supportive environment. By creating a balanced diet that aligns with personal preferences and lifestyle, men can navigate the challenges of andropause while promoting weight management and overall health.

Portion Control and Mindful Eating

Portion control and mindful eating are essential strategies for men facing andropause who want to manage weight effectively. As hormonal changes occur during andropause, metabolic rates may decrease, leading to potential weight gain. Understanding how to regulate portion sizes and develop a mindful approach to eating can significantly impact overall health and well-being. These techniques can help in making more conscious food choices, reducing overeating, and fostering a healthier relationship with food.

Portion control involves being aware of serving sizes and understanding the energy content of different foods. Men often underestimate the amount of food they consume, particularly when dining out or snacking. By using smaller plates, measuring servings, and being mindful of calorie-dense foods, individuals can better regulate their intake. It is important to educate oneself on appropriate portion sizes, as this can help prevent unintentional weight gain. Simple adjustments, like serving a portion of protein that is roughly the size of a deck of cards or filling half the plate with vegetables, can make a significant difference.

Mindful eating complements portion control by encouraging individuals to pay attention to their eating habits and the sensory experiences associated with food. This practice involves slowing down during meals, savouring each bite, and recognizing hunger and fullness cues. By being present during meals, men can develop a deeper awareness of their body's signals and reduce the likelihood of emotional or mindless eating. This approach can also help individuals enjoy their food more and make healthier choices, ultimately leading to better weight management.

Moreover, involving partners in the process of portion control and mindful eating can enhance the experience and support success. Couples can work together to prepare meals, make healthier food choices, and hold each other accountable. Sharing the journey creates a supportive environment that can make transitioning into healthier habits more enjoyable and sustainable. Open communication about dietary goals and challenges can strengthen partnerships and foster a collaborative approach to weight management.

In conclusion, incorporating portion control and mindful eating into daily routines is crucial for men approaching andropause. By understanding portion sizes and practicing mindfulness while eating, individuals can effectively manage their weight and enhance their overall quality of life. These strategies not only contribute to physical health but also promote a positive mindset regarding food and eating. As men and their partners navigate this transitional phase, focusing on these practical techniques can pave the way for lasting wellness and vitality.

Exercise Strategies for Weight Management

Importance of Physical Activity

Physical activity plays a crucial role in managing weight, particularly for men approaching andropause. As testosterone levels fluctuate during this transitional phase, men may experience an increase in body fat and a decrease in lean muscle mass. Engaging in regular physical activity can help counteract these changes by promoting muscle preservation and fat loss. It is essential for both men and their partners to understand that incorporating exercise into daily routines can significantly contribute to maintaining a healthy weight and overall well-being during this period.

In addition to aiding weight management, physical activity has numerous health benefits that are particularly relevant during andropause. Regular exercise has been shown to improve cardiovascular health, enhance metabolic function, and reduce the risk of chronic diseases such as diabetes and hypertension. For men experiencing the symptoms of andropause, such as fatigue, depression, or decreased libido, physical activity can serve as a natural mood booster and energy enhancer. The release of endorphins during exercise can alleviate feelings of stress and anxiety, making it a vital tool for mental health management.

Moreover, engaging in physical activity can foster social connections and support networks, which are essential during life transitions like andropause. Group exercises, such as fitness classes or sports clubs, provide opportunities for men to bond with others facing similar challenges. This sense of community can enhance motivation and accountability, making it more likely that individuals will stick to their exercise regimens. Partners can also participate in physical activities together, strengthening their relationship while promoting mutual health benefits.

It is important to highlight that the type and intensity of physical activity can vary based on individual fitness levels and health conditions. Men approaching andropause should aim for a balanced approach that includes cardiovascular exercises, strength training, and flexibility activities. Cardiovascular exercises, such as walking, cycling, or swimming, help burn calories and improve cardiovascular health. Strength training is vital for building and maintaining muscle mass, which can decline with age. Flexibility exercises, such as yoga or stretching, can enhance mobility and prevent injuries, contributing to a well-rounded fitness routine.

In conclusion, the importance of physical activity cannot be overstated for men facing andropause. As a critical component of weight management, exercise offers a multitude of health benefits that extend beyond mere physical appearance. By embracing an active lifestyle, men can better navigate the challenges of andropause, improve their physical and mental well-being, and foster supportive relationships with their partners. Encouraging a commitment to regular physical activity is essential for promoting a healthier and more fulfilling life during this transitional phase.

Types of Exercises Beneficial for Men

Strength training is one of the most beneficial types of exercise for men facing andropause. As testosterone levels begin to decline, maintaining muscle mass becomes increasingly important. Strength training not only helps in building and preserving muscle but also increases metabolism, which can counteract weight gain. Exercises such as weightlifting, resistance band workouts, and body-weight exercises like push-ups and squats are particularly effective. Engaging in strength training two to three times a week can lead to improvements in body composition, strength, and overall well-being.

Cardiovascular exercise is another essential component for men dealing with andropause. Activities such as walking, jogging, cycling, or swimming can boost heart health, enhance endurance, and aid in weight management. These exercises promote calorie burning, which is vital as metabolism tends to slow with age. Aiming for at least 150 minutes of moderate-intensity aerobic activity each week can help mitigate some of the physical changes associated with andropause, including weight gain and decreased energy levels.

Flexibility and balance exercises are equally important, especially as men age. Incorporating activities like yoga or Pilates can improve flexibility, enhance joint health, and reduce the risk of injuries. These exercises also promote relaxation and stress relief, which can be beneficial during periods of hormonal transition. Additionally, balance exercises, such as tai chi or simple balance drills, can help prevent falls, which is crucial as muscle strength and coordination may decline with age.

High-Intensity Interval Training (HIIT) has gained popularity for its efficiency and effectiveness in burning fat and improving cardiovascular fitness. HIIT involves short bursts of intense exercise followed by rest or low-intensity periods. This type of training can be particularly advantageous for men facing weight management issues related to andropause. Incorporating HIIT sessions into a weekly routine can lead to improved metabolic health and aid in fat loss, making it a valuable option for those looking to maintain a healthy weight.

Finally, incorporating functional exercises into a fitness regime can significantly benefit men during andropause. Functional exercises mimic everyday activities and help improve overall physical performance. Movements such as kettlebell swings, lunges, and step-ups enhance strength, coordination, and stability, allowing for better performance in daily tasks. This is particularly important as maintaining independence and quality of life becomes a priority. By combining various types of exercises, men can effectively manage weight and improve their physical health during this transitional phase.

Developing a Sustainable Exercise Routine

Developing a sustainable exercise routine is crucial for men experiencing andropause, as it not only aids in weight management but also enhances overall well-being. As testosterone levels fluctuate during this life stage, men may notice changes in muscle mass, energy levels, and metabolism. This makes regular physical activity even more important in counteracting weight gain and maintaining a healthy lifestyle. A well-structured exercise regimen that incorporates various types of activities can provide significant benefits, including improved mood, enhanced energy, and better body composition.

To create a sustainable exercise routine, it is essential to start with realistic goals. Setting specific, measurable, achievable, relevant, and time-bound (SMART) objectives can help maintain motivation and track progress. For instance, a man might aim to lose a certain number of pounds within a set timeframe or to exercise a specific number of days per week. These targets should take into account individual fitness levels and personal preferences, ensuring that the routine is enjoyable rather than a chore. Engaging in activities that one finds pleasurable increases the likelihood of sticking with the routine long-term.

Incorporating a variety of exercise types can enhance the effectiveness of an exercise regimen. A balanced approach should include cardiovascular exercises, strength training, and flexibility workouts. Cardiovascular activities, such as walking, jogging, cycling, or swimming, are effective for burning calories and improving heart health. Strength training helps combat muscle loss associated with andropause by building lean muscle mass, which can boost metabolism. Meanwhile, flexibility exercises, such as stretching or yoga, promote mobility and can help prevent injuries. A combination of these activities not only targets different aspects of fitness but also keeps the routine fresh and engaging.

Consistency is key to developing a sustainable exercise routine. Establishing a regular schedule and sticking to it can lead to long-term success. It may be beneficial to enlist the support of a workout partner, such as a friend or a partner, to enhance accountability and motivation. Additionally, tracking progress through journals or fitness apps can help reinforce commitment and celebrate milestones. For those who find it challenging to maintain motivation, varying the workout environment, such as exercising outdoors or trying new fitness classes, can also provide a refreshing change.

Lastly, it is important to listen to one's body and adjust the routine as necessary. Men facing andropause may experience fluctuations in energy levels, so being flexible with the exercise plan can help prevent burnout and injury. Incorporating rest days is crucial, allowing the body to recover and adapt to the demands placed upon it. By fostering a positive relationship with exercise and acknowledging the changes that come with andropause, men can develop a sustainable routine that not only aids in weight management but also enhances their quality of life.

Psychological Aspects of Weight Management

Motivation and Goal Setting

Motivation and goal setting are critical components for men facing the challenges of andropause, particularly when it comes to weight management. As men experience hormonal changes during this life transition, they may find it harder to maintain their weight or even lose excess pounds. Understanding the psychological aspects that drive motivation can empower individuals to take control of their health. Establishing clear, attainable goals is essential for creating a structured path toward achieving desired weight outcomes and enhancing overall well-being.

First, it is important to recognize the unique motivations that may arise during andropause. Many men may feel a loss of vitality or face body image concerns as they notice changes in their physique. These feelings can serve as powerful motivators for change. Additionally, the desire to maintain energy levels, improve physical health, and enhance self-esteem can all drive men to pursue healthier lifestyles. By identifying these motivations, individuals can create a personal connection to their weight management journey, making the process feel more relevant and necessary.

Setting specific, measurable, achievable, relevant, and time-bound (SMART) goals is an effective strategy for weight management during andropause. This approach allows individuals to break down larger objectives into smaller, more manageable tasks. For instance, rather than setting a broad goal of "losing weight," a SMART goal might be "to lose five pounds in two months by exercising three times a week and reducing portion sizes at meals." This level of specificity helps maintain focus and provides a clear framework for tracking progress, which is crucial for sustained motivation.

Support systems play a vital role in the motivation and goal-setting process. Engaging partners, friends, or health care professionals can provide encouragement and accountability. By discussing goals openly with others, men can foster a sense of community and shared purpose, which can be particularly beneficial during times of transition. Furthermore, regular check-ins with a support system can help individuals stay committed to their goals and adjust strategies as needed, ensuring that they remain on track despite potential setbacks.

Finally, it is essential to celebrate small victories along the way. Acknowledging achievements, no matter how minor, can boost motivation and reinforce positive behaviours. For example, if a man successfully incorporates more physical activity into his routine or makes healthier food choices for a week, celebrating these milestones can instil a sense of accomplishment. This practice fosters a positive mindset, encourages continued effort, and ultimately contributes to long-term success in weight management during andropause.

Addressing Emotional Eating

Emotional eating is a common challenge faced by many individuals, particularly during transitional periods such as andropause. Men may experience various emotional and physical changes during this phase, leading to increased stress, anxiety, and depression. These feelings can trigger a desire to seek comfort in food, often resulting in unhealthy eating patterns and weight gain. Addressing emotional eating requires a multifaceted approach that combines awareness, coping strategies, and support from partners and healthcare practitioners.

Understanding the triggers for emotional eating is the first step in addressing this behaviour. For many men, feelings of inadequacy, frustration, or loss of identity can arise during andropause. These emotions may lead to cravings for high-calorie, comfort foods that provide temporary relief but contribute to long-term weight gain. Keeping a food diary can help individuals identify specific situations or emotions that lead to overeating, allowing them to recognize patterns and develop healthier responses.

Incorporating mindfulness techniques can be beneficial in managing emotional eating. Mindfulness encourages individuals to focus on the present moment and acknowledge their feelings without judgment. Techniques such as deep breathing, meditation, or even brief physical activity can help men process emotions more constructively. By learning to differentiate between emotional hunger and physical hunger, individuals can make more conscious choices about their eating habits and reduce the likelihood of turning to food for comfort.

Support from partners and healthcare practitioners is crucial in addressing emotional eating. Open communication about feelings and challenges can foster a supportive environment where men feel understood and encouraged. Partners can play a significant role by participating in healthy activities together, such as cooking nutritious meals or engaging in physical exercise. Healthcare practitioners can provide resources, such as counselling or support groups, to help men explore underlying emotional issues and develop effective coping strategies.

Finally, developing a personalized action plan can help men combat emotional eating. This plan may include setting realistic goals for weight management, identifying alternative coping mechanisms, and incorporating regular physical activity into their routines. By establishing a structured approach, men can create a sense of accountability and progress. Over time, these strategies can contribute to healthier eating habits, improved emotional well-being, and successful weight management during and after the andropause transition.

Building a Support System

Building a support system is essential for men navigating the challenges of andropause, particularly in relation to weight management. As hormonal changes occur, many men experience shifts in metabolism, energy levels, and body composition, which can complicate efforts to maintain a healthy weight. Establishing a robust support network can provide the encouragement and accountability needed to make sustainable lifestyle changes. This support system can include family members, friends, healthcare professionals, and even online communities that focus on health and fitness.

Family and friends play a crucial role in providing emotional support and practical assistance. Spouses or partners can help create an environment that promotes healthy eating and physical activity, making it easier to adopt new habits together. Engaging in activities like cooking healthy meals or exercising side by side can strengthen relationships while fostering accountability. Moreover, friends who share similar goals can motivate men to stay committed to their weight management plans, whether through regular check-ins or by participating in group workouts.

Healthcare practitioners, including dietitians, personal trainers, and therapists, also form an important part of the support system. These professionals can provide tailored advice based on individual health status and goals. Dietitians can help design meal plans that accommodate changes in metabolism and nutritional needs during andropause. Personal trainers can create exercise regimens that consider any physical limitations, while therapists can address emotional or psychological factors that may influence eating behaviours and self-image during this transitional phase.

In addition to personal connections, many men find value in joining support groups or online forums that focus on andropause and weight management. These platforms allow individuals to share their experiences, challenges, and successes, fostering a sense of community and reducing feelings of isolation. By connecting with others who understand the specific struggles associated with andropause, men can gain insights and strategies that have worked for others, enriching their own journey toward better health.

Ultimately, building a support system is about creating a comprehensive network that addresses the various aspects of weight management during andropause. By surrounding themselves with understanding individuals and professionals, men can enhance their resilience, boost their motivation, and increase their chances of achieving lasting weight management. This collaborative approach not only aids in physical health but also contributes to emotional well-being, making the transition through andropause a more manageable and fulfilling experience.

Practical Tips for Everyday Life

Meal Planning and Preparation

Meal planning and preparation are crucial components in managing weight, especially for men approaching andropause. During this transition, men often experience hormonal changes that can lead to increased body fat, particularly around the abdomen. By focusing on balanced meals and strategic planning, individuals can better control their weight and enhance their overall health. This proactive approach not only aids in weight management but also helps in maintaining energy levels, improving mood, and supporting muscle mass.

The foundation of effective meal planning involves understanding nutritional needs. Men experiencing andropause may require adjustments in their dietary intake to accommodate changes in metabolism and energy expenditure. A diet rich in lean proteins, healthy fats, whole grains, and plenty of fruits and vegetables is essential. By prioritizing nutrient-dense foods, men can foster an environment conducive to maintaining muscle mass and reducing fat gain. Incorporating foods high in antioxidants and omega-3 fatty acids can also support hormonal balance and overall well-being.

When it comes to meal preparation, organization is key. Setting aside time each week to plan meals can alleviate the stress of last-minute food choices that often lead to unhealthy eating. Creating a weekly menu allows individuals to thoughtfully select recipes that align with their nutritional goals. Additionally, preparing meals in bulk can save time and ensure that healthy options are readily available during busy days. This strategy not only promotes consistency in dietary choices but also reduces reliance on processed foods that may hinder weight management efforts.

Portion control is another vital aspect to consider during meal preparation. As men transition through andropause, they may find that their caloric needs shift. It becomes essential to listen to hunger cues and adjust portion sizes accordingly. Utilizing measuring tools or visual cues can help maintain appropriate serving sizes, preventing overeating. Moreover, mindful eating practices, such as savouring each bite and minimizing distractions during meals, can enhance satisfaction and promote healthier eating behaviours.

Lastly, involving partners in meal planning and preparation can foster a supportive environment, making the journey towards weight management more enjoyable. Collaborating on meals encourages accountability and allows for shared responsibility in maintaining a healthy lifestyle. Couples can explore new recipes together, try cooking classes, or even visit local farmers' markets to select fresh ingredients. By engaging in this process together, couples not only strengthen their relationship but also promote a healthier lifestyle that benefits both individuals as they navigate the challenges of andropause.

Navigating Social Situations

Navigating social situations can be particularly challenging for men experiencing andropause, especially when weight gain is a concern. The psychological and emotional impact of this transitional phase can lead to feelings of self-consciousness and anxiety in social settings. It is essential to develop strategies that not only facilitate comfortable interactions but also promote positive body image and self-esteem. Understanding the dynamics of social environments can empower men to engage more fully, regardless of their physical changes.

One effective approach is to prepare mentally for social events. Before attending gatherings, men can benefit from visualizing themselves in positive and successful interactions. This mental rehearsal can reduce anxiety and increase confidence. Additionally, discussing concerns with a partner can provide emotional support and reassurance. Partners can play a crucial role by encouraging open dialogue about feelings related to weight gain and the changes associated with andropause, thereby fostering a supportive environment.

Eating habits in social situations also merit careful consideration. Men should feel empowered to make informed choices about food and drink at gatherings. This might involve selecting healthier options, such as salads or grilled proteins, while being mindful of portion sizes. It is equally important to enjoy treats in moderation without guilt. Practicing mindful eating can enhance the experience, allowing men to savor their food while maintaining control over their dietary choices. By prioritizing health-conscious decisions, men can navigate social situations without compromising their weight management goals.

Physical activity is another crucial component to consider when engaging in social settings. Participating in active social events, such as group sports or hiking, can create a fun atmosphere while promoting fitness. These activities not only help manage weight but also foster camaraderie and connection with friends and family. Men can suggest active outings to their social circles, transforming gatherings into opportunities for exercise and socialization, which can alleviate the focus on weight-related insecurities.

Lastly, developing a supportive network can significantly enhance the experience of navigating social situations during andropause. Whether through friends, family, or support groups, having a community that understands the challenges of weight gain and hormonal changes can provide encouragement and accountability. Sharing experiences and coping strategies can foster a sense of belonging and reduce feelings of isolation. By cultivating supportive relationships, men can navigate the complexities of social interactions with increased confidence and resilience, ultimately leading to a healthier and more fulfilling lifestyle during andropause.

Tracking Progress and Adjustments

Tracking progress in weight management during andropause is crucial for understanding how lifestyle changes impact physical health and overall well-being. As men face hormonal shifts that can lead to weight gain, it becomes essential to establish a baseline for monitoring changes. This can be accomplished through regular weigh-ins, body composition assessments, and keeping a record of dietary habits and physical activity. By documenting these metrics, both men and their partners can identify trends and make informed decisions about necessary adjustments to their routines.

Regular assessments not only provide tangible data but also serve as motivational tools. Setting specific, measurable goals can help maintain focus and commitment. For instance, tracking weekly weight changes or recording the number of days spent exercising can reinforce positive behaviours. Additionally, using smartphone apps or journals can simplify this process, making it easier to visualize progress over time. Recognizing small victories along the way can boost morale and encourage adherence to a weight management plan.

Adjustments are a natural part of any weight management journey, especially during the transitions associated with andropause. As men experience fluctuations in energy levels, metabolism, and body composition, it is essential to remain flexible and willing to adapt strategies. If initial dietary choices are not yielding the desired results, it may be time to reevaluate macronutrient ratios or calorie intake. Similarly, if certain physical activities are proving to be ineffective or unenjoyable, exploring new forms of exercise can reinvigorate motivation and engagement.

Moreover, it is important to consider the role of emotional and psychological factors in tracking progress. Weight management during andropause can be accompanied by feelings of frustration or inadequacy, particularly if results do not align with expectations. Open communication between men and their partners can foster a supportive environment, where both individuals feel empowered to discuss challenges and celebrate successes. This partnership can enhance accountability and encourage a more holistic approach to health that focuses on emotional well-being alongside physical changes.

Lastly, the involvement of healthcare practitioners can provide valuable insights and guidance throughout the weight management process. Regular check-ins with a doctor or nutritionist can help ensure that any adjustments made are safe and effective. These professionals can offer personalized recommendations based on individual health profiles and may also monitor for any underlying medical conditions that could influence weight gain. By combining self-monitoring, open communication, and professional support, men can navigate the complexities of andropause with greater confidence and achieve sustainable weight management.

Partner Support and Communication

Understanding Each Other's Challenges

Understanding each other's challenges during andropause is vital for both men experiencing this transition and their partners. This period often brings about significant physical, emotional, and psychological changes that can affect relationships and individual well-being. By fostering an environment of empathy and communication, both partners can navigate these challenges more effectively. The more each party understands the other's experiences, the better they can support one another in managing the associated weight gain and lifestyle shifts.

For men, andropause can manifest in various ways, including hormonal changes that lead to weight gain, fatigue, and decreased motivation. The gradual decline in testosterone levels can influence not only physical attributes but also mental health, resulting in symptoms such as irritability or depression. Recognizing that these changes are not merely a personal failing, but a natural biological process can help alleviate feelings of shame or frustration. Men need to articulate these feelings to their partners to foster mutual understanding and support.

Partners play a crucial role in this journey. They often witness firsthand the changes their loved ones are experiencing and may feel helpless or unsure about how to offer support. It is essential for partners to educate themselves about andropause and its effects on men. This knowledge equips them to be more empathetic and proactive in encouraging healthier habits, such as engaging in physical activities together or preparing nutritious meals. Open dialogue about each person's feelings and experiences can enhance emotional intimacy and strengthen the partnership during this transitional phase.

Communication is key when addressing the challenges of andropause. Men may struggle to express their emotions or concerns, which can lead to misunderstandings or feelings of isolation. Partners should create a safe space for discussion, where men feel comfortable sharing their experiences without fear of judgment. By actively listening and validating each other's feelings, couples can build a stronger foundation to face these challenges together. This approach not only promotes understanding but also fosters a sense of teamwork in managing weight and health during this critical time.

Ultimately, understanding each other's challenges during andropause is about building resilience as a couple. By acknowledging the complexities of this transition, both men and their partners can develop a shared strategy for coping with the changes. This might involve setting mutual goals for physical activity, exploring stress-reduction techniques, or seeking professional guidance. Through collaboration and compassion, couples can transform the challenges of andropause into opportunities for growth, reinforcing their bond as they adapt to this new chapter in their lives.

Encouraging Healthy Habits Together

Encouraging healthy habits together is a critical component for men and their partners navigating the challenges of andropause. As men experience hormonal changes, they may encounter weight gain and other health issues that require a supportive environment to foster positive lifestyle changes. By working together, couples can create a balanced approach to health that emphasizes mutual support and understanding, ultimately enhancing both physical well-being and emotional connection.

One of the first steps in encouraging healthy habits is setting shared goals. Couples can sit down and discuss their individual health objectives and how these align with their collective aspirations. Whether it's aiming for a specific weight, increasing physical activity, or adopting a healthier diet, establishing common goals can create a sense of teamwork. This collaborative process not only makes the journey more enjoyable but also reinforces accountability, as each partner can motivate the other to stay committed to their health plans.

Incorporating physical activity into daily routines can also strengthen the bond between partners. Engaging in exercise together, whether it's walking, cycling, or participating in a fitness class, allows couples to share experiences while promoting physical health. Regular physical activity is known to combat weight gain associated with andropause, improve mood, and enhance overall well-being. Additionally, couples can explore new activities together, such as hiking or dancing, which can introduce an element of fun and adventure into their fitness journey.

Nutrition plays a crucial role in managing weight during andropause. Couples should consider preparing meals together, as cooking can be a bonding experience that promotes healthier eating habits. By planning meals that are rich in whole foods, lean proteins, and healthy fats, partners can support each other in making nutritious choices. It's important to educate themselves about portion sizes and the nutritional value of different foods, fostering a shared understanding of how diet impacts their health. This cooperative approach can also make it easier to resist unhealthy temptations, as both partners can encourage one another to stick to their dietary commitments.

Lastly, open communication is essential in fostering a supportive environment for healthy habits. Partners should feel comfortable discussing their struggles and successes, celebrating milestones together, and addressing any challenges that arise. This ongoing dialogue not only strengthens their relationship but also reinforces their commitment to mutual health goals. By creating a space where both partners can express their feelings and concerns, they can navigate the complexities of andropause more effectively, ensuring that they emerge from this transition stronger and healthier together.

Open Conversations About Health

Open conversations about health play a crucial role for men and their partners facing andropause. This transitional phase can bring about various physical and emotional changes, including weight gain, hormonal fluctuations, and shifts in mental well-being. Engaging in open discussions about these issues not only normalizes the experience but also fosters a supportive environment where both partners can address their concerns and seek appropriate strategies for management. By breaking down barriers and encouraging dialogue, men can better navigate this transition while feeling understood and supported.

Weight gain during andropause is often linked to hormonal changes, particularly the decline in testosterone levels. This hormonal shift can lead to an increase in body fat and a decrease in lean muscle mass, which may compound feelings of frustration and anxiety. Men may find it challenging to maintain their previous levels of physical activity or may experience changes in their metabolism. By discussing these changes openly, men can gain insights into how their bodies are responding during this time, allowing them to develop realistic goals and strategies tailored to their new circumstances.

Partners play a significant role in this conversation, as they can provide emotional support and encouragement throughout the transition. It is essential for both partners to express their feelings and experiences openly. This can create a deeper understanding of how andropause affects not only the individual but also the relationship. By sharing their concerns and learning about each other's perspectives, couples can work together to find effective solutions, such as adopting healthier eating habits or engaging in physical activities that they can enjoy together.

Health care practitioners also have a vital part in fostering these conversations. They can create a safe space for their patients to discuss concerns related to weight gain, lifestyle changes, and emotional health. Practitioners should encourage open dialogue by asking targeted questions, providing resources, and suggesting strategies for managing symptoms associated with andropause. This proactive approach can empower men to take charge of their health while reinforcing the importance of support from their partners and healthcare teams.

Ultimately, open conversations about health can lead to better outcomes for men experiencing andropause and their partners. By addressing weight gain and other related issues transparently, individuals can work together to implement positive changes in their lives. This collaborative effort not only enhances individual health and well-being but also strengthens relationships, creating a foundation for resilience and shared growth during a challenging phase of life.

Seeking Professional Guidance

When to Consult a Health Care Practitioner

Recognizing the signs of andropause is crucial for men and their partners as they navigate this transitional phase. Andropause, often characterized by hormonal changes, can lead to various physical and emotional symptoms, including weight gain, fatigue, and mood swings. It is important for men experiencing these changes to consider consulting a health care practitioner when they notice significant shifts in their well-being. This professional guidance can provide clarity on whether these changes are typical of aging or indicative of underlying health issues.

Consultation with a health care practitioner is especially important if weight gain occurs rapidly or is accompanied by other concerning symptoms. Men should be aware of changes in their metabolism, as hormonal fluctuations during andropause can affect how the body processes food and stores fat. If a man notices that he is gaining weight despite maintaining a healthy diet and exercise routine, it may signal a need for medical evaluation to rule out conditions such as hypothyroidism or metabolic syndrome. A practitioner can conduct appropriate tests to assess hormone levels and overall health, providing a clearer picture of the situation.

Additionally, emotional health is a significant aspect of the andropause experience. Men may feel increased anxiety, depression, or irritability, which can further complicate weight management efforts. If these emotional shifts interfere with daily life or relationships, seeking help from a health care practitioner becomes vital. Mental health professionals can offer strategies and support tailored to men facing the challenges of andropause, ensuring that emotional well-being is addressed alongside physical health.

Partnership in health management is also essential during this transition. It is beneficial for partners to engage in discussions about any changes experienced, as this can foster mutual understanding and support. Health care practitioners can provide couples with valuable insights on how andropause affects both partners and suggest ways to work together in managing weight and overall health. This collaborative approach can strengthen relationships and create a supportive environment for making lifestyle changes.

Finally, proactive health care involvement can lead to better long-term outcomes. Men are encouraged to establish a relationship with a health care practitioner even before significant issues arise. Regular check-ups can help monitor hormone levels and weight, enabling early intervention if necessary. By prioritizing health consultations during this transitional period, men and their partners can navigate andropause more effectively, maintaining both physical health and emotional resilience.

Types of Professionals Who Can Help

Understanding the types of professionals who can assist in managing weight during andropause is crucial for men and their partners. As physiological changes occur, particularly hormonal shifts, men may experience weight gain that can be challenging to manage. A multidisciplinary approach can be beneficial, drawing on the expertise of various health professionals who specialize in different aspects of health and wellness. This collaborative effort can provide a comprehensive strategy for addressing the unique challenges posed by andropause.

Primary care physicians are often the first point of contact for men experiencing symptoms related to andropause. These practitioners can perform initial assessments to determine hormonal levels and assess overall health. They can help identify any underlying medical conditions that may contribute to weight gain, such as thyroid dysfunction or metabolic syndrome. Additionally, primary care providers can facilitate referrals to specialists, ensuring a coordinated approach to the management of weight and other related symptoms.

Nutritionists and dietitians play a critical role in weight management during andropause. They can provide tailored dietary plans that consider the specific metabolic changes men face during this transition. With expertise in nutrition science, they can educate individuals about the importance of balanced diets, portion control, and mindful eating practices. These professionals can also help identify food triggers that may lead to weight gain, offering strategies to make healthier food choices while still enjoying meals.

Physical trainers and exercise physiologists are instrumental in developing personalized fitness programs. Regular physical activity is essential for weight management, especially as metabolism slows during andropause. These professionals can design exercise regimens that align with individual fitness levels and goals, emphasizing strength training, cardiovascular health, and flexibility. By incorporating enjoyable and sustainable physical activities, they can help men build muscle, increase metabolism, and enhance overall well-being.

Mental health professionals, including psychologists and counsellors, should not be overlooked in the weight management equation. Emotional and psychological factors can significantly influence eating habits and motivation for physical activity. Professionals in this field can provide support through therapy, helping individuals address body image issues, emotional eating, and stress management. By fostering a positive mindset and coping strategies, they can empower men to navigate the emotional landscape of andropause, making it easier to adopt healthier lifestyles.

Integrating Professional Advice into Your Plan

Integrating professional advice into your weight management plan during andropause is essential for achieving sustainable results and maintaining overall health. As men navigate the physical and emotional changes associated with andropause, professional guidance can provide the necessary support and expertise needed to address weight gain effectively. Healthcare practitioners, including dietitians, endocrinologists, and personal trainers, can offer personalized strategies that consider individual health conditions, lifestyle factors, and specific weight management goals.

Consulting with a healthcare practitioner is a critical first step. A thorough assessment of hormone levels, metabolic health, and nutritional needs can help identify underlying issues contributing to weight gain. Blood tests to evaluate testosterone levels, thyroid function, and other hormonal imbalances can reveal valuable insights. Understanding these factors allows practitioners to tailor recommendations that not only focus on weight loss but also on restoring hormonal balance, which is crucial during andropause.

Incorporating nutritional advice from a registered dietitian can significantly enhance your approach to weight management. A dietitian can help design a balanced eating plan that emphasizes whole foods, nutrient-dense options, and appropriate portion sizes. This personalized plan should address any specific dietary restrictions or preferences, making it easier to adhere to in the long run. Additionally, a dietitian can provide education on reading food labels, understanding macronutrients, and making healthier choices when dining out or preparing meals at home.

Exercise plays a vital role in weight management, particularly as men experience the physical changes of andropause. Collaborating with a certified personal trainer can help create a structured workout regimen that incorporates both strength training and cardiovascular exercise. Strength training is particularly important, as it helps counteract muscle loss and supports metabolic function. A trainer can also ensure that exercises are performed safely and effectively, reducing the risk of injury and promoting adherence to a consistent fitness routine.

Finally, regular follow-ups with healthcare professionals can help track progress and make necessary adjustments to your plan. Weight management is not a one-size-fits-all journey; it often requires ongoing evaluation and modification based on how your body responds to dietary and lifestyle changes. Open communication with your healthcare team ensures that any concerns are addressed promptly, fostering a supportive environment that encourages long-term success. By integrating professional advice into your weight management plan, you empower yourself and your partner to navigate the challenges of andropause with confidence and resilience.

Long-term Strategies for Success

Setting Realistic Expectations

Setting realistic expectations is crucial for men and their partners as they navigate the challenges of andropause, particularly regarding weight management. This transitional phase can lead to various physiological and psychological changes, including weight gain due to hormonal fluctuations. Understanding these changes is essential for developing a practical approach to weight management. It is important to recognize that the body's metabolism may slow, leading to an increased propensity for weight gain. Therefore, setting achievable goals becomes a foundational step in this journey.

Men experiencing andropause should aim to set specific, measurable, attainable, relevant, and time-bound (SMART) goals. For instance, rather than aiming to lose a significant amount of weight in a short period, it may be more beneficial to focus on losing one to two pounds per week. This approach not only allows for a more sustainable weight loss but also helps in building confidence and motivation as progress is made. Moreover, it is essential to understand that weight loss is not always linear; fluctuations can occur due to various factors, including changes in muscle mass and water retention. Therefore, patience and consistency are key components of a successful weight management strategy.

In addition to weight loss goals, men and their partners should consider the importance of incorporating healthy lifestyle changes that promote overall well-being. This includes a balanced diet rich in whole foods, regular physical activity, and adequate sleep. By focusing on these areas, individuals can improve their health in a holistic manner rather than concentrating solely on the number on the scale. Setting realistic expectations about the pace of these changes can help prevent frustration and disappointment, fostering a more positive outlook on the journey toward weight management.

It is also crucial for partners to communicate openly about their expectations and experiences during andropause. This shared understanding can help both individuals navigate the challenges associated with weight gain and hormonal changes. Encouragement from partners can play a significant role in maintaining motivation and adherence to lifestyle changes. Establishing a supportive environment can help mitigate feelings of isolation or embarrassment that may arise during this transition, reinforcing the idea that weight management is a shared journey rather than an individual struggle.

Lastly, healthcare practitioners must play an active role in guiding men through this transition by providing education and resources to support realistic goal setting. Offering tailored advice based on individual health profiles can empower men to take charge of their weight management effectively. Moreover, addressing the psychological aspects of andropause, such as stress and emotional well-being, is equally important. By fostering a comprehensive understanding of these dynamics, both men and their partners can approach weight management with realistic expectations, ultimately leading to healthier outcomes during this significant life phase.

Maintaining Motivation Over Time

Maintaining motivation over time is crucial for men experiencing andropause, particularly when it comes to managing weight. As hormonal changes occur, many men encounter various physical and psychological challenges that can make weight management seem daunting. Understanding the factors that influence motivation can help both men and their partners create a supportive environment conducive to lasting change. Establishing clear goals, fostering accountability, and celebrating small victories can all contribute to sustained motivation throughout this transitional phase.

Setting realistic and achievable goals is the first step in maintaining motivation. Men often feel overwhelmed by the prospect of losing weight, especially when faced with other changes associated with andropause. It is essential to break larger goals into smaller, manageable milestones. This approach not only makes the process less intimidating but also provides a sense of accomplishment as each milestone is reached. Partners can play a vital role in this process by helping to set these goals and encouraging their loved ones to stay focused on them.

Accountability can significantly enhance motivation over time. Men may benefit from enlisting a support system that includes friends, family, or health care practitioners who understand the challenges posed by andropause. Regular check-ins, whether through informal conversations or structured meetings, can help keep individuals on track. Additionally, using technology such as fitness apps or online communities allows for tracking progress and sharing experiences, reinforcing the commitment to weight management through peer support.

Incorporating enjoyable activities into a weight management plan can also help maintain motivation. Exercise does not have to be a chore; finding physical activities that are enjoyable can make the process more appealing. Whether it's hiking, swimming, or participating in team sports, integrating fun into fitness can keep men engaged in their routines. Couples can also benefit from exercising together, which not only fosters a sense of partnership but also makes the journey towards better health more enjoyable.

Lastly, recognizing and celebrating small victories is vital for maintaining motivation. Each step taken towards better health should be acknowledged, whether it's losing a few pounds, increasing stamina, or simply making healthier food choices. These celebrations reinforce positive behaviour and help men stay motivated as they navigate the challenges of andropause. By cultivating a mindset that values progress over perfection, men can better manage their weight and overall health, leading to a more fulfilling life during this transitional period.

Adapting to Life Changes

Adapting to life changes is an essential aspect of navigating the complexities of andropause, a phase that many men encounter as they age. This period often brings a variety of physical and emotional changes that can impact overall health and well-being. One of the most prominent issues faced during andropause is weight gain, which can result from hormonal fluctuations, decreased metabolism, and lifestyle changes. Understanding these changes is crucial for men and their partners, as well as health care practitioners, to effectively address the challenges associated with weight management during this transitional phase.

Hormonal shifts during andropause can lead to a decrease in testosterone levels, which is closely linked to changes in body composition. Men may experience an increase in fat mass and a decrease in lean muscle mass, contributing to weight gain. Additionally, factors such as stress, decreased energy levels, and alterations in sleep patterns can further complicate weight management efforts. Recognizing the physiological changes that occur during andropause allows men to better understand their bodies and the weight gain they may be experiencing, helping to alleviate feelings of frustration and confusion.

Adaptation to these changes requires a multifaceted approach that includes dietary modifications, increased physical activity, and mental health support. Men are encouraged to adopt a balanced diet rich in whole foods, lean proteins, healthy fats, and plenty of fruits and vegetables. Such dietary changes can help mitigate weight gain and promote overall health. Furthermore, incorporating regular exercise into daily routines not only aids in weight management but also enhances mood and energy levels, counteracting some of the negative effects of andropause.

Support from partners and healthcare practitioners is vital during this transition. Open communication about the challenges faced can foster understanding and cooperation, making it easier to implement lifestyle changes together. Health care practitioners can play an instrumental role by offering guidance on effective weight management strategies and addressing any underlying health concerns. This collaborative approach promotes accountability and motivation, making the adaptation process less daunting for men experiencing andropause.

Ultimately, adapting to life changes during andropause is a journey that requires patience and resilience. By acknowledging the physical and emotional shifts that accompany this stage of life, men can take proactive steps to manage their weight and improve their quality of life. With the right strategies in place, men and their partners can navigate the challenges of andropause together, emerging stronger and more informed as they embrace this significant life transition.

Moving Forward with Confidence

Embracing Change and New Beginnings

Embracing change is a fundamental aspect of navigating the transition into andropause, a period marked by significant hormonal shifts that can influence both physical and emotional well-being. For many men, this phase brings challenges such as weight gain, reduced muscle mass, and changes in metabolism. Understanding that these changes are a natural part of aging is crucial. By acknowledging the inevitability of these shifts, men can adopt a proactive approach to their health, focusing on strategies that promote well-being rather than resisting the changes that come with age.

The onset of andropause can be a wake-up call for many men, often prompting reflections on lifestyle choices and health priorities. This period serves as an opportunity to reassess dietary habits, exercise routines, and overall wellness strategies. Incorporating a balanced diet rich in nutrients can help mitigate weight gain and support hormonal balance. Whole foods, including lean protein, healthy fats, and plenty of fruits and vegetables, play a vital role in maintaining energy levels and managing weight. This transition is not solely about losing weight but about cultivating a healthier lifestyle that can lead to improved quality of life.

Physical activity is another essential component of embracing change during andropause. Regular exercise not only helps in weight management but also enhances mood and reduces the risk of chronic diseases. Men should consider incorporating a combination of strength training, cardiovascular exercise, and flexibility workouts into their routines. Engaging in activities that are enjoyable and sustainable fosters a positive attitude toward fitness and encourages consistency. Additionally, involving partners in these activities can strengthen relationships and create a shared commitment to health and well-being.

Mental health is equally important during this transition. The psychological effects of andropause, including mood swings and feelings of inadequacy, can significantly impact weight management and overall health. It is essential for men to address these emotional aspects openly and seek support when needed. This could involve discussing feelings with partners, participating in support groups, or consulting with mental health professionals. Acknowledging and addressing these emotional changes can empower men to take charge of their health, fostering resilience and adaptability.

Finally, embracing change also means being open to new beginnings and seeking knowledge. Continuous learning about health, nutrition, and fitness can empower men and their partners to make informed decisions. Workshops, seminars, and online resources can provide valuable insights and strategies tailored to the unique challenges of andropause. By fostering a mindset of growth and adaptability, men can transform this transitional phase into a period of rejuvenation, ultimately leading to healthier lifestyles and stronger relationships.

Celebrating Achievements

Celebrating achievements during the transition of andropause is crucial for maintaining motivation and positive mental health. As men navigate the changes in their bodies, recognizing milestones can foster a sense of accomplishment and encourage continued effort toward health and wellness goals. This process is not merely about weight management; it encompasses broader aspects of well-being, such as emotional resilience, improved energy levels, and better relationships. Acknowledging these successes can help men and their partners stay engaged and committed to their health journeys.

One way to celebrate achievements is through setting realistic, achievable goals that can be measured over time. These goals should encompass various areas of health, including weight loss, increased physical activity, and improvements in dietary habits. For instance, a man might aim to reduce his body weight by a certain percentage or increase his weekly exercise duration. Each time a goal is met, it is essential to take a moment to recognize the effort that went into achieving it. This not only reinforces positive behaviour but also helps create a more profound sense of satisfaction and motivation to pursue further improvements.

Involving partners in the celebration of achievements can enhance the experience and strengthen relationships. Couples can create rituals that acknowledge progress, such as cooking a healthy meal together to reward weight loss or engaging in physical activities that both enjoy. These shared experiences can deepen emotional connections and foster a supportive environment for both partners. By celebrating achievements together, couples can build a healthier lifestyle as a team, which can be especially beneficial during the challenging times of andropause.

Tracking progress through journals or apps can also serve as a motivational tool. Documenting achievements, no matter how small, allows individuals to visualize their journey and see how far they have come. This practice helps to maintain focus on long-term objectives and provides a tangible record of successes. Regularly reviewing these accomplishments can provide encouragement during challenging periods, reinforcing the idea that setbacks are part of the journey and that progress is achievable over time.

Ultimately, celebrating achievements in the context of andropause is about more than just weight management; it encompasses the overall journey toward health and wellness. By recognizing and honouring milestones, men and their partners can cultivate a positive mindset and foster resilience in the face of challenges. This approach not only enhances individual well-being but also strengthens relationships, creating a supportive environment that encourages ongoing commitment to health goals.

Looking Ahead: A Healthier Future

Looking ahead, the conversation surrounding andropause and its associated challenges is evolving, particularly regarding weight management. As men transition through this phase of life, understanding the physiological changes that occur is crucial. Changes in hormone levels, particularly testosterone, can lead to weight gain, altered metabolism, and increased fat distribution, particularly around the abdomen. Recognizing these changes allows men and their partners to adopt proactive strategies that foster a healthier lifestyle, ultimately leading to improved overall well-being.

Incorporating physical activity into daily routines is an essential component of managing weight during andropause. Regular exercise not only helps to counteract weight gain but also boosts mood and energy levels, which can be particularly beneficial during this transitional period. Engaging in a mix of cardiovascular exercises, strength training, and flexibility routines can enhance muscle mass, which tends to decline with age. Men and their partners should work together to create an enjoyable and sustainable exercise plan that fits their lifestyles, making physical activity a shared goal rather than a chore.

Nutrition plays a pivotal role in achieving a healthier future during andropause. As metabolism slows, it becomes essential to focus on a balanced diet rich in whole foods, including fruits, vegetables, lean proteins, and healthy fats. Understanding the impact of dietary choices on weight and overall health can empower men to make informed decisions. Collaborating with healthcare practitioners can provide personalized dietary recommendations, while also addressing any specific health concerns that may arise during this transition.

Mental health is another critical aspect to consider in the journey towards a healthier future. The emotional and psychological effects of andropause can lead to stress, anxiety, and depression, which may further exacerbate weight gain. It is vital for men to engage in open conversations with their partners about their experiences and feelings. Moreover, seeking support from mental health professionals can provide valuable coping strategies and tools to navigate this challenging time. A focus on mental well-being, combined with physical health efforts, creates a more holistic approach to managing weight during andropause.

Ultimately, the path to a healthier future during andropause is one that requires commitment, education, and community support. Men and their partners must actively participate in their health journey, leveraging the resources available to them, including healthcare practitioners, support groups, and educational materials. By fostering a proactive mindset and embracing the changes that come with andropause, individuals can not only manage weight effectively but also enhance their quality of life, paving the way for a vibrant and fulfilling future.

Pause for Thought

- Andropause, the male equivalent to the menopause seen in female, typically occurs in middle aged men which is characterised by a gradual decline in testosterone levels.
- This hormonal shift leads to physiological changes such as weight gain, reduced muscle mass and altered fat distribution. Of note is a more pronounced waistline which is often linked to various health risk as cardiovascular risk and diabetes.
- Andropause affects other biological systems. There is often a decline in the production of growth hormones and insulin-like growth factor essential for muscle growth and maintenance. This decline contributes to the difficulty many men face in maintaining muscle mass as they age. As muscle mass decreases, metabolism slows down, making it easier to gain weight and harder to lose it.
- Psychological factors also play a role during this transitional phase as men may experience mood swings, fatigue, and decreased motivation. These psychological changes can influence lifestyle choices, including diet and exercise habits. Men may find themselves less inclined to engage in physical activity or may turn to comfort foods, further exacerbating weight gain.
- As men approach andropause, a variety of physiological and emotional symptoms may emerge, significantly impacting their daily lives and

relationships. Common physical symptoms include fatigue, reduced libido, and changes in body composition.

- The emotional impact of andropause extends beyond individual experiences affecting relationships with partners and families. Men may experience heightened irritability, anxiety, or sadness, which can strain communication and intimacy with significant others. Partners may feel uncertain about how to provide support or may misinterpret these emotional shifts as personal grievances, leading to misunderstandings.
- Psychological responses to andropause symptoms can lead to increased stress and even depression. Men who feel overwhelmed by their physical changes may withdraw from social interaction or activities they once enjoyed leading to feelings of isolation and dissatisfaction. This emotional toll can create a vicious cycle where declining mental health further exacerbates physical symptoms.
- Muscle mass play a critical role in the overall health and well-being of men, particularly as they approach andropause. Understanding the importance of maintaining muscle mass during this transitional phase is essential for effective weight management and overall health.
- Testosterone is closely linked to muscle growth and maintenance, as testosterone levels drop during andropause, the ability to build and maintain diminishes. This creates a cycle where reduced muscle leads to further hormonal imbalances exacerbating the symptoms of andropause.

- The psychological benefits of maintaining muscle mass should also not be overlooked. Engaging in strength training can boost self esteem and confidence which may be challenged during andropause. The physical changes that accompany this life stage can affect how men perceive themselves leading to issues such as anxiety and depression. By focusing on building and maintaining muscle , men can foster a sense of accomplishment and control over their bodies, which can significantly improve mental health and emotional resilience.

Take Home Nuggets

- Muscle mass serves as a protective factor against chronic diseases. Research indicates higher muscle mass is associated with a lower risk of conditions such as type 2 diabetes, cardiovascular disease, and osteoporosis. Targeted exercise and proper nutrition prioritizing muscle maintenance can lead to long-term health benefits. So with protective steps to preserve muscle mass, men can improve both their physical and enhance their quality of life during this transitional period and beyond.

- Motivation and goal setting are critical components for men facing the challenges of andropause particularly as it relates to weight management, establishing clear, attainable goals is essential for creating a structured path toward achieving desired weight outcomes and enhancing overall well-being.

- Embracing change is a fundamental aspect of navigating the transition into andropause, a period marked by significant hormonal shifts that can influence both physical and emotional well-being.
- Maintaining motivation over time is crucial but can be quite challenging for men experiencing andropause as hormonal changes occur, many men encounter various physical and psychological challenges that may make weight management daunting.
- Establishing clear goals, fostering accountability, and celebrating small victories can all contribute to sustained motivation throughout this transitional phase.
- Setting achievable and realistic goals is a necessary step in maintaining motivation, men are often overwhelmed by the prospect of losing weight particularly when faced with other changes associated with andropause. It is essential to break larger goals into smaller, manageable milestones.
- Adopting life changes is an essential aspect of navigating the complexities of andropause. This period often brings a variety of physical and emotional changes that can impact overall health and wellbeing.
- The onset of andropause can be a wake-up call for many men, often prompting reflections on lifestyle choices and health priorities.
- Mental health is equally important during andropause. The psychological effects of andropause, including mood swings and feelings of inadequacy can significantly impact on management and overall health.

- The celebration of achievements during the transition of andropause is crucial for maintaining motivation and positive mental health. One way to celebrate achievements is to recognise the effort that went into achieving it, the involvement of partners in celebrations can both enhance the experience and strengthen relationships.

Chapter 4
The Science of Bone Health in Andropause

Bone Density Explained

Bone density refers to the amount of mineral matter per square centimetre of bones, serving as a crucial indicator of bone strength and overall skeletal health. In men, particularly as they age and enter andropause, bone density can significantly decline due to hormonal changes, lifestyle factors, and nutritional deficiencies. This decline can lead to conditions such as osteoporosis, characterized by fragile bones that are more susceptible to fractures. Understanding bone density is essential for men and healthcare practitioners to develop effective strategies for maintaining bone health throughout the aging process.

Several factors influence bone density, including genetics, age, hormonal levels, nutrition, and physical activity. Testosterone, the primary male hormone, plays a critical role in maintaining bone density. As men transition into andropause, testosterone levels typically decline, leading to an increased risk of bone loss. Additionally, lifestyle choices such as smoking, excessive alcohol consumption, and a sedentary lifestyle can further exacerbate the decline in bone density. Conversely, engaging in weight-bearing exercises and ensuring adequate intake of calcium and vitamin D can help mitigate these risks.

The process of bone remodelling is a natural cycle where old bone tissue is replaced with new tissue. This cycle is influenced by various cells, including osteoblasts, which build new bone, and osteoclasts, which break down old bone. In healthy individuals, these processes are balanced, maintaining optimal bone density. However, in men experiencing andropause, this balance can shift, leading to bone resorption outpacing bone formation. This imbalance underscores the importance of monitoring bone health during this transitional phase of life.

Healthcare practitioners should prioritize routine bone density screenings for men, especially those over the age of 50 or those with risk factors for osteoporosis. Dual-energy X-ray absorptiometry (DEXA) scans are the gold standard for assessing bone density, providing valuable insights into a patient's bone health. Based on the results, practitioners can recommend personalized interventions, such as dietary adjustments, lifestyle changes, and potentially pharmacological treatments, to help maintain or improve bone density.

In conclusion, understanding bone density is vital for men navigating the challenges of andropause. By recognizing the factors that affect bone health and the importance of proactive measures, men can take control of their skeletal health. Healthcare practitioners play a key role in guiding men through this process, ensuring they have the knowledge and resources to support their bone density and overall vitality as they age. Promoting awareness of bone density issues can lead to healthier outcomes and an improved quality of life for men in this demographic.

Factors Affecting Bone Health

Bone health is influenced by a myriad of factors that can significantly impact the strength and density of bones, particularly in men experiencing andropause. One of the primary factors is age, as bone density naturally decreases with advancing years. The process of bone remodelling, where old bone is replaced by new bone, becomes less efficient, leading to a gradual loss of bone mass. This decline can be exacerbated during andropause, a phase marked by hormonal changes, particularly the decrease in testosterone levels, which plays a crucial role in maintaining bone density.

Nutrition is another vital element in supporting bone health. A diet rich in calcium and vitamin D is essential for maintaining bone strength. Calcium is the primary mineral found in bones, while vitamin D helps the body absorb calcium effectively. Men should focus on incorporating dairy products, leafy greens, and fortified foods into their diets. Additionally, protein intake is important as it provides the necessary building blocks for bone tissue. However, a balanced diet is key; excessive intake of sodium, caffeine, or alcohol can negatively affect calcium absorption and bone health.

Physical activity is crucial for maintaining and improving bone density. Weight-bearing exercises, such as walking, running, or resistance training, stimulate bone formation and help preserve bone mass. Engaging in regular physical activity not only strengthens bones but also improves overall health and vitality, which can be particularly beneficial during andropause. Men should aim for a mix of aerobic and strength-training exercises to optimize their bone health and reduce the risk of osteoporosis.

Hormonal balance also plays a significant role in bone health. Testosterone is important for bone density, and its decline during andropause can lead to increased bone fragility. Men experiencing symptoms of low testosterone may benefit from discussing hormone replacement therapy with their healthcare providers. Monitoring other hormones, such as parathyroid hormone and oestrogen, is equally important, as imbalances can contribute to bone loss. Regular health check-ups can help identify hormonal issues that may affect bone health.

Lastly, lifestyle choices and environmental factors cannot be overlooked. Smoking has been linked to decreased bone density, while excessive alcohol consumption can impair bone formation and increase the risk of fractures. Furthermore, certain medications and chronic health conditions, such as diabetes or rheumatoid arthritis, can adversely affect bone health. Men should be aware of these risk factors and work proactively with healthcare practitioners to develop a comprehensive approach to maintaining bone density and overall health during andropause.

The Aging Process and Bone Loss

The aging process brings about a multitude of physiological changes, one of the most significant being bone loss. As men age, particularly during andropause, their bodies undergo hormonal shifts that can negatively impact bone density. Testosterone, which plays a vital role in maintaining bone health, tends to decline during this period. This decline can lead to an increase in bone resorption, where the body breaks down bone tissue faster than it can be rebuilt, resulting in a net loss of bone density over time.

Bone loss is not a uniform process; it can be influenced by a variety of factors including genetics, lifestyle choices, and overall health. Men with a family history of osteoporosis or fractures may be at a greater risk of experiencing significant bone loss as they age. Additionally, sedentary lifestyles, poor nutrition, and smoking can exacerbate these effects. Health care practitioners often emphasize the importance of a proactive approach to maintaining bone health through lifestyle modifications that can mitigate the risk of osteoporosis and related complications.

Vitamin D and calcium are essential nutrients that play a crucial role in maintaining bone health. As men age, their ability to absorb these nutrients can diminish, leading to further declines in bone density. It is essential for men, especially those in their middle to later years, to ensure they are receiving adequate amounts of these vitamins either through diet or supplementation. Regular check-ups and blood tests can help identify deficiencies early, allowing for timely intervention to prevent further bone loss.

Physical activity is another critical factor in combating age-related bone loss. Weight-bearing exercises, such as walking, jogging, and resistance training, stimulate bone formation and improve overall bone strength. Health care practitioners often recommend incorporating a structured exercise program that includes both strength training and cardiovascular components to promote optimal bone health. This not only helps in maintaining bone density but also enhances balance and coordination, reducing the risk of falls and fractures.

Finally, understanding the connection between hormonal changes and bone health is vital for men experiencing andropause. Health care practitioners should engage in discussions about the impact of hormonal therapy options, such as testosterone replacement therapy, which may help in preserving bone density in men with low testosterone levels. By addressing the aging process and its effects on bone health, men can take proactive steps to maintain their vitality and overall well-being as they navigate the challenges of aging.

The Importance of Calcium and Vitamin D

Calcium and vitamin D play critical roles in maintaining bone health, particularly for men experiencing andropause. This life phase is often accompanied by hormonal changes that can adversely affect bone density. As testosterone levels decline, the risk of osteoporosis and fractures increases. Adequate intake of calcium and vitamin D becomes essential to mitigate these risks and support overall skeletal strength. Both nutrients work synergistically to enhance calcium absorption and bone mineralization, making them vital for maintaining optimal bone health.

Calcium is the primary mineral found in bones and is essential for their structure and strength. Men typically need about 1,000 to 1,200 milligrams of calcium daily, depending on age and specific health conditions. While dairy products are well-known sources of calcium, other foods, such as leafy greens, nuts, seeds, and fortified products, can also contribute to the daily requirement.

For men in andropause, ensuring adequate calcium intake is crucial to prevent bone loss that can lead to debilitating fractures later in life.

Vitamin D is equally important, as it facilitates the absorption of calcium in the intestines and helps maintain adequate serum calcium and phosphate levels. The recommended daily allowance for vitamin D varies, but many health experts suggest that men should aim for about 600 to 800 IU daily, especially if they have limited sun exposure. Sunlight is a natural source of vitamin D; however, factors such as geographical location, skin colour, and season can influence synthesis. As a result, dietary sources like fatty fish, egg yolks, and fortified foods become necessary to meet these needs.

The interplay between calcium and vitamin D is particularly significant during andropause, as hormonal changes can lead to increased bone turnover and reduced bone formation. Insufficient levels of either nutrient can exacerbate bone density loss, leading to an increased risk of osteoporosis. Healthcare practitioners should emphasize the importance of routine screenings for vitamin D levels and encourage men to consider supplementation if dietary intake is inadequate or if they have risk factors for deficiency. This proactive approach can help in early intervention and management of bone health issues.

Incorporating adequate calcium and vitamin D into the daily regimen not only supports bone health but also contributes to overall vitality and well-being. Men seeking to maintain their strength and reduce the risk of fractures should prioritize these nutrients in their diet. Alongside lifestyle modifications such as regular weight-bearing exercise and avoiding smoking, a focus on calcium and vitamin D can empower men to navigate the challenges of andropause effectively. As knowledge about the importance of these nutrients spreads, men and healthcare practitioners can work collaboratively to foster healthier aging and improved quality of life.

The Connection Between Andropause and Bone Health

Hormonal Changes and Bone Density

Hormonal changes in men, particularly during andropause, have a significant impact on bone density. As men age, testosterone levels gradually decline, often leading to a range of physiological changes. Testosterone plays a crucial role in maintaining bone health by promoting bone formation and inhibiting bone resorption. Lower levels of testosterone can result in decreased bone mineral density, increasing the risk of fractures and osteoporosis. Understanding the relationship between these hormonal shifts and bone density is essential for both men navigating this life stage and healthcare practitioners advising them.

The decline in testosterone levels typically begins in a man's late 30s and continues at an approximate rate of one percent per year. This gradual decrease can create a cumulative effect on bone density over time. In addition to testosterone, other hormones such as oestrogen, which is also present in men albeit in lower levels, contribute to bone health. Oestrogen helps to regulate bone remodelling, balancing the processes of bone resorption and formation. As testosterone decreases, the body may experience an imbalance in these processes, leading to a net loss of bone density.

Additionally, the interplay between hormonal changes and lifestyle factors cannot be overlooked. Physical activity, nutrition, and body composition all influence bone health. Weight-bearing exercises are particularly beneficial, as they stimulate bone formation. Men experiencing andropause should focus on maintaining an active lifestyle that includes strength training and aerobic exercise. A balanced diet rich in calcium and vitamin D is also crucial for supporting bone density during this phase. Healthcare practitioners should encourage their patients to adopt these lifestyle changes as part of a comprehensive approach to maintaining bone health.

Moreover, the psychological aspects of hormonal changes can also affect bone health indirectly. Men undergoing andropause may experience mood swings, depression, or decreased motivation, which can lead to a sedentary lifestyle and poor dietary choices. Addressing these mental health concerns is vital for promoting an active lifestyle and ensuring adherence to bone health practices. Healthcare providers must take a holistic approach, considering both the physical and psychological impacts of hormonal changes on men's overall well-being and bone density.

In conclusion, hormonal changes during andropause have profound implications for bone density in men. The decline in testosterone and its influence on oestrogen levels play a critical role in the maintenance of bone health. By understanding these changes, men can take proactive measures to support their bone density through lifestyle modifications. Healthcare practitioners play a key role in guiding men through this transition, emphasizing the importance of physical activity, nutrition, and mental well-being in preserving bone health during and beyond andropause.

The Impact of Testosterone on Bone Health

Testosterone plays a crucial role in maintaining bone health, particularly in men, as it influences bone density and strength. As men age, testosterone levels naturally decline, which can lead to a decrease in bone mineral density and an increased risk of fractures. This relationship is especially important during andropause, a phase characterized by hormonal changes that can significantly affect overall health. Understanding the impact of testosterone on bone health is essential for both men and healthcare practitioners, as it enables proactive measures to mitigate the risks associated with low testosterone levels.

Research indicates that testosterone has a direct effect on bone tissue by stimulating bone formation and reducing bone resorption. Osteoblasts, the cells responsible for bone formation, are influenced by testosterone, which enhances their activity and promotes the deposition of minerals in the bone matrix. Conversely, testosterone inhibits the activity of osteoclasts, the cells that break down bone tissue. This balance between bone formation and resorption is critical for maintaining bone density and preventing osteoporosis, a condition that can lead to debilitating fractures.

The decline of testosterone during andropause can lead to significant skeletal changes. Studies show that men with lower testosterone levels have a higher incidence of osteoporosis and fragility fractures. This is particularly concerning considering that men are often diagnosed with osteoporosis later than women, leading to more severe outcomes. Healthcare practitioners should be vigilant in monitoring testosterone levels in aging men and evaluating their bone health through appropriate screening methods, such as bone density tests, to identify those at risk early.

Lifestyle factors also play a significant role in the relationship between testosterone and bone health. Regular weight-bearing exercises, a balanced diet rich in calcium and vitamin D, and maintaining a healthy body weight can all contribute to improved bone density. Additionally, avoiding excessive alcohol consumption and smoking can help mitigate the adverse effects of declining testosterone levels. Men should be encouraged to adopt healthy habits that support both their hormonal balance and bone health.

The interplay between testosterone and bone health underscores the importance of a holistic approach to men's health during andropause. Healthcare practitioners should not only focus on testosterone replacement therapy when appropriate but also educate men about lifestyle modifications that can enhance bone density. By fostering awareness of the impact of testosterone on bone health, men can take proactive steps to preserve their skeletal integrity, thus enhancing their vitality and overall well-being as they age.

Risk Factors for Osteoporosis in Men

Osteoporosis is often perceived as a condition that primarily affects women, yet men are also at significant risk, especially as they age. Understanding the risk factors for osteoporosis in men is crucial for prevention and management. Age is one of the most prominent risk factors; as men reach their 50s and beyond, bone density naturally declines due to decreased testosterone levels. This hormonal change leads to a reduction in bone mass, making it essential for men to monitor their bone health as they age.

Another critical risk factor is lifestyle choices. Diet plays a significant role in bone health, and men who consume inadequate amounts of calcium and vitamin D are at a heightened risk for osteoporosis. Foods rich in these nutrients are vital for maintaining bone density. Additionally, excessive alcohol consumption and smoking are detrimental to bone health. Alcohol can interfere with the body's ability to absorb calcium, while smoking has been linked to lower bone density and increased fracture risk. Men should be encouraged to adopt healthier lifestyle habits to mitigate these risks.

Medical history is also a key consideration. Men with a history of certain medical conditions, such as rheumatoid arthritis, chronic kidney disease, or hormonal disorders, are more susceptible to osteoporosis. Furthermore, medications like corticosteroids, often prescribed for inflammation and autoimmune diseases, can weaken bones over time. Healthcare practitioners should take a comprehensive medical history when assessing a man's risk for osteoporosis, ensuring that all potential contributing factors are considered.

Family history is another important risk factor that should not be overlooked. Men with a family history of osteoporosis or fractures have a greater likelihood of developing the condition themselves. Genetic factors play a role in bone density, and understanding familial patterns can aid both men and their healthcare providers in identifying individuals at higher risk. Genetic testing may be an option for some, providing deeper insights into personalized risk assessments.

Finally, physical inactivity is a significant contributor to osteoporosis risk in men. Regular weight-bearing exercise is essential for maintaining bone strength and density. Men who lead sedentary lifestyles are more likely to experience bone loss. Incorporating activities such as walking, running, or resistance training can help strengthen bones and improve overall health. Encouraging men to engage in regular physical activity is vital for osteoporosis prevention and can enhance their quality of life as they age.

Prevention Strategies

Prevention strategies for andropause and bone health are essential for men as they age, especially considering the physiological changes that occur during this phase of life. Andropause, often characterized by a gradual decline in testosterone levels, can lead to various health issues, including decreased bone density. Implementing effective prevention strategies is crucial for maintaining vitality and ensuring a better quality of life as men navigate these changes.

One of the primary strategies for preventing the negative effects of andropause is to maintain a balanced diet rich in nutrients that support hormonal health and bone density. Foods high in calcium, vitamin D, and magnesium are particularly important. Incorporating dairy products, leafy greens, fatty fish, and nuts into daily meals can help bolster bone strength. Additionally, a diet that includes healthy fats, lean proteins, and a variety of fruits and vegetables can support overall hormonal balance and physical well-being, reducing the risk of complications associated with andropause.

Regular physical activity plays a significant role in preventing the adverse effects of andropause and promoting bone health. Weight-bearing exercises, such as walking, jogging, and resistance training, are particularly beneficial for improving bone density. Engaging in strength training not only helps to build muscle but also stimulates the production of testosterone, which can counteract some of the hormonal declines experienced during andropause. Furthermore, incorporating flexibility and balance exercises, like yoga or tai chi, can enhance overall physical function and reduce the risk of falls and fractures.

Another critical aspect of prevention is routine health screenings and consultations with healthcare practitioners. Regular check-ups can help identify early signs of hormonal imbalance or bone density loss, allowing for timely interventions. Men should discuss their risk factors with their healthcare provider, including family history, lifestyle choices, and any symptoms they may be experiencing. This proactive approach enables tailored recommendations for supplementation, lifestyle modifications, or prescription therapies that can be pivotal in maintaining health during andropause.

Lastly, addressing mental and emotional health is vital for holistic prevention strategies. The changes associated with andropause can lead to anxiety, depression, and reduced motivation, which can further complicate physical health. Engaging in stress-reducing activities such as mindfulness, meditation, or hobbies can enhance mental well-being and encourage a more active lifestyle. Building a strong support network of family, friends, or support groups can also foster resilience and provide encouragement as men navigate the challenges of aging, ultimately leading to better health outcomes.

Nutrition for Optimal Health

Essential Nutrients for Bone and Hormonal Health

Bone and hormonal health are critical components of overall well-being, particularly for men experiencing andropause. This transitional phase often leads to hormonal imbalances that can affect bone density, muscle mass, and energy levels. To mitigate these effects, it is essential to focus on a diet rich in essential nutrients that support both bone and hormonal health. Key nutrients include calcium, vitamin D, magnesium, zinc, and vitamin K, each playing a unique role in maintaining strong bones and balanced hormones.

Calcium is perhaps the most recognized nutrient for bone health. It is the primary mineral found in bones and is crucial for maintaining their strength and structure. Men aged 50 and older should aim for a calcium intake of about 1,200 milligrams per day. Dairy products, leafy greens, and fortified foods are excellent sources of calcium. However, calcium alone is not enough; it requires adequate vitamin D for proper absorption. Vitamin D can be synthesized through sun exposure and is also found in fatty fish, egg yolks, and fortified foods. Ensuring sufficient vitamin D levels is vital for maintaining optimal calcium levels and supporting bone mineralization.

Magnesium is another mineral that plays a significant role in bone health and hormonal balance. It helps convert vitamin D into its active form, which in turn aids calcium absorption. Additionally, magnesium is involved in over 300 biochemical reactions in the body, including those that regulate hormone production. Foods high in magnesium include nuts, seeds, whole grains, and green leafy vegetables. A balanced intake of magnesium not only supports bone density but also contributes to overall hormonal balance, making it an essential nutrient for men experiencing andropause.

Zinc and vitamin K are also pivotal for maintaining both bone integrity and hormonal health. Zinc assists in testosterone production, which is crucial for muscle mass and bone density. It can be found in foods such as meat, shellfish, legumes, and seeds. Vitamin K, on the other hand, plays a role in bone mineralization and helps prevent fractures. Green leafy vegetables and fermented foods are rich in vitamin K. Together, these nutrients help to create a balanced environment for hormonal function and bone maintenance, reducing the risk of osteoporosis and other age-related conditions.

In conclusion, a diet rich in essential nutrients is fundamental for men navigating the challenges of andropause. By focusing on calcium, vitamin D, magnesium, zinc, and vitamin K, men can promote better bone density and hormonal balance, ultimately enhancing their vitality and quality of life. Health care practitioners should encourage men to incorporate these nutrients into their diets, along with regular physical activity and lifestyle changes, to create a holistic approach to maintaining health during this critical phase of life.

Dietary Recommendations

Dietary recommendations for men experiencing andropause and concerns about bone health are crucial for maintaining vitality and overall well-being. A balanced diet rich in essential nutrients can help manage the symptoms of andropause while also supporting bone density. Key elements such as adequate protein, healthy fats, vitamins, and minerals should be prioritized to ensure both hormonal balance and skeletal health.

Protein plays a vital role in maintaining muscle mass and supporting bone structure. Men should aim to include a variety of protein sources, such as lean meats, fish, legumes, and dairy products, in their daily diet. Adequate protein intake not only helps in muscle preservation but also contributes to the production of hormones like testosterone, which can decline during andropause. It is recommended that men consume protein with every meal to promote muscle repair and growth, ultimately aiding in maintaining strength and reducing the risk of osteoporosis.

Healthy fats are another important aspect of dietary recommendations. Incorporating sources of omega-3 fatty acids, such as fatty fish, walnuts, and flaxseeds, can help reduce inflammation and support heart health. Additionally, monounsaturated fats from sources like avocados and olive oil are beneficial for overall hormonal balance. It is essential for men to limit saturated and trans fats, which can negatively impact both heart health and hormonal levels. By focusing on healthy fats, men can enhance their overall vitality while supporting their bone density.

Vitamins and minerals are critical for bone health, with calcium and vitamin D being the most prominent. Calcium is the primary building block of bones, and men should aim to consume adequate amounts through dairy products, leafy greens, and fortified foods. Vitamin D, on the other hand, is essential for calcium absorption and can be obtained through sunlight exposure and dietary sources such as fatty fish and fortified foods. It is advisable for men to have their vitamin D levels checked, as deficiency can lead to decreased bone density and increased fracture risk.

Finally, hydration and moderation in alcohol intake are vital components of a healthy diet. Staying adequately hydrated supports all bodily functions, including muscle and bone health. Men should aim to drink plenty of water throughout the day and limit sugary beverages. Furthermore, while moderate alcohol consumption may have some health benefits, excessive intake can lead to weakened bones and hormonal imbalances. By adhering to these dietary recommendations, men can take proactive steps towards managing andropause symptoms and enhancing their bone health, ultimately fostering a more vibrant and fulfilling life.

Supplements: What Works?

Supplements play a crucial role in supporting men's health, particularly during andropause when hormonal changes can impact vitality and bone density. Understanding which supplements are effective can empower men to make informed decisions about their health. Not all supplements are created equal; scientific evidence varies widely regarding their efficacy. Focusing on those with proven benefits can help combat the challenges posed by aging, including reduced testosterone levels and increased risk of osteoporosis.

Vitamin D is one of the most critical supplements for men, especially in relation to bone health. It aids in calcium absorption, which is vital for maintaining strong bones. Studies have shown that adequate levels of vitamin D can not only bolster bone density but also contribute to overall hormonal balance. Many men, particularly those living in northern latitudes or who spend limited time outdoors, may have suboptimal levels of vitamin D. Supplementation can help mitigate these deficiencies and promote better health outcomes during andropause.

Calcium is another essential supplement for men concerned about bone density. As men age, their ability to absorb calcium diminishes, making supplementation important to prevent osteoporosis. The recommended dietary allowance for calcium varies by age and health status, but many men find it challenging to meet these needs through diet alone. A combination of calcium and vitamin D supplements can create a synergistic effect, enhance bone health and reducing the risk of fractures, which is particularly important as men navigate the changes associated with aging.

Omega-3 fatty acids also warrant attention when considering supplements for men's health. These essential fats have anti-inflammatory properties and are linked to numerous health benefits, including improved cardiovascular health and potentially enhanced testosterone levels. Research suggests that omega-3 supplementation may support overall vitality and well-being during andropause. Regular consumption of these fatty acids, whether through fish oil supplements or dietary sources, can promote not only bone health but also overall physical and mental health.

Lastly, it is important for men to approach supplementation with a critical eye. Consulting with healthcare practitioners before starting any new supplement regimen is essential, as individual health needs can vary significantly. Some supplements may interact with medications or may not be suitable for men with specific health conditions. By working with healthcare professionals, men can develop a personalized plan that incorporates effective supplements, dietary adjustments, and lifestyle changes to support their health during andropause and promote optimal bone density.

Hydration and Its Importance

Hydration is a critical component of overall health, particularly for men experiencing andropause, a phase marked by hormonal changes that can influence various bodily functions. Adequate hydration plays a vital role in maintaining optimal physiological processes, including metabolism, thermoregulation, and joint lubrication. As men age, their body's ability to conserve water declines, making it essential to understand the significance of hydration and its impact on bone health and vitality.

Water is essential for the transportation of nutrients and oxygen throughout the body. It aids in the digestion and absorption of food, ensuring that vital minerals such as calcium and magnesium are delivered to bones effectively. During andropause, men may experience changes in appetite or digestive efficiency, which can affect nutrient intake. Proper hydration can help mitigate these issues, facilitating better nutrient absorption and supporting bone density. This is particularly important as men face an increased risk of osteoporosis and fractures as they age.

In addition to its role in nutrient transport, hydration is crucial for maintaining joint health. Dehydration can lead to joint stiffness and discomfort, which may exacerbate conditions such as arthritis. For men, especially those engaged in physical activities or strength training, maintaining joint health is essential for sustaining an active lifestyle. Drinking sufficient water helps to keep synovial fluid at optimal levels, cushioning the joints and reducing the risk of injury. This is particularly relevant for men undergoing changes in hormone levels during andropause, as they may be more susceptible to joint-related issues.

Moreover, hydration is linked to energy levels and cognitive function. Dehydration can lead to fatigue, decreased concentration, and mood disturbances, which can be particularly problematic for men navigating the complexities of andropause. Maintaining hydration not only supports physical performance but also enhances mental clarity and emotional well-being. For health care practitioners, emphasizing the importance of hydration in their patients' routines can be a simple yet effective strategy to improve overall quality of life.

Finally, it is important to recognize that hydration needs can vary individually based on activity level, climate, and overall health. Men should aim to drink water consistently throughout the day, rather than waiting until they feel thirsty. Incorporating hydrating foods such as fruits and vegetables can also contribute to overall fluid intake. Health care practitioners should encourage their patients to monitor their hydration status by observing signs such as urine color and frequency, ensuring that they remain adequately hydrated for optimal health during andropause and beyond.

Exercise and Physical Activity

The Role of Exercise in Managing Andropause

The role of exercise in managing andropause is crucial for maintaining overall health and well-being during this transitional phase of life. As men age, hormonal changes can lead to symptoms such as fatigue, mood swings, decreased libido, and reduced muscle mass. Engaging in regular physical activity can mitigate these effects by enhancing hormonal balance, boosting energy levels, and improving mental health. Exercise serves not only to counteract the physical changes associated with andropause but also as a holistic approach to promote vitality and longevity.

Resistance training plays a significant role in maintaining muscle mass and bone density, both of which can decline during andropause. As testosterone levels decrease, men may experience a reduction in muscle strength and an increased risk of osteoporosis. Incorporating weight-bearing exercises can stimulate bone formation and enhance bone density, reducing the likelihood of fractures. Additionally, resistance training promotes the production of growth hormone, which can further support muscle retention and overall metabolic health.

Cardiovascular exercise is equally important for men experiencing andropause. Regular aerobic activity, such as brisk walking, cycling, or swimming, can improve cardiovascular health, enhance mood, and boost energy levels. This type of exercise increases blood flow and oxygen delivery to tissues, which can help combat fatigue and improve overall stamina. Furthermore, cardiovascular workouts have been shown to help regulate hormonal fluctuations, contributing to better emotional stability and resilience against stress.

Flexibility and balance exercises also play a vital role in the management of andropause. Practices such as yoga or tai chi not only improve physical flexibility but also promote mental clarity and stress relief. As men age, the risk of falls and injuries increases, making balance training essential. Incorporating flexibility and balance exercises into a regular fitness routine can enhance mobility, reduce the risk of injury, and foster a greater sense of well-being, which is particularly beneficial during times of hormonal change.

In conclusion, exercise is a powerful tool in managing the symptoms of andropause and promoting overall health. A well-rounded fitness program that includes resistance training, cardiovascular activities, and flexibility exercises can address the physical and emotional challenges men face during this period. Healthcare practitioners should encourage their patients to adopt an active lifestyle as part of a comprehensive approach to andropause management. By prioritizing exercise, men can enhance their vitality, improve bone health, and embrace this new stage of life with confidence and resilience.

Weight-Bearing Exercises for Bone Health

Weight-bearing exercises play a crucial role in enhancing bone health, particularly for men experiencing andropause. As testosterone levels decline with age, the risk of osteoporosis and bone density loss increases. Engaging in regular weight-bearing activities can stimulate bone formation and slow down the loss of bone mass. These exercises force the body to work against gravity, which is essential for maintaining the structural integrity of bones. By understanding the importance of these exercises, men can take proactive steps to protect their skeletal health and overall vitality.

The primary mechanism behind weight-bearing exercises is their ability to create mechanical stress on bones. When muscles contract during these activities, they pull on the bones, promoting a process called bone remodelling. This process involves the breakdown of old bone tissue and the formation of new, stronger bone. High-impact activities like running, jumping, and resistance training are particularly effective in this regard. They not only enhance bone density but also improve muscle strength and balance, which are vital for reducing the risk of falls and fractures.

Incorporating a variety of weight-bearing exercises into a fitness regimen is essential for maximizing bone health benefits. Activities such as walking, jogging, dancing, and hiking can be easily integrated into daily routines. Additionally, resistance training using free weights, resistance bands, or body weight exercises like push-ups and squats can further enhance bone strength. It's important for men to choose exercises that they enjoy, as this increases the likelihood of long-term adherence to an active lifestyle, ultimately supporting sustained bone health.

For men in the andropause stage, the intensity and frequency of weight-bearing exercises should be carefully considered. While it is important to challenge the body, overexertion can lead to injury, particularly in older adults. It is advisable to start with moderate-intensity exercises and gradually increase the intensity as strength and endurance improve. Consulting with a healthcare practitioner or a certified fitness trainer can help in designing a safe and effective exercise program tailored to individual needs and capabilities.

In conclusion, weight-bearing exercises are an essential component of maintaining bone health during andropause. By engaging in these activities regularly, men can combat the effects of aging on bone density and improve their overall physical well-being. It is never too late to start incorporating these exercises into daily life, and the benefits extend beyond just bone health, positively impacting muscle strength, balance, and overall vitality. Embracing weight-bearing exercises can lead to a healthier, more active lifestyle, enhancing quality of life as men age.

Strength Training and Its Benefits

Strength training is an essential component of maintaining overall health and wellness, particularly for men experiencing andropause. As testosterone levels decline with age, men may face various health challenges, including decreased muscle mass, increased fat accumulation, and lower bone density. Engaging in strength training can counteract these age-related changes, helping to preserve muscle function and promote a healthier body composition. Regular strength training helps increase muscle strength, improves metabolism, and enhances physical performance, making it a vital practice for men in this phase of life.

One of the primary benefits of strength training is its positive impact on bone density. Resistance exercises stimulate bone formation and help prevent osteoporosis, a condition characterized by weak and brittle bones. This is particularly crucial for older men who are at a higher risk of bone fractures and injuries. Studies have shown that weight-bearing exercises can lead to significant gains in bone mineral density, especially in the spine and hip, which are common sites for fractures. Therefore, incorporating strength training into a regular exercise routine can effectively mitigate the risks associated with declining bone health in men.

Moreover, strength training has been linked to improved hormonal balance, which is especially beneficial during andropause. As men age, testosterone levels typically decline, leading to various physical and emotional symptoms. Engaging in regular resistance training has been shown to stimulate testosterone production, contributing to enhanced mood, increased energy levels, and improved libido. This hormonal boost can greatly enhance the quality of life for men experiencing the effects of andropause, providing a natural way to combat some of the associated challenges.

In addition to its physical benefits, strength training can also have significant mental health advantages. Exercise, particularly resistance training, has been shown to reduce symptoms of anxiety and depression. For men navigating the emotional fluctuations that can accompany andropause, strength training can serve as a powerful outlet for stress relief and empowerment. The discipline and routine involved in a strength training program can foster a sense of accomplishment and improved self-esteem, further enhancing mental well-being during this transitional period.

Finally, strength training promotes functional fitness, which is crucial for maintaining independence as men age. By improving strength, balance, and coordination, resistance exercises can help prevent falls and injuries, allowing men to remain active and engaged in their daily lives. This functional aspect of strength training is particularly important for older adults, as it enables them to perform everyday activities with greater ease and confidence. In conclusion, integrating strength training into a regular fitness routine is vital for men facing andropause, offering a plethora of benefits that enhance both physical and mental health, ultimately contributing to a more vibrant and active lifestyle.

Flexibility and Balance

Flexibility and balance are crucial components of overall health, especially as men age and experience changes associated with andropause. These physical attributes not only enhance daily functioning but also significantly contribute to preventing injuries and maintaining bone density. As testosterone levels decline, men may experience stiffness in joints and reduced muscle mass, making it imperative to incorporate flexibility and balance exercises into their routines. By doing so, men can counteract some of the physical changes that occur during andropause and promote a healthier, more active lifestyle.

Flexibility exercises, such as stretching, yoga, and Pilates, help improve the range of motion in joints and promote better posture. These activities can alleviate discomfort from stiffness and tension associated with aging. Regular stretching can also increase blood flow to the muscles, enhancing recovery and reducing the risk of injury during other forms of physical activity. For men experiencing muscle tightness or pain, incorporating flexibility training into their weekly regimen can lead to significant improvements in mobility and overall quality of life.

Balance exercises play a vital role in maintaining stability and preventing falls, which are critical concerns as men age. Activities such as tai chi, balance boards, and single-leg stands can help improve core strength and coordination. These exercises not only enhance physical stability but also engage the mind, as they require focus and concentration. Improved balance can lead to greater confidence in movement, allowing men to participate in various physical activities without fear of injury. This confidence is particularly important in promoting an active lifestyle, which is essential for maintaining bone health.

Furthermore, the relationship between flexibility, balance, and bone density cannot be overstated. Engaging in regular physical activity, including flexibility and balance training, helps stimulate bone remodelling and increases bone density. As men experience hormonal changes during andropause, maintaining bone strength becomes increasingly important. Weight-bearing exercises, combined with flexibility and balance practices, create a comprehensive approach to bone health. This holistic strategy not only supports bone density but also enhances overall vitality, making it essential for men to prioritize these components in their fitness routines.

In conclusion, flexibility and balance are indispensable for men navigating the challenges of andropause and striving to maintain optimal bone health. By integrating flexibility and balance exercises into their lifestyle, men can improve their overall physical capacity, reduce the risk of injury, and foster a sense of well-being that transcends age. Health care practitioners should encourage their patients to adopt these practices, emphasizing their importance in promoting longevity, vitality, and a high quality of life. Embracing flexibility and balance as essential elements of fitness can empower men to take control of their health as they age.

Lifestyle Modifications

Managing Stress and Mental Health

Managing stress and mental health is a crucial aspect of overall well-being, particularly for men experiencing andropause. This transitional phase, often marked by a decline in testosterone levels, can lead to various physical and emotional challenges. Stress management strategies can significantly impact mental health, aiding in the navigation of these changes. Understanding how stress affects the body and mind is essential for both men and healthcare practitioners as they work together to develop effective coping mechanisms.

The physiological changes during andropause can lead to increased stress levels. Symptoms such as fatigue, mood swings, and decreased libido are not only frustrating but can also contribute to a heightened state of anxiety. It is vital for men to recognize these symptoms as interconnected rather than isolated issues. Regular physical activity, such as strength training and cardiovascular exercises, can serve as a natural stress reliever, improving both mood and bone density. Practicing mindfulness techniques, such as meditation and deep-breathing exercises, can also be beneficial in managing stress and enhancing mental clarity.

Social support plays a significant role in mental health during andropause. Men often face societal pressures to remain stoic, which can lead to isolation and exacerbated stress. Encouraging open dialogue about mental health among peers can help dismantle the stigma surrounding vulnerability. Support groups, whether informal among friends or structured within healthcare settings, provide a platform for men to share experiences and coping strategies. Healthcare practitioners should promote the importance of community and connection, helping their patients build strong support networks.

Nutrition is another critical element in managing stress and mental health. A well-balanced diet rich in vitamins and minerals can positively influence mood and cognitive function. Nutrients such as omega-3 fatty acids, found in fish, and antioxidants from fruits and vegetables can help reduce inflammation and support brain health. Men should be encouraged to adopt dietary habits that not only promote vitality but also provide the necessary fuel for managing stress. Healthcare practitioners can offer tailored nutritional advice to meet the specific needs of men undergoing andropause.

Finally, seeking professional help when necessary is an integral part of stress management. Mental health professionals can provide valuable support and guidance, particularly for those experiencing significant anxiety or depression related to andropause. Therapy options, including cognitive-behavioural therapy (CBT), can equip men with tools to better cope with stressors and improve their overall mental health. Healthcare practitioners should remain vigilant in assessing their patients' mental health and be proactive in recommending appropriate resources. By fostering an environment where mental health is prioritized, men can navigate the complexities of andropause with resilience and strength.

The Importance of Sleep

The role of sleep in overall health cannot be overstated, particularly for men experiencing andropause. As testosterone levels decline, the body's physiological processes can become disrupted, leading to various health challenges. Quality sleep is essential for hormone regulation, muscle recovery, and maintaining bone density. Studies indicate that inadequate sleep can exacerbate symptoms of andropause, such as fatigue, mood swings, and decreased libido, making it imperative for men to prioritize restful nights.

Sleep is a critical factor in the body's ability to repair and regenerate. During deep sleep, the body undergoes essential restorative processes, including muscle growth and tissue repair. This is particularly relevant for men in their middle age and beyond, as maintaining muscle mass becomes increasingly challenging. Additionally, sleep promotes the release of growth hormone, which plays a vital role in maintaining bone density. A lack of sleep can hinder these processes, leading to a decline in both muscle and bone health.

Furthermore, sleep impacts mental health and cognitive function, areas that can suffer significantly during andropause. Many men report increased anxiety and depression during this transition, which can be linked to poor sleep quality. Chronic sleep deprivation can lead to cognitive decline, affecting memory and decision-making abilities. For healthcare practitioners, addressing sleep issues is crucial in developing comprehensive treatment plans for men dealing with andropause and associated health concerns.

The relationship between sleep and metabolic health is also significant. Insufficient sleep is associated with an increased risk of obesity and metabolic syndrome, conditions that can further complicate the health of men in andropause. Disrupted sleep patterns can lead to hormonal imbalances that increase appetite and cravings, making it challenging to maintain a healthy weight. By improving sleep hygiene, men can enhance their metabolic health, thereby supporting their overall vitality and well-being.

In summary, the importance of sleep for men experiencing andropause cannot be overlooked. Quality sleep supports hormone regulation, muscle recovery, mental health, and metabolic function, all critical elements in maintaining health during this life stage. Men and healthcare practitioners should prioritize sleep as a foundational aspect of health management, recognizing that improving sleep quality can lead to significant enhancements in overall health outcomes and quality of life.

Avoiding Harmful Habits

Avoiding harmful habits is critical for men navigating the challenges of andropause and maintaining optimal bone health. As men age, hormonal changes can lead to a decline in testosterone levels, which in turn can affect bone density and overall vitality. It is essential to recognize and eliminate behaviours that could exacerbate these issues. Engaging in a proactive approach to health can significantly mitigate the risks associated with aging, particularly in the context of bone strength and hormonal balance.

One of the most detrimental habits to avoid is smoking. Research has consistently shown that smoking is linked to lower bone density and increased fracture risk. The chemicals in cigarettes can interfere with the body's ability to absorb calcium and other essential nutrients that are crucial for bone health. For men experiencing andropause, quitting smoking can lead to improvements in overall hormonal levels and bone mineral density. Support systems and resources are available to assist those looking to quit, making it a vital step toward better health.

Excessive alcohol consumption is another habit that can have severe repercussions on bone health and hormonal balance. While moderate drinking may have some health benefits, heavy drinking can lead to osteoporosis and other bone-related issues. Alcohol can also disrupt testosterone production, compounding the effects of andropause. Men should aim to limit their alcohol intake and seek healthier alternatives that promote vitality and well-being. This shift not only benefits bone density but also enhances overall health.

Poor dietary choices can also contribute to harmful habits that negatively impact bone health. Diets low in essential nutrients, such as calcium and vitamin D, can lead to weakened bones and increased susceptibility to fractures. Men should prioritize a balanced diet rich in whole foods, including leafy greens, lean proteins, and fortified foods. Additionally, staying hydrated is crucial for overall health and can aid in the absorption of nutrients necessary for maintaining bone density. Working with a nutritionist can provide personalized guidance on optimizing dietary habits.

Lastly, a sedentary lifestyle can have dire consequences for both hormonal levels and bone health. Regular physical activity helps to strengthen bones and maintain muscle mass, which is essential as men age. Weight-bearing exercises, in particular, are beneficial for stimulating bone growth and density. It is advisable for men to incorporate a mix of cardiovascular, strength, and flexibility training into their routines. Engaging in consistent physical activity not only combats the effects of andropause but also enhances overall vitality and well-being. By replacing harmful habits with healthier alternatives, men can foster a more robust foundation for their health as they age.

Building a Support System

Building a supportive network is crucial for men experiencing andropause and related health issues, including bone density concerns. This support system can encompass family, friends, health care professionals, and community resources. Each component plays a distinct role in fostering emotional resilience, providing practical advice, and facilitating access to information and treatment options. Men often face societal pressures that discourage open discussions about health, particularly those related to aging. Establishing a strong support system can help break down these barriers and create an environment where men feel comfortable sharing their experiences and seeking assistance.

Family and friends are often the first line of support. They can offer emotional encouragement and practical help, especially during challenging times. Engaging loved ones in conversations about andropause and its effects can foster understanding and empathy. It is essential for men to communicate openly about their feelings and health concerns, as this can strengthen relationships and create a sense of solidarity. Friends and family can also encourage healthy lifestyle changes, such as participating in physical activities together or preparing nutritious meals, which can significantly impact overall health and vitality.

Healthcare practitioners play a pivotal role in a man's support system. Regular check-ups and consultations can help identify early signs of andropause and monitor bone density levels. A knowledgeable practitioner will not only provide medical advice but also serve as a resource for education about lifestyle modifications, nutritional guidance, and treatment options. Men should feel empowered to ask questions and express their concerns during medical appointments. Building a trusting relationship with healthcare providers can lead to better health outcomes and a more proactive approach to managing andropause effects.

Community resources can further enhance a support system. Local support groups, fitness classes, and wellness programs specifically geared towards men's health can provide invaluable connections. These resources offer opportunities to meet others facing similar challenges, share experiences, and learn from one another. Engaging in community activities not only promotes physical health through exercise and socialization but also helps combat feelings of isolation that can accompany andropause. Men should seek out organizations or groups focused on men's health to find additional support and encouragement.

Ultimately, building a robust support system involves a combination of emotional, practical, and informational resources. Men experiencing andropause and concerns about bone health should actively seek out and nurture their support networks. By fostering open communication with loved ones, maintaining relationships with healthcare providers, and engaging with community resources, men can navigate this life stage with greater confidence and improved health outcomes. A well-rounded support system is not just beneficial; it is essential for fostering resilience and promoting vitality during and beyond andropause.

Medical Interventions and Treatments

Hormone Replacement Therapy

Hormone Replacement Therapy (HRT) has gained considerable attention as an intervention for men experiencing andropause, a phase marked by a decline in testosterone levels that can affect physical, mental, and emotional health. This therapy aims to restore hormonal balance, alleviating symptoms such as fatigue, decreased libido, depression, and reduced bone density. For men facing these challenges, understanding the role of HRT can be pivotal in navigating this stage of life effectively.

Testosterone replacement therapy, a common form of HRT, can be administered via injections, transdermal patches, gels, or pellets. Each method has its advantages and drawbacks, with factors such as patient preference, convenience, and potential side effects guiding the choice of administration. Regular monitoring is essential to ensure that hormone levels are maintained within a therapeutic range, minimizing risks while maximizing benefits. This careful management plays a crucial role in enhancing quality of life and overall vitality.

Research indicates that HRT may have a positive impact on bone density, a significant concern for aging men. Low testosterone levels are associated with an increased risk of osteoporosis and fractures. By restoring testosterone, HRT can help improve bone mineral density, reducing the likelihood of fractures and promoting overall skeletal health. Additionally, the therapy may enhance muscle mass and strength, further supporting bone health by providing the necessary mechanical loading required to maintain bone integrity.

While HRT offers potential benefits, it is not without risks. Side effects may include acne, sleep apnoea, and an increased risk of cardiovascular issues and prostate health concerns. Therefore, comprehensive evaluation and ongoing supervision by healthcare practitioners are critical. A thorough assessment of medical history, current health status, and individual patient concerns can help mitigate risks while tailoring the therapy to meet specific needs.

In conclusion, Hormone Replacement Therapy can be a valuable tool for men experiencing the effects of andropause, particularly regarding bone health and overall vitality. By understanding the mechanisms, benefits, and risks associated with HRT, men and healthcare practitioners can make informed decisions that promote long-term health and wellness. As research advances, the potential for personalized approaches to HRT may further enhance its effectiveness, ensuring that men navigate this life stage with resilience and vitality.

Medications for Bone Health

Medications for maintaining and enhancing bone health play a crucial role in managing conditions such as osteoporosis, particularly in men experiencing andropause. During andropause, hormonal changes can lead to a decrease in bone density, raising the risk of fractures and other complications. To combat these effects, healthcare practitioners often recommend a variety of pharmacological options. Understanding the types of medications available, their mechanisms of action, and potential side effects is essential for men seeking to optimize their bone health during this life stage.

Bisphosphonates are among the most prescribed medications for bone health. These drugs work by inhibiting osteoclast activity, which are the cells responsible for bone resorption. By slowing down the breakdown of bone, bisphosphonates help increase bone density and reduce the risk of fractures. Medications such as alendronate, risedronate, and zoledronic acid have demonstrated effectiveness in improving bone mineral density in men, particularly those with low testosterone levels. While generally well-tolerated, they can cause gastrointestinal side effects and, in some cases, may be associated with rare but serious complications such as osteonecrosis of the jaw.

Another class of medications, selective oestrogen receptor modulators (SERMs), offers an alternative approach to bone health management. Raloxifene, a SERM, mimics oestrogen's beneficial effects on bone without some of the risks associated with hormone replacement therapy. By acting on oestrogen receptors in bone tissue, raloxifene helps reduce bone resorption and increase bone density. This medication is particularly appealing for men who may be concerned about the side effects of traditional hormone therapies. However, potential side effects such as hot flashes and an increased risk of thromboembolic events should be discussed with a healthcare provider.

For men with severe osteoporosis or those who do not respond to other treatments, parathyroid hormone (PTH) analogues, such as teriparatide, may be considered. PTH analogues stimulate new bone formation and have been shown to significantly increase bone density and reduce the risk of fractures. This treatment is typically reserved for individuals at high risk or those with a history of fractures, as it is administered through daily injections. While effective, the cost and the need for ongoing monitoring can be barriers for some patients, making it essential for healthcare providers to assess the appropriateness of this option on a case-by-case basis.

In addition to these medications, vitamin D and calcium supplementation are vital components of a comprehensive approach to bone health. Ensuring adequate levels of these nutrients supports the efficacy of medications and promotes overall bone strength. Men experiencing andropause should undergo regular assessments of their bone health, including bone density tests, to monitor changes and adjust treatment as necessary. Collaborative discussions between patients and healthcare practitioners about medication options, lifestyle changes, and nutritional needs will empower men to take proactive measures in maintaining their bone health throughout the andropause transition.

Monitoring and Regular Check-Ups

Monitoring and regular check-ups are essential components of maintaining men's health, particularly as they transition into andropause. This phase, often marked by hormonal fluctuations, can have significant implications for overall well-being. Regular monitoring allows individuals to identify and address changes in their health status early, thereby mitigating potential complications associated with andropause. Health care practitioners should emphasize the importance of routine assessments, including hormonal evaluations and metabolic screenings, to track changes over time and tailor interventions accordingly.

Bone density is a critical area of focus during andropause, as men are at increased risk for osteoporosis and related fractures. Regular bone density screenings, typically conducted through dual-energy X-ray absorptiometry (DEXA), provide valuable insights into bone health. These assessments help identify individuals who may benefit from preventive measures or treatments aimed at preserving bone mass. Health care practitioners should recommend these screenings based on age, family history, and other risk factors, ensuring men are aware of their bone health status as they age.

In addition to bone density, monitoring other health markers is crucial. Testosterone levels, for instance, can fluctuate during andropause, affecting mood, energy levels, and muscle mass. Regular blood tests to evaluate testosterone and other hormone levels can guide treatment decisions, such as hormone replacement therapy, lifestyle modifications, or nutritional interventions. Men should be encouraged to maintain open communication with their healthcare providers, discussing any symptoms or concerns they may have, which can lead to timely and effective management of hormonal changes.

Lifestyle factors play a significant role in overall health and can greatly influence outcomes related to andropause and bone health. Regular check-ups provide an opportunity for healthcare practitioners to discuss dietary habits, exercise routines, and other lifestyle choices that impact bone density and hormone levels. Engaging in weight-bearing exercises, for instance, is essential for maintaining bone strength, while a balanced diet rich in calcium and vitamin D supports bone health. Regular monitoring allows for the adjustment of lifestyle recommendations based on individual progress and needs.

Ultimately, fostering a proactive approach to health through monitoring and regular check-ups can empower men to take charge of their well-being during the andropause transition. By prioritizing routine assessments and maintaining open lines of communication with healthcare practitioners, men can effectively manage the challenges associated with hormonal changes and optimize their bone health. This collaborative effort between men and their healthcare providers is vital for achieving sustained vitality and quality of life as they age.

Alternative Therapies

Alternative therapies have gained popularity in recent years as men seek holistic approaches to address issues related to andropause and bone health. These therapies often focus on enhancing overall well-being and promoting natural healing processes. Among the various alternative therapies available, acupuncture, herbal medicine, and nutritional supplementation have shown promise in alleviating symptoms associated with andropause, such as fatigue, mood swings, and decreased libido. By understanding these therapies, men can make informed decisions about their health and explore options that complement conventional treatments.

Acupuncture, an ancient practice rooted in Traditional Chinese Medicine, involves inserting thin needles into specific points on the body. This technique is believed to stimulate the body's energy flow, or "qi," and can help relieve symptoms associated with andropause. Research suggests that acupuncture may improve hormone balance, reduce anxiety, and enhance overall vitality. For men experiencing issues such as erectile dysfunction or low energy levels, regular acupuncture sessions may serve as a beneficial adjunct to more traditional medical approaches.

Herbal medicine offers another avenue for men looking to manage andropause symptoms and support bone health. Certain herbs, such as ashwagandha and ginseng, are traditionally used to bolster energy levels and enhance sexual function. Additionally, herbs like red clover and saw palmetto may help alleviate hormonal imbalances. It is crucial for men to consult with healthcare practitioners before incorporating herbal remedies into their routines, as potential interactions with prescription medications should be carefully considered. When used appropriately, herbal medicine can provide a natural alternative or complement to conventional treatments.

Nutritional supplementation also plays a vital role in supporting men's health during andropause. Key nutrients, such as vitamin D, calcium, magnesium, and omega-3 fatty acids, are essential for maintaining bone density and overall vitality. Men may benefit from tailored supplement regimens that address specific deficiencies or health concerns. For instance, vitamin D is crucial for calcium absorption and bone health, while omega-3 fatty acids may help reduce inflammation and improve mood. Consulting with a knowledgeable healthcare practitioner can help men identify the most beneficial supplements based on their individual health profiles.

While alternative therapies can offer significant benefits, it is essential to approach them with caution and in conjunction with conventional medical care. Men should engage in open dialogues with their healthcare practitioners about their interest in alternative treatments, ensuring a comprehensive and coordinated approach to their health. By integrating these therapies thoughtfully, men can enhance their quality of life, support their bone health, and navigate the challenges of andropause with greater confidence and vitality.

Case Studies and Testimonials

Success Stories from Men

Success stories from men who have navigated the challenges of andropause and improved their bone health can serve as powerful testimonials for others facing similar situations. These narratives highlight the importance of proactive health management and the positive outcomes that can arise from making informed lifestyle changes. By sharing their experiences, these men offer valuable insights into what it takes to maintain vitality and well-being during this transitional phase of life.

One inspiring story comes from a 55-year-old man named Tom, who experienced significant fatigue and decreased strength due to andropause. Recognizing the need for change, Tom sought the guidance of a healthcare practitioner specializing in men's health. Together, they developed a tailored plan that included regular exercise focusing on strength training and cardiovascular activities. Alongside this, Tom made dietary adjustments, incorporating more calcium-rich foods and vitamin D supplements to enhance bone density. Within months, he reported feeling revitalized, with improved energy levels and a noticeable increase in his overall strength.

Another remarkable journey is that of Mark, a 62-year-old who faced the risk of osteoporosis after a bone density scan showed early signs of deterioration. Determined to take control of his health, Mark embraced a holistic approach that included both physical activity and nutritional changes. He joined a local fitness group that emphasized weight-bearing exercises, which are crucial for bone health. Additionally, Mark educated himself about the benefits of a balanced diet rich in fruits, vegetables, and lean proteins. His commitment paid off; subsequent scans showed marked improvements in his bone density, and he felt more confident in his physical capabilities.

David, age 58, shares a different angle on his andropause experience. Initially resistant to the idea of seeking help, he eventually attended a men's health seminar where he learned about the hormonal changes associated with aging and their impact on bone health. This newfound knowledge motivated him to consult with a healthcare professional, who recommended lifestyle modifications, including stress management techniques and regular health screenings. By becoming an active participant in his health journey, David not only improved his bone health but also fostered a supportive community with other men facing similar issues. His story emphasizes the importance of education and community support in overcoming health challenges.

Finally, there's James, a 60-year-old who transformed his life after realizing the significance of maintaining bone health as he aged. After experiencing a minor fracture, James was alarmed by the implications it had on his daily life. He sought advice from experts who introduced him to the concept of functional fitness, which emphasizes exercises that improve everyday movements. By incorporating functional training and focusing on flexibility and balance, James not only strengthened his bones but also regained his confidence in physical activities. His experience illustrates how a proactive approach to health can lead to profound lifestyle changes and enhanced quality of life.

These success stories reflect the diverse experiences of men navigating andropause and its associated health challenges. They highlight the importance of seeking professional guidance and making informed lifestyle choices. By sharing their journeys, these men inspire others to take charge of their health, encouraging a proactive approach to maintaining vitality and preventing bone-related issues as they age.

Practitioner Perspectives

The concept of andropause, often dubbed the male equivalent of menopause, has gained significant attention in recent years. Health care practitioners are increasingly recognizing the physiological and psychological changes that occur in men as they age. This transition typically involves a gradual decline in testosterone levels, which can lead to a range of symptoms including fatigue, depression, and a decrease in muscle mass. Understanding the nuances of andropause is essential for health care providers to effectively address these changes and offer appropriate interventions. It is crucial for practitioners to stay informed about the latest research, treatment options, and the holistic nature of men's health during this transitional phase.

Bone density is another critical concern for aging men, as it is closely linked to overall vitality and quality of life. Osteoporosis, often perceived as a women's issue, is increasingly recognized as a significant health risk for men as well. Practitioners must be aware of the risk factors that contribute to bone density loss in men, including lifestyle choices, dietary habits, and hormonal changes. Regular assessments of bone health, including bone density scans, are essential for early detection and intervention. By integrating bone health into routine care, practitioners can better support their male patients in maintaining strength and mobility as they age.

Nutrition plays a pivotal role in both andropause and bone health. Health care practitioners should emphasize the importance of a balanced diet rich in calcium and vitamin D, which are vital for bone health. Additionally, they should encourage patients to incorporate foods high in phytonutrients and antioxidants, which can mitigate some of the oxidative stress associated with aging. Given that lifestyle modifications can significantly impact both testosterone levels and bone density, practitioners can guide men toward healthier eating patterns and encourage physical activity as part of a comprehensive approach to health.

Mental health is often overlooked in discussions about andropause and bone health, yet it is an integral component of overall well-being. Symptoms of andropause, such as mood swings and depression, can negatively affect a man's motivation to engage in health-promoting behaviours. Practitioners should remain vigilant in assessing mental health and providing support through counselling, stress management strategies, and, when necessary, pharmacological interventions. By addressing mental health issues, practitioners can help men navigate the emotional challenges of aging and foster a more positive outlook on their health.

Collaborative care is essential in managing the complexities of andropause and bone health. Practitioners must work together across disciplines—such as endocrinology, nutrition, and mental health—to create comprehensive care plans tailored to the unique needs of aging men. This multidisciplinary approach allows for a more thorough understanding of the interplay between hormonal changes, physical health, and psychological well-being. By fostering open communication and a supportive environment, practitioners can empower men to take an active role in their health journey, ultimately enhancing their vitality and quality of life as they age.

Lessons Learned

In exploring the complexities of andropause and its impact on men's health, several key lessons have emerged that are crucial for both men experiencing these changes and health care practitioners guiding them. First and foremost, understanding andropause as a natural phase of aging rather than a medical condition requiring treatment can reshape perceptions around male health. This shift in mindset encourages men to embrace lifestyle changes that promote overall vitality rather than focusing solely on hormone replacement therapies. By recognizing that andropause does not equate to a loss of masculinity but rather a transition, men can approach this phase with a proactive attitude.

Another significant lesson learned is the critical importance of maintaining bone health throughout the aging process. Men often overlook the risks associated with decreased bone density, which can lead to osteoporosis and fractures. Education on the factors that contribute to bone health, such as nutrition, exercise, and lifestyle choices, is essential. Health care practitioners should emphasize the role of calcium and vitamin D, alongside weight-bearing exercises, in sustaining bone density. This knowledge empowers men to take charge of their health and mitigate the risks associated with aging.

Furthermore, mental health plays a pivotal role during andropause, highlighting the need for a holistic approach to well-being. Many men experience mood swings, anxiety, and depression as testosterone levels decline. Recognizing these symptoms as a common part of andropause can encourage men to seek help and support. Mental health should not be viewed in isolation; rather, it should be integrated into discussions about physical health. Practitioners should be equipped to provide resources for mental wellness, including counselling and stress management techniques, as part of a comprehensive health strategy.

Another lesson pertains to the significance of open communication between men and their health care providers. Many men are hesitant to discuss symptoms related to andropause, often due to societal stigma surrounding vulnerability. Encouraging open dialogue can lead to early intervention and better management of symptoms. Health care practitioners should foster an environment of trust, ensuring that men feel comfortable discussing their experiences. By addressing concerns related to sexual health, emotional well-being, and physical changes, practitioners can provide a more effective and supportive health care experience.

Finally, the importance of community and support networks cannot be understated. Men often benefit from sharing their experiences and challenges with peers who are navigating similar issues. Support groups, whether in-person or online, provide a platform for men to connect, share resources, and gain insights into managing andropause and maintaining bone health. Health care practitioners should facilitate these connections, guiding men toward appropriate resources and encouraging them to build supportive relationships. By fostering a sense of community, men can better navigate the complexities of aging, ensuring a more vibrant and fulfilling life during and beyond andropause.

Future Directions in Men's Health

Current Research and Innovations

Current research in andropause and bone health is revealing significant insights into how men can maintain vitality as they age. Andropause, often characterized by hormonal changes and a decline in testosterone levels, has been linked to various health issues, including decreased bone density. Recent studies have focused on the relationship between testosterone therapy and its potential benefits for bone health. Researchers are exploring safe and effective ways to administer testosterone to mitigate the risks of osteoporosis and fractures in aging men. These findings underscore the importance of individualized treatment plans that consider both hormonal levels and overall health.

Innovations in diagnostic techniques are also transforming the landscape of men's health. Advanced imaging technologies, such as dual-energy X-ray absorptiometry (DEXA) scans, allow for more accurate assessments of bone density. These tools help healthcare practitioners identify at-risk individuals earlier, facilitating prompt intervention and prevention strategies. Additionally, biomarkers for bone turnover are being studied to provide a clearer picture of bone health in men experiencing andropause. These innovations not only enhance diagnosis but also guide more targeted therapeutic approaches.

Nutritional research plays a vital role in understanding how diet impacts bone health during andropause. Recent studies have highlighted the significance of specific nutrients, such as calcium and vitamin D, in promoting bone density. Furthermore, emerging evidence suggests that certain dietary patterns, including those rich in antioxidants and omega-3 fatty acids, may contribute to improved bone health. Health practitioners are increasingly advising men to adopt balanced diets that can support bone strength, alongside traditional medical interventions. This holistic approach emphasizes the interplay between nutrition and hormonal health.

Exercise remains a cornerstone of maintaining vitality and bone density in aging men. Current research emphasizes resistance training and weight-bearing exercises as critical components of a comprehensive health strategy. Studies have shown that regular physical activity can significantly improve bone mineral density and reduce the risk of fractures. Innovative exercise programs are being developed, tailored specifically for men experiencing andropause, to ensure they can engage safely and effectively. Health care practitioners are encouraged to incorporate these exercise recommendations into their treatment plans to foster better outcomes for their patients.

In conclusion, the ongoing research and innovations in the fields of andropause and bone health are paving the way for improved strategies to enhance men's health as they age. The integration of hormonal therapy, advanced diagnostics, nutritional insights, and targeted exercise regimens represents a multifaceted approach to addressing the challenges posed by andropause. As more findings emerge, it is essential for men and health care practitioners to stay informed and adapt to these advancements, ensuring optimal health and vitality throughout the aging process.

The Role of Technology in Health Management

The integration of technology into health management has revolutionized the way individuals approach their well-being, particularly concerning andropause and bone health. Various technological advancements enable men to monitor their health metrics more effectively, allowing for proactive measures in managing conditions commonly associated with aging. Mobile applications, wearable devices, and telehealth services offer unprecedented convenience and accessibility, empowering men to take charge of their health and make informed decisions based on real-time data.

Wearable technology, such as fitness trackers and smartwatches, plays a crucial role in promoting physical activity and monitoring vital signs. These devices can track daily steps, heart rate, and even sleep patterns, providing men with valuable insights into their overall health. For instance, maintaining regular physical activity is essential for bone density, and wearables can help establish and sustain fitness goals. Moreover, many of these devices now include features specifically designed to monitor factors related to andropause, such as energy levels and hormonal fluctuations, thereby facilitating a more comprehensive understanding of one's health status.

Telehealth has emerged as a vital resource in health management, particularly during times when in-person visits may be challenging. Through virtual consultations, healthcare practitioners can provide personalized guidance to men experiencing andropause symptoms or concerns related to bone health. This accessibility not only enhances patient engagement but also allows for timely interventions that can prevent the progression of health issues. Moreover, telehealth can facilitate continuous monitoring and follow-up, ensuring that men receive the support they need as they navigate changes associated with aging.

Artificial intelligence (AI) and machine learning are also beginning to play a significant role in health management. These technologies can analyse vast amounts of health data to provide tailored recommendations for lifestyle changes, dietary adjustments, and exercise regimens that cater to individual needs. For men dealing with andropause and bone health issues, AI-driven platforms can suggest specific supplements or therapies based on personal health profiles. This data-driven approach enhances the ability to create customized health plans that address unique challenges and promote overall vitality.

Finally, the role of technology in health management extends to education and awareness. Online resources, webinars, and health-focused apps provide men and healthcare practitioners with access to the latest research and information regarding andropause and bone health. By fostering a culture of learning and self-awareness, technology empowers men to better understand their health challenges and make informed choices. As these technological tools continue to evolve, they will undoubtedly play an increasingly integral role in enhancing the well-being and vitality of men as they age.

Advocacy and Awareness

Advocacy and awareness play a crucial role in addressing the challenges associated with andropause and bone health. As men age, they may experience hormonal changes that can lead to a range of physical and psychological effects. These changes often go unrecognized or misunderstood, leading to a lack of appropriate support and treatment. By promoting awareness of andropause, men can better understand their health needs and seek timely interventions. Healthcare practitioners also have a vital role in educating their patients about these issues, ensuring that they are equipped with the necessary knowledge to navigate the complexities of aging.

Raising awareness about andropause is essential for dispelling myths and stereotypes that often surround male aging. Many men feel reluctant to discuss their symptoms due to societal expectations of masculinity, which can hinder their willingness to seek help. Advocacy efforts should focus on creating a safe space for men to share their experiences and seek advice without stigma. This can be achieved through community programs, health seminars, and online platforms that foster open discussions about male health concerns, including the physiological and emotional impacts of andropause.

Bone health is another critical aspect that deserves attention in the context of men's health advocacy. Osteoporosis and low bone density are often perceived as issues primarily affecting women, yet men are also at significant risk, particularly as they age. Educating men about the importance of maintaining bone density through lifestyle choices, such as diet and exercise, is essential.

Furthermore, healthcare practitioners should emphasize routine screenings and risk assessments for osteoporosis in men, helping to create a proactive approach to bone health management.

Leveraging the influence of social media and digital platforms can enhance advocacy efforts significantly. Online campaigns can spread awareness about andropause and bone health, reaching a broader audience and encouraging men to prioritize their well-being. Sharing personal stories, expert insights, and practical health tips on these platforms can empower men to take charge of their health. Healthcare practitioners can utilize these tools to connect with patients, providing valuable resources and support that encourage lifestyle changes conducive to better health outcomes.

Ultimately, fostering a culture of advocacy and awareness surrounding andropause and bone health can lead to improved quality of life for men. It is essential for health care practitioners to lead by example, prioritizing continuous education and open communication with their patients. By addressing misconceptions, advocating for routine health assessments, and promoting healthy lifestyle choices, the medical community can significantly impact how men approach their health as they age. The combined efforts of individuals and practitioners can create a more informed society that values men's health and encourages proactive management of andropause and bone health issues.

Creating a Personalized Health Plan

Assessing Individual Needs

Assessing individual needs is a crucial step in understanding the complex landscape of men's health, particularly as it pertains to andropause and bone density. For men experiencing andropause, the transition can significantly affect both physical and mental well-being. Hormonal changes during this period may lead to symptoms such as fatigue, mood swings, and decreased libido. These changes can also impact bone density, making it essential to assess individual needs to create tailored health strategies. A comprehensive evaluation that includes medical history, lifestyle factors, and specific health concerns is vital to identifying the unique challenges faced by each man.

To effectively assess individual needs, healthcare practitioners should begin with a thorough medical history. This includes not only current health issues but also past medical conditions, family history of osteoporosis or other bone-related diseases, and any previous experiences with hormonal therapies. Understanding these aspects allows for a clearer picture of how andropause may be affecting the individual's health. Additionally, inquiries about lifestyle choices—such as diet, exercise, and smoking habits—provide insight into factors that may contribute to bone density and overall vitality.

Moreover, utilizing standardized assessment tools can enhance the evaluation process. Tools such as the Androgen Deficiency in Aging Males (ADAM) questionnaire can help identify symptoms related to low testosterone levels, while bone density tests like dual-energy X-ray absorptiometry (DEXA) scans can provide objective data on bone health. These assessments allow healthcare providers to pinpoint specific areas of concern and to monitor changes over time, ensuring that interventions can be adjusted as necessary. Regular screenings are especially important as men age, given the increased risk of osteoporosis and fractures.

In addition to physical assessments, understanding the psychological and emotional aspects of andropause is equally important. Mood swings, anxiety, and depression can accompany hormonal changes, impacting a man's motivation and ability to engage in healthy behaviours. Mental health screenings and discussions about emotional well-being should be integrated into the overall assessment process. Addressing these psychological factors can lead to more effective treatment plans that encompass both physical and mental health needs.

Finally, creating a personalized health plan based on the assessment findings is essential for promoting vitality and overall well-being. This plan should include recommendations for nutritional adjustments, exercise routines tailored to improve bone density, and potential hormonal therapies if deemed necessary. Collaboration between the patient and healthcare provider is crucial for setting realistic health goals and ensuring adherence to the plan. By effectively assessing individual needs, men can navigate the challenges of andropause and maintain their bone health and vitality well into their later years.

Setting Realistic Goals

Setting realistic goals is crucial for men navigating the complexities of andropause and maintaining bone health. As men age, they may experience a variety of hormonal changes, diminished energy levels, and potential bone density loss. Understanding how to set achievable goals can empower men to take control of their health, enhance their vitality, and mitigate the impact of these changes. Goals should be specific, measurable, attainable, relevant, and time-bound to ensure they are practical and effective.

When establishing goals related to andropause symptoms, men should first assess their current health status. This can involve consulting with healthcare practitioners to understand hormone levels, bone density, and overall physical fitness. For example, if a man discovers that his testosterone levels are lower than optimal, a realistic goal could be to increase testosterone through lifestyle changes such as diet, exercise, and stress management. These goals should be framed within a reasonable timeline, allowing for gradual improvement rather than overnight transformation.

In terms of bone health, setting goals might involve incorporating weight-bearing exercises into a weekly routine. Men can aim to engage in activities like walking, running, or weightlifting for at least 150 minutes each week. By breaking down this goal into smaller, manageable sessions—such as 30 minutes of activity five times a week—men can create a sustainable plan that fits into their daily lives. This approach not only improves bone density but also contributes to overall physical vitality, making it easier to stick with the program.

Nutrition also plays a pivotal role in achieving health-related goals. Men should focus on a balanced diet rich in calcium and vitamin D to support bone health. Setting a goal to include specific food groups—such as leafy greens, dairy products, or fortified foods—on a daily or weekly basis can help ensure that nutritional needs are met. Collaborating with a healthcare practitioner or nutritionist can provide additional guidance on meal planning, allowing men to make informed choices that support their health objectives.

Lastly, it is essential for men to recognize the importance of monitoring progress towards their goals. Regular check-ins with healthcare professionals can help evaluate the effectiveness of the strategies employed, making it possible to adjust goals as needed. This ongoing evaluation fosters a sense of accountability and encourages men to stay committed to their health journey. By setting realistic, attainable goals, men can navigate the challenges of andropause and maintain optimal bone health, ultimately enhancing their overall quality of life.

Tracking Progress

Tracking progress is an essential component of managing health during andropause, particularly regarding bone density and overall vitality. As men age, physiological changes can impact their bone health, leading to increased risk of osteoporosis and fractures. Monitoring these changes through regular assessments allows individuals and healthcare practitioners to make informed decisions about lifestyle adjustments, dietary changes, and medical interventions. A structured approach to tracking progress not only empowers men to take charge of their health but also helps healthcare providers tailor their guidance based on specific needs.

One effective method for tracking progress in bone health is through regular bone density screenings. Dual-energy X-ray absorptiometry (DEXA) scans are the gold standard for measuring bone mineral density. These scans provide a clear picture of bone health and can identify early signs of osteopenia or osteoporosis. Men should begin discussing the timing and frequency of these screenings with their healthcare providers, especially if they have risk factors such as a family history of bone disease, a sedentary lifestyle, or a history of smoking or excessive alcohol consumption.

In addition to medical screenings, self-monitoring can play a significant role in tracking health during andropause. Men can keep a journal detailing their dietary intake, exercise routines, and any symptoms they experience. This method not only fosters awareness but also helps identify patterns that may correlate with changes in bone density or overall vitality. Regularly assessing factors such as calcium and vitamin D intake, physical activity levels, and weight can provide valuable insights into how lifestyle choices affect bone health.

Incorporating technology can further enhance tracking progress. Various apps and wearable devices can help monitor physical activity, dietary habits, and even mood changes. These tools often provide reminders for exercise and nutrient intake, fostering a proactive approach to health maintenance. Moreover, some applications allow users to set goals and track achievements over time, creating a sense of accountability and motivation. By leveraging technology, men can gain a more comprehensive view of their health and make data-driven decisions.

Finally, communicating progress with healthcare practitioners is crucial for optimal health management. Regular check-ins can facilitate discussions about the effectiveness of current strategies and the necessity for adjustments. Healthcare providers can interpret tracking data to recommend personalized interventions, whether through nutritional counselling, exercise programs, or pharmacological treatments. By fostering an open dialogue and sharing progress, men can work collaboratively with their healthcare teams to enhance their bone health and overall vitality during andropause, ensuring a healthier future.

Resources and Support Networks

Resources and support networks play a crucial role in navigating the complexities of andropause and maintaining bone health. As men age, they may experience a range of physical and emotional changes that can impact their overall well-being. Understanding these changes and accessing the right resources can empower men to take charge of their health. Healthcare practitioners can also benefit from being aware of these resources to better support their patients during this life transition.

One of the primary resources available to men dealing with andropause is educational materials. Books, articles, and reputable online resources can provide valuable information about the symptoms, causes, and management strategies associated with andropause. Organizations such as the American Urological Association and the International Society for Men's Health offer guidelines and research findings that can help both men and healthcare providers understand the implications of hormonal changes on health. These materials can serve as a foundation for discussions between men and their healthcare practitioners.

Support groups are another vital resource for men experiencing andropause and bone health issues. Connecting with peers who share similar experiences can foster a sense of community and understanding. Support groups can be found both in-person and online, offering men a platform to share their challenges, seek advice, and exchange coping strategies. Organizations focused on men's health often facilitate these groups, providing a safe environment for open dialogue and emotional support. This connection can alleviate feelings of isolation and empower men to address their health proactively.

Healthcare practitioners can further enhance support networks by integrating multidisciplinary approaches in their practice. Collaborating with nutritionists, physical therapists, and mental health professionals can provide men with comprehensive care tailored to their unique needs. For instance, nutritionists can offer dietary recommendations to support bone density, while physical therapists can design exercise regimens that enhance strength and balance. Practitioners should also encourage open communication about mental health, as emotional well-being is intricately linked to physical health during andropause.

Lastly, technology has become an invaluable resource in promoting men's health. Mobile applications and online platforms can track health metrics, provide reminders for medication, and facilitate communication with healthcare providers. Additionally, telehealth services have made it easier for men to access medical consultations from the comfort of their homes. These technological advancements not only foster convenience but also encourage men to take a proactive approach to their health by utilizing tools that facilitate ongoing management of andropause and bone health.

Pause for thought

- Bone density refers to the amount of mineral matter per square centimetre of bone which is a crucial indication of bone strength and overall health.
- As men age and enter the andropause, bone density can significantly decline due to hormonal changes, lifestyle factors and nutritional deficiencies. This decline can lead to conditions such as osteoporosis, characterised by fragile bones that are more susceptible to fractures.
- Several factors influence bone density, among them are genetics, age, hormonal levels, nutrition, and physical activity. Testosterone is the primary male hormone which plays a critical role in maintaining bone density.
- Lifestyle choices such as smoking, excessive alcohol consumption, and a sedentary lifestyle can further exacerbate the decline in bone density. Engaging in weight-bearing exercises and ensuring adequate intake of calcium and vitamin D can help mitigate the risk of fractures.
- Bone texture is maintained by a balance between osteoblasts (bone forming cells) and osteoclasts (bone resorption cells). In healthy individuals the process is balanced, maintaining optimal bone density.

However, in men experiencing andropause, the balance is lost, leading to bone resorption outpacing bone formation. This therefore necessitates the importance of monitoring bone health during this transitional phase of life.

- Men over the age of 50 or those with risk factors for osteoporosis should have routine bone density screening. Dual energy X-ray absorptiometry scars (DEXA) scans are the gold standard for assessing bone density and provides valuable insights into a partner's bone health. Knowledge of the results of these investigations can inform personalised interventions such as dietary adjustments, lifestyles changes and potentially pharmacologically treatments to help maintain or improve bone density.
- Hormonal balance plays a significant role in bone health. Testosterone is important for bone density, and its decline during andropause can lead to increase bone fragility. Men experiencing symptoms of low testosterone may benefit from discussing hormone replacement therapy with their health care providers. Other hormones such as parathyroid hormone and oestrogen are equally important as imbalances can contribute to bone loss.
- Apart from age and its reduced levels of the primary male sex hormone-testosterone which promotes the activity of osteoblasts while it has an inhibitory role on osteoclasts, a balance that is reversed on aging. Family history is also important as genetic factors plays a role in influencing

bone density, thus genetic testing can provide deeper insights into personalised risks assessments and so inform management.

- Minerals such as calcium, magnesium, and Zinc are integral in maintaining bone density. Men aged 50 and older should aim for a calcium intake of about 1,200mg/day. Calcium can be obtained from fatty foods, dairy products, leafy green vegetables and fortified foods. Magnesium helps in vitamin D metabolism and can be obtained from nuts, seeds, whole grains and green leafy vegetables. Zinc on the other hand is involved in testosterone production. It can be found in foods such as meat, shellfish, legumes and seeds. Vitamin K plays a role in bone mineralisation, thus helping to prevent fractures.
- Supplement such as vitamin D and calcium are essential supplements for men concerned about bone density. These work synergistically to enhance bone health and reduce the risk of fractures. Before taking any supplements, we recommend consulting with your healthcare practitioner, as individual health needs can vary.

Take Home Nuggets

- Hydration is critical component of overall health particularly for men experiencing andropause. As men age, the body's ability to conserve water declines, it is therefore essential to understand the significance of hydration and its impact on bone health and vitality.

- As men age, hormonal changes can lead to symptoms such as fatigue, mood swings, decreased libido, and reduced muscle mass. Engaging in regular physical activity can mitigate these effects by enhancing hormonal balance, boosting energy levels and improving mental health. Exercise serves not only counteract the physical changes associated with andropause but also as a holistic approach to promote vitality and longevity.
- Cardio-vascular workouts have been shown to help regulate hormonal fluctuation, thus contributing to better emotional stability and resilience against stress.
- Practices like yoga or tai chi not only improve physical flexibility but also promote mental clarity. As men age, the risk of falls and injuries increases, hence the importance of balance training. Thus, incorporating flexibility and balance exercises into a regular fitness routine can enhance mobility, reduce the risk of injury and foster a greater sense of wellbeing, which is particularly beneficial during times of hormonal change.
- As men age, they may face various health challenges including decreased muscle mass, increased fat accumulation and lower bone density. Engaging in strength training can counteract these age related changes helping to preserve muscle function and promote a healthier body composition. Regular strength training help increase muscle

strength, improves metabolism and enhances physical performance, making it a vital practice for men in this phase of life.

- One of the primary benefits of strength training is its positive impact on bone density. Resistance exercises stimulate bone formation and help prevent osteoporosis, a condition characterised by weak and brittle bone. This is particularly important for older men who are at higher risk for bone fractures and osteoporosis.
- Managing stress and mental health is a crucial aspect of overall wellbeing, particularly for men experiencing andropause. The physiological changes during andropause can lead to increased stress levels. Symptoms such as fatigue, mood swings, and decreased libido are not only frustrating but can also contribute to a heightened state of anxiety. It is important to recognise these symptoms as being interconnected rather than isolated issues.
- Social support plays a significant role in mental health during andropause. Men often face societal pressures to remain stoic, which can lead to isolation and exacerbated stress. Encouraging open dialogue about mental health among peers can help dismantle the stigma surrounding vulnerability
- Inadequate sleep can exacerbate symptoms of andropause such as fatigue, mood swings, and decreased libido, making it imperative for men to prioritise restful nights.

- Testosterone replacement therapy has gained considerable attention as an intervention for men going through andropause. Testosterone therapy can be administered as injections transdermal patches, gels or pellets. The choice of administration is guided by patient's choice convenience and potential side effects. Regular monitoring to ensure the hormonal levels remain in the therapeutic range, thus minimising risk while maximising benefits.

Chapter 5
The Andropause Effect

Stages of Andropause

The stages of andropause can be categorized into three distinct phases. The first stage involves a gradual decrease in testosterone levels, which generally begins in a man's late 30s or early 40s. During this phase, men may not notice significant changes, but subtle shifts in mood, energy, or libido can be present. It is crucial for healthcare workers to recognize that these early symptoms may be dismissed as normal aging, making early diagnosis challenging.

As men transition into the second stage of andropause, the decline in testosterone becomes more pronounced. Symptoms such as fatigue, decreased muscle mass, increased body fat, and changes in hair patterns may start to manifest. Hair loss, particularly male pattern baldness, can accelerate during this time, affecting self-esteem and body image. Healthcare providers should be vigilant in assessing these changes and offering guidance on management strategies, which may include lifestyle modifications or hormone replacement therapy.

The final stage of andropause involves more significant systemic changes and a potential increase in associated health risks. Men may experience emotional fluctuations, depression, or anxiety, alongside physical symptoms like osteoporosis and cardiovascular concerns. The culmination of these effects can lead to a diminished sense of well-being. It is important for healthcare professionals to address these issues holistically, considering both the physical and mental health of the patient, and to provide support for coping strategies.

In conclusion, andropause is a multifaceted process that can deeply affect men's health, particularly in relation to hair loss and overall vitality. As testosterone levels decline, understanding the stages of andropause can empower both men and healthcare workers to recognize symptoms early and take proactive measures. By fostering open dialogues about these changes, healthcare providers can play a pivotal role in improving men's health outcomes during this natural transition. Awareness and education about andropause will ultimately enhance quality of life for many men facing these challenges.

Symptoms and Signs

The symptoms and signs of andropause can vary significantly among individuals, but several commonalities exist that can help in identifying this phase in men's lives. One of the most prominent symptoms is a noticeable decrease in testosterone levels, which may manifest as fatigue, reduced libido, and loss of muscle mass. Men may also experience mood swings, irritability, and even symptoms resembling depression. These psychological changes can be just as impactful as physical symptoms, affecting interpersonal relationships and overall quality of life.

Another common sign of andropause is hair loss, which is often linked to hormonal changes. Many men may find that their hair thins or recedes more rapidly during this period, leading to a sense of decreased self-esteem or anxiety about aging. Along with hair loss, grey hair can emerge more prominently, signalling not only a natural aging process but also the influence of hormonal fluctuations. The emotional response to these visible changes can be profound, often leading men to seek solutions that address both the physical and psychological aspects of their appearance.

Cognitive changes are also reported during andropause, with difficulties in concentration, memory lapses, and an overall sense of mental fog being quite common. These cognitive symptoms can be troubling, particularly for men who are used to maintaining a sharp and active mind. As testosterone levels decline, the brain's neuroplasticity may be affected, leading to challenges in learning and memory retention. Recognizing these symptoms early can help in developing strategies to manage them effectively.

In addition to the more commonly recognized symptoms, men may also experience physiological changes such as increased body fat, particularly around the abdomen. This shift in body composition can contribute to a host of health concerns, including cardiovascular issues and metabolic syndrome. Weight gain can further exacerbate feelings of unattractiveness and contribute to a cycle of low self-esteem and mental health challenges. Awareness of these physical changes is essential for both men and healthcare workers in promoting healthy lifestyle choices during this transitional phase.

Finally, it is important to note that the experience of andropause can vary widely among individuals, influenced by factors such as genetics, lifestyle, and overall health. Understanding the diverse symptoms and signs associated with andropause allows men and healthcare professionals to approach this life stage with greater insight and compassion. It also underscores the importance of seeking medical advice when experiencing these changes to ensure that any underlying health issues are addressed and managed effectively.

Hormonal Changes and Their Effects

Hormonal changes during andropause significantly impact various aspects of men's health, including hair loss and the greying of hair. As men age, particularly after the age of 40, testosterone levels gradually decline. This decrease can lead to several physiological changes, including a shift in hair follicle dynamics. Hair follicles are sensitive to hormonal fluctuations, and the reduction in testosterone can result in a higher ratio of dihydrotestosterone (DHT), a potent androgen that is linked to hair thinning and loss.

The role of hormones extends beyond just testosterone and DHT. Other hormones, such as oestrogen and cortisol, also play a crucial part in the aging process. As men experience hormonal changes, the balance between testosterone and oestrogen may shift, potentially leading to increased body fat and changes in hair distribution. Elevated cortisol levels, often associated with stress, may further exacerbate hair loss by shortening the hair growth cycle, leading to thinning hair and increased shedding.

Furthermore, the impact of hormonal changes on hair pigmentation is notable. The greying of hair is primarily influenced by a decrease in melanin production, which is regulated by hormonal levels. As testosterone diminishes, the melanocytes responsible for hair colour may also decline in function, resulting in the loss of pigmentation. This process is not only a cosmetic concern for many men but also can be indicative of broader hormonal imbalances that may require attention.

Understanding the interplay between hormones and hair health is essential for both individuals and healthcare providers. An awareness of how andropause affects hormone levels can aid in identifying potential treatment options for hair loss and greying. Lifestyle modifications, such as improved diet and exercise, can help mitigate some of these hormonal changes, while medical interventions, including hormone replacement therapy, may also be considered for those experiencing significant symptoms.

Addressing hormonal changes during andropause is not just about managing hair loss and grey hair but also encompasses overall well-being. By recognizing the effects of hormonal fluctuations, men can take proactive steps to maintain their health, hair, and confidence. Healthcare providers play a vital role in guiding patients through this transition, emphasizing the importance of a comprehensive approach that includes hormonal assessment, lifestyle management, and potential therapeutic options.

The Science of Hair Loss

Types of Hair Loss

Hair loss can manifest in various forms, each with distinct characteristics and underlying causes. The most common type is androgenetic alopecia, often referred to as male or female pattern baldness. This genetic condition typically begins with a receding hairline or thinning at the crown in men, while women usually experience a broader part and overall thinning. The role of androgens, particularly testosterone and its derivative dihydrotestosterone (DHT), is critical in this process, as they affect hair follicle sensitivity and growth cycles. Understanding this type of hair loss is vital for developing effective treatment strategies.

Telogen effluvium is another prevalent type of hair loss that occurs when a significant number of hair follicles enter the resting phase of the hair growth cycle prematurely. This can be triggered by various factors, including stress, hormonal changes, nutritional deficiencies, or medical conditions. Unlike androgenetic alopecia, telogen effluvium is often reversible, and addressing the underlying cause can lead to regrowth. Recognizing the signs of this condition can help individuals and healthcare professionals implement timely interventions that promote hair regrowth.

Alopecia areata is an autoimmune disorder characterized by sudden hair loss in patches. It occurs when the immune system mistakenly attacks hair follicles, leading to hair loss in various areas of the scalp and body. This condition can affect individuals at any age, but it often presents in younger adults. While the exact cause remains unclear, factors such as genetics and environmental triggers may play a role. Treatment options include corticosteroids and other immunosuppressive agents, making awareness of this type of hair loss crucial for timely diagnosis and management.

Traction alopecia is another form of hair loss that results from prolonged tension on the hair follicles, often due to certain hairstyles like tight ponytails, braids, or extensions. This type of hair loss is particularly common among individuals who frequently wear such styles. The damage caused by traction can lead to irreversible hair loss if not addressed early. Educating patients about the importance of choosing hairstyles that minimize tension on the hair can help prevent this avoidable condition.

Lastly, scarring alopecia's, also known as cicatricial alopecia's, encompass a group of disorders that cause permanent hair loss due to inflammation and scarring of the hair follicles. Conditions such as lichen planopilaris and frontal fibrosing alopecia fall under this category. These disorders can arise from various factors, including autoimmune conditions and infections. Early recognition and intervention are crucial, as the scarring process can lead to irreversible hair loss. Understanding the diverse types of hair loss not only aids in diagnosis but also empowers individuals and healthcare providers to approach treatment more effectively.

Causes of Hair Loss in Men

Hair loss in men is a multifaceted issue influenced by a range of factors, one of the most prominent being genetics. Male pattern baldness, or androgenetic alopecia, is the most common cause of hair loss in men. This hereditary condition is linked to the presence of androgens, particularly dihydrotestosterone (DHT), which affects hair follicles by shortening their growth cycle and ultimately leading to miniaturization. Men with a family history of baldness are at a higher risk of experiencing this condition, making genetics a critical aspect to consider when addressing hair loss.

Hormonal changes also play a significant role in hair loss among men. As men age, they undergo changes in hormone levels, particularly a decrease in testosterone. This decline can lead to an increase in the level of DHT, which, as previously mentioned, contributes to hair follicle shrinkage and loss. Additionally, imbalances in other hormones, such as thyroid hormones, can lead to hair thinning or shedding. Understanding the hormonal landscape is vital for both men and healthcare providers when diagnosing and treating hair loss.

Medical conditions can further exacerbate hair loss in men. Conditions such as alopecia areata, which causes sudden hair loss in patches, and scalp infections like tinea capitis can lead to significant hair thinning. Chronic illnesses, including diabetes and lupus, can also impact hair health. Certain medications used to treat these conditions, such as blood thinners and antidepressants, may have side effects that include hair loss. Therefore, it is essential for healthcare professionals to conduct thorough assessments to identify any underlying medical issues contributing to hair loss.

Lifestyle factors are another crucial element influencing hair loss in men. Stress, whether acute or chronic, can trigger a type of hair loss known as telogen effluvium, where hair follicles prematurely enter the resting phase of the growth cycle. Poor nutrition, particularly deficiencies in vitamins and minerals such as iron, zinc, and biotin, can also lead to weakened hair and increased shedding. Additionally, habits such as smoking and excessive alcohol consumption have been linked to hair loss, emphasizing the importance of a healthy lifestyle in maintaining hair health.

Finally, environmental factors cannot be overlooked when discussing the causes of hair loss in men. Exposure to pollutants, harsh chemicals, and extreme weather conditions can damage hair and scalp health, leading to thinning or loss. Prolonged sun exposure can also degrade hair proteins, making hair more susceptible to breakage. For healthcare workers addressing hair loss in men, considering these environmental influences is essential in providing comprehensive care and guidance for patients seeking solutions.

The Role of Hormones in Hair Health

Hormones play a crucial role in the health and vitality of hair, influencing various aspects from growth to pigmentation. The primary hormones associated with hair health include androgens, oestrogens, and thyroid hormones. Androgens, such as testosterone and its derivative dihydrotestosterone (DHT), are particularly significant in men, as they can contribute to hair loss due to their effects on hair follicles. DHT can shrink hair follicles, leading to thinning hair and eventual baldness, a condition known as androgenetic alopecia. Understanding the hormonal balance is essential for addressing hair loss and managing its effects during andropause.

Oestrogens, while primarily associated with female biology, also play a role in men's hair health. They have been shown to promote hair growth by counteracting the effects of androgens. As men age and experience changes in their hormonal profile, particularly during andropause, the decrease in oestrogen levels can exacerbate hair loss. Additionally, the relationship between oestrogen and testosterone can also affect hair pigmentation, contributing to the greying process that many adults experience. Maintaining a balance between these hormones is crucial for promoting healthier hair outcomes.

Thyroid hormones are another critical factor in hair health. An underactive thyroid, or hypothyroidism, can lead to hair thinning and loss, while an overactive thyroid may cause hair to become brittle and fall out more easily. During andropause, men may experience fluctuations in thyroid function, which can further complicate issues related to hair loss and greying. Regular monitoring of thyroid levels, alongside hormonal assessments, can provide valuable insights into the root causes of hair-related concerns and allow for targeted treatment options.

Moreover, lifestyle factors such as diet, stress, and overall health can influence hormone levels and, consequently, hair health. A diet rich in vitamins and minerals, particularly B vitamins, zinc, and iron, supports hormonal balance and hair growth. Stress management techniques, including exercise and mindfulness practices, can help regulate cortisol levels, which may otherwise negatively impact hair health. Health care workers should educate patients about these lifestyle choices, emphasizing that hormonal health is intertwined with overall well-being and can significantly affect hair condition.

In conclusion, understanding the role of hormones in hair health is vital for adults experiencing hair loss and greying during andropause. By recognizing the interplay between androgens, oestrogens, and thyroid hormones, individuals can take proactive steps in managing their hair health. Health care workers can play a pivotal role in guiding patients through this complex relationship, offering insights into treatment options and lifestyle modifications that can help mitigate the effects of hormonal changes on hair. Ultimately, a comprehensive approach to hair health that includes hormonal assessment and lifestyle adjustment can lead to better outcomes for those facing these challenges.

The Connection Between Andropause and Hair Loss

How Testosterone Affects Hair Growth

Testosterone plays a significant role in hair growth and maintenance, influencing various stages of the hair cycle. It affects both the quantity and quality of hair, particularly in men, where it is often linked to patterns of hair loss. Understanding how testosterone interacts with hair follicles can provide insight into conditions such as andropause, which typically involves fluctuations in hormone levels that can lead to noticeable changes in hair density and texture.

The relationship between testosterone and hair follicles is complex, as testosterone itself is converted into dihydrotestosterone (DHT) by the enzyme 5-alpha reductase. DHT is more potent than testosterone and has a profound impact on hair follicles, particularly in the scalp. While testosterone can stimulate hair growth in certain areas, such as the beard and body, elevated levels of DHT can lead to miniaturization of hair follicles on the scalp, resulting in thinning hair and eventual hair loss, a condition commonly known as androgenetic alopecia.

During andropause, which typically occurs in men as they age, testosterone levels can decline, leading to an array of symptoms, including changes in hair growth. As testosterone levels decrease, the balance between testosterone and DHT may shift, potentially exacerbating hair loss. This hormonal imbalance can contribute to an increase in grey hair as well, as lower testosterone levels are associated with a decrease in melanin production, the pigment responsible for hair color.

In addition to its direct effects on hair follicles, testosterone also influences overall health, which can indirectly impact hair growth. Factors such as stress, nutrition, and lifestyle choices, all of which can be affected by hormonal changes, play a role in hair health. For instance, high levels of stress can elevate cortisol, a hormone that can further disrupt the balance of testosterone and DHT, leading to accelerated hair loss. Maintaining a healthy lifestyle, including a balanced diet and regular exercise, can help mitigate these effects.

Understanding the role of testosterone in hair growth is essential for both patients and healthcare providers when addressing issues related to hair loss and greying. Awareness of these hormonal dynamics can guide treatment options, ranging from lifestyle modifications to medical interventions that target hormonal imbalances. By recognizing the influence of testosterone and DHT on hair health, individuals can make informed decisions and adopt strategies to maintain their hair during the andropause transition.

The Impact of Dihydrotestosterone (DHT)

Dihydrotestosterone (DHT) is a potent androgen derived from testosterone, playing a crucial role in various physiological processes. Its impact on hair follicles is particularly significant, as DHT is widely recognized as a primary factor in androgenetic alopecia, commonly known as male or female pattern baldness. This condition affects a large proportion of adults, especially those experiencing andropause, where hormonal changes can exacerbate hair loss. Understanding the relationship between DHT and hair follicles is essential for both individuals and healthcare providers aiming to address hair loss effectively.

DHT binds to androgen receptors in hair follicles, leading to a reduction in hair growth. In genetically predisposed individuals, this binding can trigger a process known as follicular miniaturization, where hair follicles shrink over time, producing thinner and shorter hair strands. This process can ultimately lead to complete follicle shutdown, resulting in baldness. For healthcare workers, recognizing the signs of androgenetic alopecia and its link to DHT is vital for providing informed treatment options to patients experiencing hair loss during and after andropause.

Moreover, DHT's influence extends beyond hair loss, impacting other aspects of health during andropause. Elevated levels of DHT are often associated with benign prostatic hyperplasia (BPH), a condition that affects many older men, leading to urinary issues. The dual role of DHT in hair follicle health and prostate enlargement illustrates the importance of monitoring DHT levels in aging adults. For healthcare professionals, understanding these associations can facilitate comprehensive patient care, addressing both hair loss and prostate health concerns simultaneously.

Interventions targeting DHT have become a focal point in treating hair loss. Medications such as finasteride and dutasteride work by inhibiting the enzyme responsible for converting testosterone to DHT, thereby reducing DHT levels in the scalp and potentially reversing hair loss. While these treatments can be effective, they may also come with side effects that need to be carefully considered. It is essential for healthcare providers to discuss the benefits and risks of DHT-targeting therapies with patients, ensuring they make informed decisions regarding their treatment options.

In conclusion, DHT has a profound impact on hair health, particularly for adults experiencing andropause. Understanding its role in hair loss and related health issues allows both patients and healthcare workers to navigate the complexities of treatment more effectively. As research continues to evolve, new insights into DHT's effects will likely lead to more targeted and effective interventions for managing hair loss and promoting overall well-being during the aging process.

Psychological Effects of Hair Loss During Andropause

Hair loss during andropause can have significant psychological effects on men, often leading to decreased self-esteem and a negative self-image. As men transition through this stage of life, they may confront changes in their physical appearance that are difficult to accept. The visibility of thinning hair or greying can serve as a constant reminder of aging, fostering feelings of vulnerability and insecurity. This psychological burden may not only affect how men perceive themselves but also how they believe they are perceived by others, leading to social withdrawal or avoidance of situations where they feel their appearance may be judged.

The impact of hair loss extends beyond individual self-perception; it can also influence interpersonal relationships. Men experiencing hair loss may feel less attractive to their partners, which can lead to anxiety and stress within romantic relationships. These feelings can create a vicious cycle, where the stress of perceived unattractiveness leads to further emotional distress, potentially exacerbating the issue of hair loss itself. Open communication with partners about these feelings is crucial, as it can foster understanding and support, helping to mitigate some of the psychological effects.

Moreover, hair loss can trigger or intensify feelings of depression and anxiety in some men. The societal emphasis on youth and virility often places undue pressure on men to maintain a certain image, and losing hair can be perceived as a sign of diminished masculinity. This perception can lead to a sense of loss not only regarding physical appearance but also concerning identity and personal worth. Addressing these emotions through counselling or therapy can be beneficial for men struggling with these feelings, providing them with coping strategies to deal with the challenges of andropause.

Social stigma surrounding hair loss can compound these issues, as men may feel judged or ridiculed because of their changing appearance. This stigma can lead to isolation, as men might avoid social situations or activities where they feel their hair loss will be noticed. Such behaviour can further entrench feelings of loneliness and despair, as the lack of social interaction can prevent them from receiving support from friends and family. Awareness and education about hair loss and andropause can help reduce stigma and encourage more open discussions about these experiences.

Ultimately, understanding the psychological effects of hair loss during andropause is essential for both men and healthcare workers. By recognizing the emotional struggles associated with this transition, effective support systems can be established. Healthcare professionals can play a pivotal role in providing not only medical advice but also psychological support, helping men navigate the complexities of aging and its impact on self-image. Creating an environment where men feel comfortable discussing their experiences can lead to better mental health outcomes and a more positive approach to dealing with hair loss.

Understanding Grey Hair

The Biology of Hair Colour

Hair colour is primarily determined by the presence and type of pigments in the hair follicles. The two main types of pigments responsible for hair colour are eumelanin and pheomelanin. Eumelanin is responsible for darker shades, including black and brown, while pheomelanin contributes to lighter shades, such as blonde and red. The ratio of these pigments varies among individuals and influences not only the colour of hair but also its texture and thickness. The production of these pigments is controlled by a complex interplay of genetic factors and environmental influences.

Genetics plays a crucial role in determining hair colour. Specific genes, such as the MC1R gene, are known to influence the type and amount of melanin produced in hair follicles. Variations in these genes can lead to a diversity of hair colours within families and populations. Furthermore, hair colour can be affected by other genetic factors that regulate the function of melanocytes, the cells responsible for pigment production. These genetic predispositions can manifest as a range of hair colours, from the deepest black to the lightest blonde, and can change over an individual's lifetime due to various factors, including hormonal changes and aging.

Hormonal changes, particularly during andropause, can significantly impact hair colour. Andropause, characterized by a decline in testosterone levels, can lead to changes in hair follicles. These hormonal fluctuations may cause a decrease in melanin production, resulting in the greying of hair. This process is often gradual and can be influenced by an individual's overall health, diet, and stress levels. As testosterone levels decline, the balance of hormones affecting hair follicles shifts, potentially leading to both hair loss and changes in hair pigmentation.

Environmental factors also contribute to hair colour changes over time. Exposure to sunlight can lighten hair due to the breakdown of melanin by ultraviolet (UV) rays. Additionally, chemical exposure from hair treatments, such as dyes and bleaches, can alter the natural pigmentation of hair. These external influences can interact with genetic predispositions, sometimes exacerbating the natural greying process or triggering hair loss. Understanding these environmental contributors can help individuals make informed choices about hair care and maintenance.

In summary, the biology of hair colour is a multifaceted subject intertwined with genetics, hormones, and environmental factors. For adults experiencing andropause, the interplay of these elements can lead to significant changes in hair pigmentation and density. By understanding the biological mechanisms behind hair colour, individuals and healthcare workers can better address concerns related to hair loss and greying, fostering a proactive approach to hair health during this transitional life stage.

Factors Contributing to Grey Hair

Grey hair is a common phenomenon that many adults experience as they age. The primary factor contributing to grey hair is the natural aging process, which affects the hair follicles. As individuals age, melanocytes, the cells responsible for producing melanin—the pigment that gives hair its colour—gradually diminish in number and activity. This reduction leads to less melanin being deposited in the hair shaft, resulting in grey or white hair. While genetics play a crucial role in determining when an individual will start to grey, lifestyle choices and environmental factors also contribute significantly to this process.

Genetics is one of the most significant determinants of when and how quickly a person will develop grey hair. Research indicates that if one or both parents experienced premature greying, their children are more likely to follow suit. Specific genes have been identified that influence melanin production and the aging of hair follicles. Understanding these genetic factors can help individuals better anticipate the onset of grey hair, allowing them to make informed decisions about hair care and potential treatments.

In addition to genetics, lifestyle factors such as diet, stress, and smoking can also influence the greying process. A diet lacking in essential nutrients, particularly those rich in vitamins B12, D3, and minerals like copper and zinc, can contribute to premature greying. Stress is another significant factor; chronic stress can lead to the depletion of melanocytes in hair follicles. Studies have shown that individuals experiencing high levels of stress may notice an acceleration in the greying of their hair. Furthermore, smoking has been linked to an increased risk of premature greying, suggesting that lifestyle choices can have a direct impact on hair pigmentation.

Environmental factors, including exposure to pollutants and harsh chemicals, can also contribute to the greying of hair. Environmental stressors may damage hair follicles and accelerate the aging process of hair. For instance, exposure to certain chemicals in hair products or environmental toxins can lead to oxidative stress, which negatively affects hair health. Protecting hair from these elements through careful product selection and minimizing exposure to pollutants can help mitigate some of the effects that contribute to grey hair.

Finally, hormonal changes associated with andropause can influence the onset of grey hair in men. As testosterone levels fluctuate during this stage of life, there can be a corresponding impact on various bodily functions, including hair growth and pigmentation. Hormonal imbalances may disrupt the normal functioning of hair follicles, further contributing to changes in hair colour. Understanding these hormonal influences can provide essential insights for healthcare workers and adults looking to address concerns related to grey hair and overall hair health.

The Role of Genetics and Aging

Genetics plays a crucial role in determining the onset and progression of various aging-related changes, including hair loss and greying. Research indicates that hereditary factors significantly influence an individual's susceptibility to conditions such as androgenetic alopecia, commonly known as male or female pattern baldness. This condition is often linked to the presence of specific genes that affect hair follicle sensitivity to androgens, leading to miniaturization of hair follicles and subsequent hair loss. Understanding these genetic predispositions can help individuals anticipate changes in their hair and seek proactive measures to manage them.

In addition to hair loss, genetics also affects the greying of hair, a process that often accompanies aging. The production of melanin, the pigment responsible for hair colour, diminishes as one age, and genetic factors can determine the rate at which this occurs. Certain gene variants have been identified as influencing the timing of grey hair onset, suggesting that some individuals may experience significant greying earlier than others due to their genetic makeup. This process is not solely cosmetic; it can impact self-esteem and perceptions of age, making awareness of genetic influences particularly pertinent in discussions surrounding aging.

Aging itself is a complex biological process influenced by genetics, with implications for overall health and well-being. As individuals age, the cumulative effects of genetic predispositions manifest in various ways, including changes in skin elasticity, muscle mass, and hair density. The interplay between genetics and environmental factors, such as lifestyle choices and exposure to toxins, further complicates the aging process. For healthcare professionals, understanding this interplay is essential for providing effective guidance to patients experiencing hair loss or changes in hair colour during andropause.

Moreover, the role of epigenetics in aging is an emerging area of research that highlights how environmental factors can influence gene expression related to hair health. Lifestyle choices, such as diet, stress management, and sun exposure, can modify the way genes are expressed, potentially impacting hair growth and pigmentation. Educating patients about these factors can empower them to adopt healthier lifestyles that may mitigate some of the genetic predispositions they face, ultimately leading to improved hair health and overall quality of life.

In conclusion, the intersection of genetics and aging is a critical aspect of understanding hair loss and greying, particularly during andropause. For adults and healthcare workers, recognizing the genetic factors at play allows for more informed discussions about prevention and treatment options. By integrating knowledge of genetics with lifestyle interventions, individuals can better navigate the challenges of aging, fostering a sense of agency over their appearance and well-being.

Lifestyle Factors Influencing Hair Health

Nutrition and Diet

Nutrition plays a critical role in maintaining overall health, particularly during the andropause phase, which can significantly impact hair health and appearance.

A balanced diet rich in essential nutrients can help mitigate some of the changes associated with aging, including hair loss and greying. Key nutrients such as vitamins, minerals, and proteins contribute to the health of hair follicles, and deficiencies in these areas can exacerbate the effects of andropause. Understanding the importance of nutrition can empower individuals to make informed dietary choices that promote healthier hair and overall well-being.

Protein is one of the most vital components for hair growth. Hair is primarily made of a protein called keratin, and without adequate protein intake, the body may struggle to produce new hair strands. Sources of high-quality protein include lean meats, fish, eggs, legumes, and dairy products. For those following a plant-based diet, incorporating a variety of plant proteins such as quinoa, lentils, and nuts can also provide the necessary building blocks for hair health. Ensuring sufficient protein intake is essential, especially for men experiencing andropause, who may notice changes in hair density and texture.

Vitamins and minerals also play a significant role in hair health. B vitamins, particularly biotin, are known for their contribution to hair growth and strength. Deficiencies in biotin can lead to hair thinning and loss. Additionally, vitamins A, C, D, and E are crucial for maintaining a healthy scalp and promoting hair follicle function. Minerals such as zinc and iron are also essential; zinc supports hair tissue growth and repair, while iron helps carry oxygen to hair follicles. A varied diet rich in fruits, vegetables, nuts, and whole grains can help ensure that individuals receive these important nutrients.

Healthy fats, particularly omega-3 fatty acids, are another important aspect of nutrition that supports hair health. These essential fats help nourish the hair and support its growth by promoting scalp health and reducing inflammation. Sources of omega-3s include fatty fish like salmon, walnuts, flaxseeds, and chia seeds. Incorporating these foods into the diet can not only benefit hair health but also contribute to overall cardiovascular health, which is particularly relevant for men undergoing andropause.

In conclusion, adopting a nutritious diet rich in protein, vitamins, minerals, and healthy fats can significantly influence hair health during andropause. As men navigate the changes associated with this life stage, being mindful of their dietary choices can help mitigate hair loss and greying. Health care workers play a vital role in educating patients about the importance of nutrition, encouraging them to take proactive steps toward maintaining healthy hair and overall bodily function. By emphasizing the connection between diet and hair health, individuals can feel empowered to make choices that support their well-being during this transitional period.

Exercise and Its Benefits

Exercise plays a crucial role in maintaining overall health, particularly during the andropause period—a phase characterized by hormonal changes in men that can lead to various physical and psychological challenges. Regular physical activity can significantly mitigate some of these effects, especially in relation to hair loss and greying hair. Engaging in regular exercise helps improve circulation, which is essential for delivering vital nutrients to hair follicles, promoting healthier hair growth. Furthermore, exercise can help regulate hormone levels, including testosterone, which can impact hair health and contribute to the onset of andropause symptoms.

One of the most notable benefits of exercise is its ability to reduce stress levels. Stress has been linked to hair loss, particularly conditions such as telogen effluvium and alopecia areata. By incorporating activities such as aerobic exercise, yoga, or even strength training, individuals can lower their stress hormones, such as cortisol. This reduction can lead to improved hair health, as lower stress levels may help prevent premature greying and hair thinning. Additionally, exercise often encourages mindfulness and relaxation, further enhancing emotional well-being during the challenging andropause years.

Exercise also plays a pivotal role in improving metabolic health, which can be particularly beneficial during andropause. As men age, they may experience changes in body composition, including an increase in body fat and a decrease in muscle mass. Regular physical activity helps counteract these changes by promoting weight management and improving insulin sensitivity. A healthier metabolism can lead to better overall hormonal balance, which is essential for maintaining not only physical health but also the vitality of hair follicles. Maintaining a healthy weight can also reduce the risk of conditions that may exacerbate hair loss, such as diabetes and cardiovascular disease.

In addition to physical benefits, exercise has profound effects on mental health, which cannot be overlooked. The andropause period is often accompanied by mood swings, anxiety, and depression. Engaging in regular physical activity has been shown to boost mood and increase feelings of well-being through the release of endorphins, often referred to as "feel-good" hormones. This emotional uplift can significantly affect self-esteem, particularly in men dealing with hair loss or changes in appearance due to greying hair. A positive mental state can foster a healthier approach to dealing with the physical changes that occur during andropause.

Lastly, community and social aspects of exercise can provide additional support during the andropause period. Joining exercise groups, classes, or clubs can create a sense of belonging and camaraderie, which is important for psychological well-being. The social interactions gained through collective exercise not only enhance motivation but also provide an avenue for sharing experiences related to hair loss and aging. This support network can be invaluable for men navigating the challenges of the andropause effect, making exercise not just a physical activity but a vital component of a holistic approach to health during this transitional phase.

Stress Management Techniques

Stress management is a crucial aspect of maintaining overall health and well-being, particularly for adults experiencing andropause. This transitional phase often brings about various physical and emotional changes, including hair loss and premature greying. Understanding effective stress management techniques can significantly mitigate these effects and contribute to healthier aging. Recognizing the sources of stress in one's life is the first step towards managing it. Common stressors during andropause may include changes in relationships, body image concerns, and the pressures of career and family responsibilities.

One effective technique for managing stress is mindfulness meditation. This practice encourages individuals to focus on the present moment, promoting relaxation and reducing anxiety. Regular mindfulness sessions can help decrease the impact of stress on the body and mind, leading to improved emotional regulation and a greater sense of control. For those dealing with hair loss or grey hair, mindfulness can foster a more positive self-image, allowing individuals to accept changes with grace and resilience.

Physical activity is another powerful stress-relief tool. Engaging in regular exercise, whether through running, yoga, or strength training, can release endorphins, the body's natural mood lifters. Exercise not only combats stress but also improves circulation, which can be beneficial for hair health. For adults facing andropause, incorporating physical activity into daily routines can enhance both mental and physical well-being, helping to counteract the effects of stress on hair loss and greying.

Additionally, maintaining a healthy diet plays a pivotal role in stress management. Nutrient-rich foods can strengthen the body's ability to cope with stress while also supporting hair health. Foods high in omega-3 fatty acids, antioxidants, and vitamins can combat oxidative stress and promote healthier hair. A balanced diet, combined with adequate hydration, can improve energy levels and mood, making it easier to manage the stressors associated with andropause.

Lastly, fostering social connections is vital for stress management. Support from friends, family, and peers can provide emotional relief and practical advice for navigating the challenges of andropause. Engaging in social activities, whether in person or through virtual platforms, can help alleviate feelings of isolation and anxiety. Building a strong support network not only enhances resilience against stress but also encourages healthier lifestyle choices that can positively impact hair health and overall well-being during this transitional phase.

Treatment Options for Hair Loss

Over-the-Counter Solutions

Over-the-counter solutions for hair loss and grey hair have gained popularity as men navigate the challenges associated with andropause. These products range from topical treatments to dietary supplements, offering various approaches to combat the signs of aging. Understanding these solutions can empower individuals to make informed decisions regarding their hair health. While results can vary, these options provide accessible alternatives for those who may not yet be ready to pursue more invasive treatments.

Minoxidil is one of the most recognized over-the-counter treatments for hair loss. Originally developed as a medication for high blood pressure, it was discovered that minoxidil promotes hair growth as a side effect. Available in liquid or foam formulations, it is applied directly to the scalp. Clinical studies have shown that consistent use can help stimulate hair regrowth in individuals experiencing androgenetic alopecia. It is important to note that results may take several months, and ongoing use is necessary to maintain any benefits. Users should also be aware of potential side effects, including scalp irritation and unwanted facial hair growth.

Another popular category of over-the-counter solutions involves dietary supplements designed to support hair health from within. These supplements often contain a blend of vitamins, minerals, and herbal ingredients that claim to promote hair growth and reduce greying. Biotin, zinc, and saw palmetto are among the common constituents found in these formulations. While some users report positive effects, scientific evidence supporting the efficacy of these supplements can be mixed. Consulting with a healthcare professional before starting any new supplement regimen is advisable, particularly for individuals with underlying health conditions or those taking other medications.

Additionally, topical products such as shampoos and conditioners infused with active ingredients can aid in managing hair health. Formulations that contain ketoconazole or caffeine are gaining traction for their reported benefits in reducing hair loss and improving scalp health. These products work by addressing potential underlying issues such as fungal infections or poor circulation to the hair follicles. When selecting a shampoo or conditioner, consumers should look for formulations specifically targeting thinning hair, as they often contain nourishing ingredients that support overall hair vitality.

In conclusion, over-the-counter solutions for hair loss and grey hair present a variety of options for adults facing the effects of andropause. From topical treatments like minoxidil to dietary supplements and specialized hair care products, individuals have the opportunity to explore methods that align with their personal needs and preferences. While these solutions can provide benefits, it is essential to approach them with realistic expectations and a comprehensive understanding of their potential outcomes. Engaging with healthcare professionals can further enhance the journey toward effective hair health management during this transitional phase of life.

Prescription Medications

Prescription medications play a significant role in managing the symptoms associated with andropause, including hair loss and premature greying. As men age, hormonal changes can lead to a decrease in testosterone levels, which may contribute to various physical and psychological effects. It is essential for healthcare professionals and patients alike to understand the available prescription options that can address these specific concerns. By recognizing the connection between hormonal shifts and hair health, individuals can make informed decisions regarding their treatment plans.

One common category of prescription medications used to combat hair loss is 5-alpha reductase inhibitors, with finasteride being the most well-known example. This medication works by blocking the conversion of testosterone to dihydrotestosterone (DHT), a hormone linked to hair follicle shrinkage and eventual hair loss. Clinical studies have shown that finasteride can effectively slow hair loss and even promote regrowth in some men, making it a popular choice for those experiencing androgenetic alopecia. Healthcare providers must evaluate each patient's medical history and potential side effects before prescribing this medication, as individual responses can vary.

Another option for managing hair loss is the use of minoxidil, a topical solution that promotes hair growth by increasing blood flow to the hair follicles. Though not a prescription medication in many regions, it is often recommended alongside prescription treatments for enhanced efficacy. Minoxidil may be used by individuals at any stage of hair loss and can be particularly beneficial for those who prefer a non-systemic approach to treatment. Healthcare professionals should educate patients on the proper application techniques and the importance of consistency in using minoxidil to achieve optimal results.

In addition to addressing hair loss, some prescription medications can indirectly influence the greying of hair. Certain hormone replacement therapies (HRT) may help restore hormonal balance and mitigate some effects of andropause, potentially impacting hair pigmentation. While research is still emerging in this area, anecdotal evidence suggests that restoring testosterone levels can lead to improved overall hair health. Healthcare workers should remain vigilant about the potential benefits and risks associated with HRT, ensuring that patients are well-informed before starting any new therapy.

Finally, it is crucial to recognize that prescription medications, while effective, are just one part of a comprehensive approach to managing andropause symptoms. Patients should be encouraged to adopt a holistic lifestyle that includes a balanced diet, regular exercise, and stress management techniques. These factors can enhance the effectiveness of medications and contribute to overall well-being. Healthcare professionals must work collaboratively with patients to create individualized treatment plans that address both the physical and emotional aspects of andropause, leading to improved quality of life and hair health.

Surgical Options

Surgical options for addressing hair loss in men experiencing andropause have evolved significantly over the years. These procedures offer solutions for individuals who seek a more permanent resolution compared to non-surgical treatments. Two of the most common surgical techniques are hair transplantation and scalp reduction. Hair transplantation involves relocating hair follicles from a donor site, typically the back of the head, to areas experiencing thinning or baldness. This method has gained popularity due to its natural-looking results and the fact that transplanted hair is generally resistant to the hormonal changes associated with andropause.

FUE (Follicular Unit Extraction) and FUT (Follicular Unit Transplantation) are the primary methods used in hair transplantation. FUE involves the extraction of individual hair follicles, which are then implanted into the thinning areas. It is less invasive, leaving minimal scarring and allowing for a quicker recovery. On the other hand, FUT involves removing a strip of scalp from the donor area, which is then dissected into individual grafts for transplantation. While this method may result in a more noticeable scar, it can yield a higher number of grafts in a single session, making it suitable for those with extensive hair loss.

Scalp reduction is another surgical option that involves the removal of bald scalp areas, followed by the stretching of the hair-bearing scalp to cover the excised area. This procedure is less common than hair transplantation but can be effective for certain individuals, particularly those with a significant amount of baldness. Scalp reduction is often combined with hair transplantation to achieve the best possible aesthetic outcome. However, candidates for this procedure should be evaluated carefully, as it may not be suitable for all individuals due to factors like scalp laxity and the extent of hair loss.

Post-operative care is crucial for the success of any surgical intervention for hair loss. Patients are typically advised to avoid strenuous activities and direct sunlight for a period following the surgery. Additionally, following the surgeon's aftercare instructions regarding washing and caring for the scalp is essential to prevent complications such as infections or poor hair growth. Regular follow-up appointments are also necessary to monitor the healing process and assess the results of the procedure.

While surgical options can be effective for restoring hair, they are not without risks. Potential complications include infection, scarring, and unnatural-looking hairlines. Therefore, individuals considering these procedures should thoroughly discuss their expectations, potential outcomes, and risks with a qualified healthcare provider. A well-informed decision can lead to satisfactory results and a renewed sense of confidence for those experiencing the effects of andropause.

Coping with Changes in Appearance

Psychological Impacts of Hair Loss and Greying

Hair loss and greying are common experiences that many adults face, particularly as they navigate through andropause. These physical changes can evoke a range of psychological responses that significantly impact self-esteem and body image. For many individuals, hair is closely tied to identity and youthfulness. The perception of losing hair or noticing grey strands can trigger feelings of inadequacy, anxiety, and even depression. Understanding these psychological impacts is essential for both individuals experiencing these changes and healthcare workers who support them.

Research has shown that hair loss, particularly male pattern baldness, can lead to increased social anxiety and diminished self-worth. Men often associate a full head of hair with virility and attractiveness. When confronted with thinning hair or baldness, they may feel less confident in social situations, leading to avoidance behavior. This shift in self-perception can create a cycle of withdrawal and isolation, further exacerbating feelings of inadequacy. Educating healthcare workers about these psychological aspects can help them provide better support and resources to patients experiencing similar feelings.

Similarly, greying hair can also influence psychological well-being, particularly for women, who may face societal pressures related to aging and beauty. The cultural stigma surrounding grey hair can lead women to feel less attractive or relevant. This societal bias can intensify the emotional burden of aging, leading to a preoccupation with appearance that distracts from other important aspects of life. Healthcare providers should be aware of these societal pressures and encourage open discussions about aging gracefully and redefining beauty standards.

Moreover, the emotional effects of hair loss and greying can extend beyond individual self-esteem issues. Relationships can also be affected, as partners might not understand the deep psychological toll that these changes can bring. Open communication about feelings associated with hair loss and greying can foster understanding and support within relationships. Healthcare professionals can play a pivotal role in facilitating these conversations, helping to bridge the gap between partners and promote a healthier dialogue about aging and appearance.

In conclusion, the psychological impacts of hair loss and greying during andropause are significant and multifaceted. It is crucial for individuals experiencing these changes to recognize their feelings and seek support. Healthcare workers should be equipped with knowledge about these psychological effects to provide empathetic care and appropriate resources. By addressing the emotional ramifications of hair loss and greying, both individuals and healthcare providers can work towards fostering a more positive outlook on aging and self-acceptance.

Strategies for Building Self-Esteem

Building self-esteem is a crucial aspect of navigating the physical and emotional changes associated with andropause, such as hair loss and greying. Self-esteem influences how individuals perceive themselves and their worth, particularly in a society that often emphasizes youthful appearance. Men experiencing andropause may find their self-image impacted by these changes, leading to feelings of inadequacy or depression. Therefore, implementing effective strategies to bolster self-esteem is essential for enhancing overall well-being during this transitional phase.

One effective strategy for building self-esteem is fostering self-acceptance. Individuals amid andropause should focus on recognizing and accepting the natural aging process. Understanding that hair loss and greying are common experiences can help normalize these changes. Engaging in positive self-talk and challenging negative thoughts about appearance is vital. By reframing the narrative around aging, individuals can cultivate a more positive self-image, embracing the wisdom and experience that come with maturity.

Another important strategy involves setting realistic and achievable goals. Individuals can enhance their self-esteem by identifying personal goals that are not solely focused on appearance but also on health and personal development. For example, pursuing new hobbies, improving physical fitness, or dedicating time to relationships can provide a sense of accomplishment and fulfilment. When individuals focus on their strengths and achievements beyond their looks, they reinforce a more holistic view of self-worth.

Social support plays a significant role in boosting self-esteem, particularly for men during andropause. Connecting with peers who share similar experiences can provide a sense of community and understanding. Support groups, whether in-person or online, can facilitate discussions about the challenges of hair loss and aging, allowing individuals to express their feelings and receive encouragement. Building strong relationships with family and friends who appreciate them for who they are, rather than how they look, can further enhance self-esteem.

Lastly, considering professional support from therapists or counsellors can be invaluable for those struggling with self-esteem issues related to andropause. Professional guidance can offer individuals tailored strategies to manage their feelings effectively. Therapy can provide a safe space to explore underlying issues related to self-image and develop coping mechanisms. Additionally, professionals can help individuals navigate the emotional complexities of aging, creating a more resilient self-view and improving overall mental health. By employing these strategies, individuals can foster a healthier self-esteem that thrives despite the physical changes associated with andropause.

Support Systems and Community Resources

Support systems and community resources play a crucial role in addressing the challenges associated with andropause, particularly concerning issues like hair loss and greying hair. Understanding the psychological and emotional implications of these changes can significantly enhance an individual's experience during this transitional phase of life. Support groups, both in-person and online, offer a space for men to share their experiences, learn from one another, and find comfort in knowing they are not alone. These groups can provide valuable insights into coping mechanisms, lifestyle changes, and practical solutions that have worked for others facing similar challenges.

Healthcare professionals also serve as an essential support system for individuals navigating the effects of andropause. Regular check-ups and consultations can help identify underlying health issues that may contribute to hair loss or accelerated greying. These professionals can offer tailored advice on nutrition, exercise, and stress management techniques that can mitigate some of the physical and emotional symptoms associated with andropause. Additionally, they can provide referrals to specialists such as dermatologists or endocrinologists who can help manage specific concerns related to hair health.

Community resources, including local wellness programs and educational workshops, can also be beneficial. These initiatives often focus on holistic approaches to health, combining physical fitness, mental well-being, and nutritional education. Participating in such programs can empower individuals to take control of their health and appearance during andropause. Moreover, engaging in community activities fosters social connections, reducing feelings of isolation that may arise from changes in personal appearance and self-esteem.

Another vital aspect of support systems is the role of family and friends. Open communication about the physical and emotional challenges associated with andropause can strengthen relationships and create a more supportive environment. Encouraging loved ones to participate in discussions about hair loss and related concerns can help demystify these changes and promote understanding. This familial support not only helps individuals cope with their experiences but also reinforces the importance of seeking help and sharing feelings, which is essential for emotional well-being.

Finally, online resources and forums dedicated to andropause can serve as additional support systems. These platforms provide access to a wealth of information, including articles, expert advice, and personal stories. Online communities allow individuals to connect with others who understand their struggles and can share coping strategies. Furthermore, these resources often include information on available treatments for hair loss and greying hair, empowering individuals to make informed decisions about their health and appearance. By leveraging both online and offline support systems, individuals can navigate the complexities of andropause with greater confidence and resilience.

Future Research and Innovations

Advances in Hair Restoration Technology

Advancements in hair restoration technology have significantly transformed the landscape of treatment options available for individuals experiencing hair loss, particularly during andropause. These innovations are not only improving the efficacy of existing methods but also expanding the possibilities for those seeking to restore their hair. One of the notable advancements is the development of minimally invasive techniques, such as follicular unit extraction (FUE). This method allows for the harvesting of individual hair follicles without the need for large incisions, resulting in less scarring and a faster recovery time. As a result, patients can achieve natural-looking results with minimal discomfort and downtime.

Another promising area of advancement is the use of platelet-rich plasma (PRP) therapy. This treatment involves drawing a small amount of the patient's blood, processing it to concentrate the platelets, and then injecting it into the scalp. The growth factors in PRP have been shown to stimulate hair follicles, promoting hair regrowth and thickening existing hair. Clinical studies have demonstrated positive outcomes, making PRP a popular choice for both men and women experiencing androgenetic alopecia and other types of hair loss. As research continues, the potential for PRP therapy to be combined with other treatments may lead to even more effective hair restoration protocols.

Furthermore, the advent of advanced laser therapies has brought a new dimension to hair restoration. Low-level laser therapy (LLLT) utilizes specific wavelengths of light to stimulate cellular activity in the hair follicles. This non-invasive approach is designed to increase blood circulation and encourage hair growth. Studies have indicated that LLLT can be effective in slowing down hair loss and promoting regrowth, making it an appealing option for individuals at various stages of hair loss. With the development of portable devices for home use, patients now have greater accessibility to this technology, allowing them to incorporate treatment into their daily routines.

In addition to these techniques, researchers are exploring the potential of regenerative medicine in hair restoration. Stem cell therapy is being investigated as a method to rejuvenate hair follicles and promote new hair growth. This approach leverages the body's natural healing processes to address hair loss at a cellular level. Although still in the experimental stages, early findings are encouraging, and continued research may soon make stem cell therapy a viable option for those facing hair loss. Such innovations reflect a broader trend toward personalized medicine, where treatments can be tailored to the individual's unique biological makeup.

As these advances in hair restoration technology continue to evolve, it is essential for both patients and healthcare professionals to stay informed about the latest developments. Understanding the range of available options allows individuals experiencing hair loss during andropause to make educated decisions regarding their treatment plans. Additionally, healthcare workers play a crucial role in guiding patients through the multitude of choices and helping them navigate their specific needs. The integration of advanced technologies into hair restoration not only offers hope for regrowth but also enhances the overall quality of life for those affected by hair loss.

Understanding the Genetic Basis of Hair Loss

Hair loss is a complex condition influenced by a multitude of genetic factors. Understanding the genetic basis of hair loss is crucial for identifying the underlying causes and developing effective treatments. Research has shown that certain genes are linked to the predisposition for androgenetic alopecia, commonly known as male or female pattern baldness. This condition is characterized by a progressive thinning of hair, and its hereditary nature is evident in families where multiple members experience similar patterns of hair loss.

The primary gene associated with androgenetic alopecia is the androgen receptor gene located on the X chromosome. This gene plays a pivotal role in how hair follicles respond to androgens, particularly dihydrotestosterone (DHT). DHT is a derivative of testosterone and is believed to shrink hair follicles, leading to shorter hair growth cycles and ultimately hair loss. Individuals with a family history of hair loss are more likely to carry variations of this gene, making them more susceptible to the effects of DHT.

In addition to the androgen receptor gene, several other genetic markers have been identified that contribute to hair loss. Genome-wide association studies (GWAS) have revealed multiple loci that harbour genes influencing hair follicle development and cycling. These findings underscore the polygenic nature of hair loss, indicating that multiple genes interact in complex ways to determine an individual's risk of experiencing hair thinning or baldness. Understanding these genetic interactions is essential for developing targeted therapies that can address the specific pathways involved in hair loss.

Furthermore, epigenetic factors can also influence hair loss, adding another layer of complexity to its genetic basis. Environmental factors such as stress, diet, and exposure to toxins can modify gene expression without altering the underlying DNA sequence. This means that even individuals with a genetic predisposition to hair loss may experience varying degrees of hair thinning depending on their lifestyle and environmental exposures. Recognizing the role of epigenetics in hair loss can help healthcare providers offer more personalized treatment options that consider both genetic and environmental influences.

In conclusion, understanding the genetic basis of hair loss is critical for both individuals experiencing this condition and healthcare workers seeking to provide effective interventions. Continued research into the genetic and epigenetic factors contributing to hair loss will likely yield new insights and treatment options. By addressing the complex interplay of genetics, hormones, and environmental influences, we can develop a more comprehensive approach to managing hair loss, particularly during andropause when hormonal changes can exacerbate these issues.

The Future of Hormonal Treatments

The future of hormonal treatments for conditions related to andropause, such as hair loss and grey hair, is poised for significant advancements, driven by ongoing research and technological innovations. As our understanding of hormonal changes in aging men continues to evolve, so too does the potential for tailored therapies that specifically address the multifaceted symptoms associated with andropause. Current treatments often involve testosterone replacement therapy or medications that influence hormone levels, but emerging strategies may offer more personalized and effective solutions.

One area of focus is the development of selective androgen receptor modulators (SARMs). These compounds are designed to selectively target androgen receptors in specific tissues, potentially minimizing side effects commonly associated with traditional hormone replacement therapies. By promoting hair growth through localized action while reducing systemic exposure, SARMs may provide a promising alternative for men experiencing hair loss during andropause. Research is ongoing to assess their efficacy and safety, but early studies suggest they could revolutionize treatment options in this field.

Additionally, advancements in genetic and molecular research are shedding light on the underlying causes of hair greying and loss. Understanding the genetic factors that contribute to these changes can lead to targeted therapies that address the root causes rather than merely treating symptoms. Gene therapy, for example, holds potential for reversing the effects of aging on hair follicles by repairing or modifying genetic pathways involved in hair pigmentation and growth. As these technologies become more refined, they may offer new hope for those affected by the visible signs of andropause.

Furthermore, the integration of lifestyle modifications with hormonal treatments is likely to become increasingly important. A holistic approach that combines hormone therapy with nutritional support, exercise, and stress management can enhance the effectiveness of treatments. Research indicates that lifestyle factors significantly influence hormonal balance, and addressing these elements can lead to improved outcomes for individuals dealing with hair loss and greying hair. Healthcare providers will need to adopt comprehensive treatment plans that take into account the individual's overall health and lifestyle.

Finally, as public awareness of andropause grows, so does the demand for effective treatments. This increasing interest is likely to drive innovation within the pharmaceutical industry, resulting in a wider array of options for men experiencing these changes. Continued collaboration between researchers, healthcare professionals, and patients will be essential in shaping the future of hormonal treatments. By fostering dialogue and promoting education around andropause, we can ensure that advancements in treatment not only address the physical symptoms but also support the overall well-being of aging men.

Conclusion and Moving Forward

Embracing Change

Embracing change during the andropause is an essential aspect of understanding and addressing the physical and emotional transformations that men experience in middle age. This period is often marked by a decline in testosterone levels, which can lead to various changes, including hair loss and the greying of hair. Acknowledging these changes rather than resisting them is crucial for both men and those who care for them. This acceptance can foster a healthier mindset and encourage proactive measures to manage these transitions.

Hair loss and greying are often viewed negatively, associated with aging and a loss of vitality. However, reframing this perspective can lead to a more positive experience. For many, hair loss can signal a new chapter in life, one that offers opportunities for personal growth and self-acceptance. Health care workers and caregivers can play a pivotal role in guiding individuals through this process, helping them understand that such changes are a natural part of aging and not a reflection of their worth or masculinity.

Embracing change also involves educating oneself about the physiological aspects of andropause. Understanding the hormonal shifts and their implications can empower individuals to take control of their health. For instance, research indicates that lifestyle modifications, such as improved diet, regular exercise, and stress management, can mitigate some effects of andropause. By promoting awareness and providing practical solutions, health care professionals can enhance the quality of life for their patients during this transitional phase.

Moreover, emotional support is vital as men navigate these changes. Many may experience feelings of inadequacy or anxiety related to their physical appearance. Open communication between patients and their healthcare providers can facilitate discussions about emotional well-being. Encouraging men to express their feelings and seek support can lead to better outcomes and a more holistic approach to health that encompasses both mental and physical aspects.

Ultimately, embracing change during andropause is about fostering resilience and adaptability. By cultivating a positive outlook on hair loss and greying, men can enhance their self-image and confidence. Health care workers can aid in this journey by providing resources, support, and encouragement. Together, they can navigate this life stage with an understanding that change, while challenging, can also lead to new beginnings and a deeper appreciation for the journey of life.

Importance of Awareness and Education

Awareness and education play a crucial role in understanding the complexities of andropause, particularly regarding its physical manifestations such as hair loss and grey hair. As men age, they may experience a decline in testosterone levels, which can significantly impact their overall health and well-being. By fostering awareness of andropause, both adults and healthcare workers can better recognize the symptoms and address the emotional and psychological effects associated with these changes. Understanding the biological processes underlying andropause can demystify the experience and encourage individuals to seek appropriate support and treatment.

Education about the connection between andropause and hair changes is essential for promoting informed discussions surrounding male health. Many men may not realize that hormonal fluctuations can lead to thinning hair or premature greying, often attributing these changes to genetics or aging alone. By providing accurate information, healthcare workers can help patients understand that these physical changes are a normal part of aging, influenced by hormonal shifts that can be managed through lifestyle changes, medical interventions, or both. This knowledge can empower men to take proactive steps in addressing their hair health, leading to improved self-esteem and quality of life.

In addition to physical symptoms, the psychological impact of andropause, including changes in body image and self-perception, cannot be overlooked. Many men may feel embarrassed or ashamed about their hair loss or greying, which can lead to anxiety or depression. By increasing awareness of these emotional challenges, healthcare professionals can create a more supportive environment for their patients. Educational initiatives that focus on emotional resilience can help men navigate the psychological effects of andropause, encouraging them to engage in open conversations about their feelings and experiences.

Moreover, awareness campaigns aimed at the general public can help reduce stigma surrounding male aging and health concerns. By normalizing discussions about andropause, hair loss, and grey hair, society can foster a more accepting environment where men feel comfortable addressing these issues. Community workshops, online resources, and support groups can serve as platforms for sharing information and personal experiences, ultimately promoting a culture of understanding and support. This collective effort can lead to greater acceptance of the aging process and the challenges that come with it.

Finally, ongoing education for healthcare workers is vital to ensure that they are well-equipped to address the needs of men undergoing andropause. Training programs and resources that focus on the latest research and treatment options can enhance the ability of healthcare professionals to provide effective care. By staying informed about the latest developments in andropause management, healthcare workers can offer tailored advice and interventions, ultimately improving outcomes for their patients. The importance of awareness and education cannot be overstated, as they are key to empowering both men and healthcare providers to navigate the complexities of andropause with confidence and compassion.

Resources for Further Support and Information

When navigating the complexities of andropause, particularly in relation to hair loss and greying hair, it is crucial to have access to reliable resources that provide comprehensive information and support. A variety of organizations, websites, and literature are dedicated to educating both individuals experiencing these changes and the healthcare workers who assist them. These resources can facilitate a deeper understanding of the physiological, psychological, and social aspects of andropause, equipping readers with the knowledge necessary to make informed decisions regarding their health.

Professional medical associations, such as the American Urological Association and the Endocrine Society, offer a wealth of information on male health issues, including andropause. These organizations publish guidelines, research articles, and patient education materials that can help both men experiencing andropause and healthcare providers understand the underlying hormonal changes. Accessing these resources allows for a more nuanced approach to addressing symptoms such as hair loss and greying, emphasizing the importance of individualized care plans.

Support groups and online forums can also serve as invaluable resources for those dealing with the effects of andropause. Platforms such as the Androgen Deficiency in the Aging Male (ADAM) and similar community-focused initiatives provide a space for individuals to share their experiences, seek advice, and find emotional support. These communities often foster a sense of belonging, which can alleviate feelings of isolation that may accompany the physical changes experienced during andropause. Healthcare providers can recommend these groups to patients as a complement to clinical treatment.

In addition to professional organizations and support communities, various books and publications delve into the subject of andropause, hair loss, and grey hair. Titles authored by medical professionals or experts in the field can offer insights into the latest research, treatment options, and lifestyle modifications that can mitigate the effects of andropause. Libraries and online bookstores are excellent starting points for finding literature that discusses both the scientific and practical aspects of managing these changes.

Finally, it is essential to highlight the role of healthcare professionals in guiding individuals through the andropause experience. Physicians, dermatologists, and mental health specialists can provide tailored advice and treatment options, while also recommending additional resources. Collaboration between patients and healthcare providers can enhance understanding and management of symptoms, leading to improved quality of life. By utilizing a combination of these resources, adults experiencing the andropause effect can navigate their journey with greater confidence and support.

Pause for Thought

- Though andropause is a continuum, it can be conveniently divided into three distinct phases. The first stage of andropause, generally begins in a man's late 30's and or early 40's. Here there are subtle shifts in mood, energy and libido. Early diagnosis may be challenging, since these early symptoms may be disguised as normal aging.
- The second stage of andropause sees a more pronounced decline in testosterone leading to symptoms such as fatigue, decreased muscle mass, increased body fat and changes in hair pattern may be observed. Male pattern baldness may accelerate at this time which may affect self esteem and body image.

- The final stage of andropause involves significant systemic changes and a potential increase in associated health risks. Emotional fluctuations leading to depression and anxiety, along with physical symptoms like osteoporosis and cardiovascular concerns. This cumulatively can lead to a diminished sense of wellbeing.

- Since the andropause can affect men both physically and mentally, a multifaceted approach is essential in an effort to proactively address the challenges of andropause awareness and education about andropause will ultimately enhance quality of life for many men facing these challenges.

- Not only does andropause manifest as fatigue, reduced libido, and loss of muscle mass, men may experience mood swings, irritability and even symptoms of depression. Andropause may also manifest as hair loss, many men may find that their hair thins and or recedes rapidly during this period which affects self esteem and or anxiety about aging. In addition to the above, cognitive changes can become noticeable, such as difficulty in concentration, memory lapses, and an overall sense of mental fog being quite common. Thus, in he testosterone decline can also affect the brain's neuroplasticity leading to challenges in learning and memory retention.

- Hormonal changes extend beyond just testosterone and dihydrotestosterone. Other hormones such as oestrogen and cortisol play a crucial role in the aging process. As men experience hormonal changes, the balance between testosterone and oestrogen may shift, potentially leading to increased body fat and changes in hair distribution. Elevated cortisol level may exacerbate hair loss by shortening the hair growth cycle leading to thinning hair and increased shedding.

- Greying of hair is primarily influenced by a decrease in melanin production which is regulated by hormonal levels as testosterone diminishes, the melanocytes responsible for hair colour may also decline in function, resulting in the loss of pigmentation. This process can be indicative of broader hormonal imbalances that may require attention.
- Hair loss can manifest in various forms each with distinct characteristics and underlying causes. The most common is androgenic alopecia, also referred as male or female pattern baldness. This genetic condition typically begins with a receding hairline or thinning at the crown in men, while women usually experience a broader area of overall thinning. The role of androgens, testosterone and dihydrotestosterone are critical in this process as they affect follicle sensitivity and growth cycles
- Telgen effluvium – a type of hair loss-occurs when a significant number of hair follicles enter the resting phase of the hair growth cycle prematurely. This can be triggered by various factors, including stress, hormonal changes , nutritional deficiencies or medical conditions. Unlike androgenic alopecia, telogen effluvium is often reversible, and addressing the underlying cause can lead to regrowth.

- Alopecia Areta is an autoimmune disorder characterised by sudden hair loss in patches. It occurs when the immune system mistakenly attacks hair follicles, leading to hair loss in various areas of the scalp and body. Though it can affect individuals at any age, but it often presents in younger adults. Though the cause is unclear, factors such as genetics and environmental triggers may play a role. Treatment options include corticosteroids and other immunosuppressive agents.

Take Home Nuggets

- Other types of alopecia include traction alopecia is a form of hair loss that results from prolonged tension on the hair follicles, often due to certain hairstyles like tight ponytails, braids, or extensions. The damage here can lead to irreversible hair loss.
- Scarring alopecia, also known as cicatricial alopecia, involves a group of disorders that cause permanent hair loss due to inflammation and scarring of their hair follicles. This category includes lichen planopilaris and frontal fibrosing alopecia. This can arise from autoimmune conditions and infections.
- Hair loss in men is multifaceted, the most prominent factor being genetics male pattern baldness, or androgenic alopecia is the most common cause of hair loss in men. This heredity condition is linked to the presence of androgens, particularly dihydrotestosterone which affect hair follicles by shortening their growth cycle and ultimately leading to

miniaturisation. Men with a family history of baldness are at a higher risk of experiencing this condition, making genetics a critical aspect to consider when addressing hair loss.

- Hair loss is multifaceted, a decline in testosterone can lead to an increase in the level of dihydrotestosterone which contributes to hair follicle shrinkage and loss. Imbalances in other hormones such thyroid hormones can lead to their thinning and shredding. Medical conditions such as alopecia arreta can cause sudden hair loss in patches and scalp infections like tinea capitis can lead to significant thinning.
- Lifestyle factors also influence hair loss in men. Stress whether acute or chronic, can trigger a type of hair loss known as telogen effluvium where hair follicles prematurely enter the resting phase of their growth cycle, poor nutrition, particularly deficiencies in vitamins and minerals such as iron, zinc, and biotin, can also lead to weakened hair and increased shredding, additionally, life lifestyle factors such as excess alcohol consumption and smoking is also associated with hair loss, thus emphasizing the importance of a healthy lifestyle in maintaining hair growth.
- Dihydrotestosterone is a potent androgen derived from testosterone and plays a critical role in various physiological processes. Dihydrotestosterone binds to androgen receptors in hair follicles leading to a reduction in hair growth. This process can ultimately lead to complete follicle shutdown, resulting in baldness but not only that;

Dihydrotestosterone is associated with benign prostatic hypertrophy. The dual role of dihydrotestosterone in hair follicle health and prostate enlargement illustrates the importance of monitoring dihydrotestosterone levels in aging adults.

- Hair colour is primarily determined by the presence and type of pigments in the hair follicles. Hair pigmentation is determined by the presence and type of pigments in the hair follicles. Hair pigmentation is determined by Eumelanin and pheomelanin. Eumelanin is responsible for darker shades including black and brown while pheomelanin contributes to lighter shades such as blonde or red. The production of this pigment is controlled by a complex interplay of genetic factors and environmental influences. Genetics play a crucial role in determining hair colour. Specific genes such as MC1R gene is known to influence the type and amount of melanin produced in hair follicles.
- Environmental factors also contribute to hair colour changes over time. Exposure to sunlight can lighten hair colour due to the breakdown of melanin by u-v rays. Chemical exposure from hair treatments, such as dyes and bleaches can alter the natural pigmentation of hair. These external influences can interact with genetic predisposition and may exacerbate the natural greying process or trigger hair loss.

- Grey hair is a common phenomenon that adults may experience as they age. As individuals age, melanocytes the cells responsible for producing melanin- gradually diminish in number and activity. Over the counter solutions for hair loss and grey hair range from topical treatment to dietary supplements, offering various approaches to the management of hair loss and greying.

Chapter 6
Understanding Mental Health in Adult Men

The Importance of Mental Health Awareness

Mental health awareness plays a crucial role in fostering a supportive environment for adult men, especially those facing the unique challenges of andropause. As men navigate this transitional phase, they often encounter emotional and psychological changes that can lead to anxiety and depression. Recognizing these mental health issues is the first step toward addressing them, enabling men to seek help and support without feeling stigmatized. By promoting awareness, we can create a culture where mental health is openly discussed, helping men feel less isolated in their struggles.

Anxiety disorders are particularly prevalent among adult males, and andropause can exacerbate these conditions. Symptoms may manifest as increased stress, irritability, or overwhelming fatigue, which can significantly impact daily life. Understanding the relationship between hormonal changes and mental health is vital. Men need to be aware that seeking help for anxiety is not a sign of weakness but an essential step in managing their well-being. This awareness can lead to improved coping strategies and healthier responses to stress.

Depression can have profound effects on men's relationships, often leading to withdrawal from social interactions and a decline in communication with loved ones. Men may feel pressured to adhere to traditional masculine norms, which discourage vulnerability and emotional expression. By raising awareness about depression and its impact, we can encourage men to share their feelings and experiences, fostering deeper connections with family and friends. This shift can enhance emotional support networks that are crucial for recovery and well-being.

Substance abuse is another area where mental health awareness is essential. Many men may turn to alcohol or drugs as a coping mechanism for their mental health challenges, particularly during times of stress or emotional upheaval. Raising awareness about the link between substance abuse and mental health can help men recognize the dangers of these behaviours and seek healthier alternatives. Education on the effects of substance abuse on mental health can empower men to make informed choices and pursue recovery options.

Lastly, understanding the role of masculinity in mental health stigma is crucial for promoting awareness. Traditional notions of masculinity often discourage men from expressing vulnerability or seeking help, which can perpetuate mental health issues. By challenging these stereotypes and promoting emotional intelligence, we can help men embrace their feelings and seek support without fear of judgment. Awareness initiatives can facilitate discussions around masculinity, encouraging a more holistic approach to men's mental health that embraces vulnerability as a strength rather than a weakness.

Common Mental Health Challenges Faced by Men

Men often face unique mental health challenges that can be exacerbated during andropause, a period marked by hormonal changes that can affect emotional well-being. Anxiety disorders are particularly common, with many men experiencing heightened levels of stress and worry that can lead to significant impairment in daily functioning. The stigma surrounding mental health often discourages men from seeking help, leading to a cycle of suffering that can be difficult to break.

Depression is another prevalent issue, and its impact on men's relationships can be profound. Men may struggle to express their emotions, which can lead to misunderstandings and distance in personal connections. The societal expectation for men to be stoic often prevents them from discussing their feelings openly, causing isolation and further exacerbating depressive symptoms. This lack of communication can strain marriages, friendships, and relationships with children, making it essential for men to find healthier ways to express their emotional struggles.

Substance abuse is frequently seen as a coping mechanism for men dealing with mental health issues. Alcohol and drugs may initially provide an escape, but they often lead to worsening mental health and create additional problems in personal and professional life. Men may turn to substances when feeling overwhelmed by stress, anxiety, or depression, which can ultimately hinder their ability to cope effectively and lead to a downward spiral.

The role of masculinity in perpetuating mental health stigma cannot be overlooked. Traditional views of masculinity often equate vulnerability with weakness, making it challenging for men to acknowledge their mental health needs. This stigma can prevent them from reaching out for help, further complicating their ability to navigate challenges such as job loss, midlife crises, or the pressures of fatherhood, all of which can significantly impact mental health.

Coping strategies are essential for men to manage their mental health effectively. Techniques such as developing emotional intelligence, practicing mindfulness, and seeking social support can empower men to address their challenges constructively. Understanding the common mental health issues faced by men, including PTSD from trauma and the emotional toll of life transitions, is crucial for fostering resilience and improving overall well-being in adulthood. By breaking the silence surrounding these struggles, men can start to reclaim their mental health and enhance their quality of life.

Anxiety Disorders in Adult Males

Overview of Anxiety Disorders

Anxiety disorders are prevalent mental health challenges that significantly affect adult males, particularly those navigating the complexities of andropause. These disorders encompass a range of conditions, including generalized anxiety disorder, panic disorder, and social anxiety disorder, each characterized by excessive fear or worry that can disrupt daily functioning. For many men, the onset of anxiety can coincide with significant life changes, such as job transitions, health concerns, or shifts in family dynamics, leading to an increase in stress and emotional turmoil.

The impact of anxiety disorders on men's relationships cannot be overstated. Men often experience societal pressure to embody strength and stoicism, which can lead to a reluctance to seek help or express vulnerability. This stigma surrounding mental health can exacerbate feelings of isolation and despair, making it even more challenging for men to connect with their partners, friends, and family members. Understanding how anxiety affects communication and emotional intimacy is crucial for fostering healthier relationships during this period of life.

Substance abuse is another concern that often intertwines with anxiety disorders in adult males. Some men may turn to alcohol or drugs as a coping mechanism to alleviate their anxiety symptoms temporarily. However, this can lead to a vicious cycle, where substance abuse exacerbates mental health issues, leading to further anxiety and depression. Recognizing the signs of this pattern is essential for both men and their support systems to intervene effectively and promote healthier coping strategies.

Navigating midlife crises can also trigger or amplify anxiety disorders. As men confront their mortality, career aspirations, and personal achievements, feelings of inadequacy or failure may surface. This introspection can lead to heightened anxiety, particularly if men feel unprepared to handle these life transitions. Developing emotional intelligence and resilience is vital for managing these challenges, allowing men to address their fears constructively rather than allowing them to spiral into debilitating anxiety.

Ultimately, understanding anxiety disorders within the context of men's mental health, especially during andropause, is essential for promoting well-being and effective coping strategies. Encouraging open conversations about mental health can help dismantle the stigma surrounding these issues, empowering men to seek support and develop healthier relationships with themselves and others. By fostering a culture of openness, men can better navigate their mental health challenges and cultivate resilience in the face of life's inevitable stresses.

Symptoms and Diagnosis

As men age, particularly during andropause, they may experience a range of symptoms that can impact their mental health. These symptoms can include persistent feelings of sadness, anxiety, and irritability. Many men might dismiss these feelings as simply a part of aging but recognizing them as potential indicators of mental health challenges is crucial for early intervention and support. Understanding these symptoms is key to addressing issues such as depression and anxiety disorders, which are often prevalent during this transitional period.

In addition to emotional symptoms, physical manifestations can also signal underlying mental health issues. Changes in sleep patterns, appetite fluctuations, and decreased energy levels are common complaints among older men. These physical symptoms can exacerbate feelings of hopelessness or anxiety, creating a cycle that is difficult to break. It is essential for men to be aware of these changes and seek help, when necessary, rather than attributing them solely to aging or stress.

Diagnosis of mental health issues in adult men can often be complicated by societal perceptions of masculinity. Many men may feel pressured to portray a stoic demeanour, leading them to avoid discussing their feelings or seeking help. The stigma surrounding mental health can deter men from recognizing their symptoms as valid concerns, which can delay diagnosis and treatment. Open conversations about mental health and recognizing that seeking help is a sign of strength are vital in overcoming these barriers.

Mental health professionals utilize various methods to diagnose conditions such as depression and anxiety. These can include comprehensive assessments, interviews about symptoms, and standardized questionnaires that help gauge the severity of mental health challenges. By providing a safe space for men to express their feelings and experiences, healthcare providers can better understand the specific challenges they face and develop appropriate treatment plans.

In conclusion, acknowledging the symptoms of mental health challenges and seeking a proper diagnosis is essential for adult males experiencing andropause. By understanding the interplay between mental health and the physical, emotional, and societal factors at play, men can take proactive steps towards improving their mental well-being. This awareness helps in dismantling the stigma associated with mental health issues, promoting healthier coping strategies, and ultimately enhancing their overall quality of life.

Treatment Options

Treatment options for mental health challenges in adult men, particularly those experiencing andropause, are diverse and should be personalized. Understanding that everyone may respond differently to various therapies is crucial in crafting an effective treatment plan. Common approaches include psychotherapy, medication, and lifestyle changes, which can all contribute to improved mental health outcomes. It is important for men to seek professional guidance to identify which combination works best for their unique situations.

Psychotherapy, or talk therapy, is one of the most effective treatment modalities for addressing anxiety and depression in adult males. Cognitive Behavioural Therapy (CBT) is particularly beneficial, as it helps individuals recognize and modify negative thought patterns. This is essential for men who may struggle with traditional expressions of emotion, as it provides them with tools to articulate their feelings and cope with stress. Engaging in therapy can also dismantle the stigma surrounding mental health, encouraging more men to seek help.

Medication can be an effective adjunct to therapy, particularly for those with moderate to severe anxiety or depression. Antidepressants and anxiolytics may help alleviate symptoms, allowing men to engage more fully in their therapeutic process. It is vital that any medication is prescribed by a qualified healthcare provider who understands the potential interactions and side effects, especially considering the hormonal changes associated with andropause.

In addition to professional therapies, lifestyle changes can significantly impact mental health. Regular exercise, a balanced diet, and adequate sleep are foundational elements that contribute to emotional well-being. Furthermore, developing healthy coping strategies, such as mindfulness and stress-relief techniques, can empower men to manage their mental health more effectively. Support groups and community involvement can also provide social connections that are crucial for emotional support.

Ultimately, treatment options should be approached holistically, considering the various aspects of a man's life, including his responsibilities as a father, his career, and his personal relationships. By addressing mental health challenges comprehensively, men can navigate midlife crises and other stressors more effectively, leading to improved emotional intelligence and resilience. It is essential for adult males to recognize the importance of seeking help and engaging in conversations about mental health, breaking down the barriers of stigma and isolation.

Depression and Its Impact on Men's Relationships

Understanding Depression

Depression is a complex mental health condition that often goes unnoticed, especially among adult males. For many men, acknowledging feelings of sadness or hopelessness can be challenging due to societal expectations around masculinity. This stigma discourages open discussions about emotional struggles, leading to a cycle where men feel isolated in their suffering. Understanding depression requires recognizing its symptoms, which may manifest as changes in mood, energy levels, and even physical health, impacting a man's overall quality of life.

As men age and encounter significant life transitions such as andropause, they may experience heightened emotional challenges. The hormonal changes during this period can contribute to feelings of irritability and sadness, which may be misinterpreted as a normal part of aging. However, it is crucial for men to differentiate between age-related mood changes and clinical depression, which necessitates professional intervention. This understanding can empower men to seek help without the fear of being perceived as weak or vulnerable.

Depression not only affects the individual but also significantly impacts relationships with family, friends, and colleagues. Men struggling with depression may withdraw from social interactions, leading to strained relationships. Partners may feel neglected or confused by the changes in their loved ones, often resulting in a cycle of misunderstandings and emotional distance. Recognizing the effects of depression on interpersonal dynamics is essential for fostering supportive environments where men can express their feelings without judgment.

Substance abuse is another critical factor that intertwines with depression in men. Many adult males turn to alcohol or drugs as a means of coping with their emotional pain, leading to a detrimental cycle that exacerbates both mental health issues and substance dependence. Understanding this relationship is vital for developing effective coping strategies. Support systems that encourage healthy coping mechanisms rather than substance use can significantly improve outcomes for men struggling with depression.

Finally, coping strategies tailored to men experiencing depression are essential for recovery. Techniques such as mindfulness, physical activity, and establishing a strong support network can provide relief. Encouraging emotional intelligence and vulnerability can help men articulate their feelings and seek help when needed. By fostering an environment that normalizes discussions around mental health, adult males can navigate their struggles more effectively, ultimately enhancing their well-being and relationships during challenging times.

How Depression Affects Relationships

Depression is a powerful force that can deeply affect relationships, particularly for adult men experiencing andropause. As men face the emotional and physical changes this phase brings, they may find themselves grappling with feelings of sadness, isolation, and inadequacy. These feelings can create a barrier to communication, making it difficult for them to connect with loved ones. The inability to express emotions often leads to misunderstandings, leaving partners and friends feeling neglected or confused about the man's emotional state.

The impact of depression on relationships often manifests in withdrawal and avoidance behaviours. Men might retreat into themselves, avoiding social interactions and isolating from their support networks. This withdrawal can create a cycle of loneliness, where the lack of interaction exacerbates depressive symptoms. As friends and family notice these changes, they may respond with concern, but without clear communication, their efforts to help can sometimes feel unwelcome or intrusive to the man suffering from depression.

Moreover, the traditional expectations of masculinity can further complicate how depression affects relationships. Many men feel pressured to conform to societal norms that discourage vulnerability and emotional expression. This stigma can prevent them from seeking help or discussing their mental health struggles, leading to a facade of strength that isolates them even more. Partners may feel frustrated or helpless, as they witness the man they care for suffering in silence.

Substance abuse can also play a significant role in how depression impacts relationships. In an attempt to cope with their feelings, some men may turn to alcohol or drugs, which can lead to further deterioration of their mental health and relationships. This coping mechanism can create a toxic cycle where substance use becomes a barrier to intimacy and trust, ultimately driving a wedge between partners. The resulting conflicts and disappointments can strain relationships to a breaking point, making recovery and healing more challenging.

It is crucial for men to recognize the effects of depression on their relationships and seek appropriate support. Open communication with partners and loved ones can help bridge the emotional gap that depression creates. Emphasizing emotional intelligence and vulnerability allows for deeper connections and understanding, paving the way for healthier relationships. By addressing these challenges head-on, men can not only improve their mental health but also foster stronger, more fulfilling relationships with those around them.

Communication and Support Strategies

Effective communication is a cornerstone of addressing mental health challenges, especially for adult males navigating the complexities of andropause. Open dialogue about feelings and struggles can foster deeper connections with friends and family. Encouraging men to share their experiences not only helps reduce the stigma surrounding mental health but also provides a support network that is crucial during difficult times. Creating a safe space for honest conversations is essential for emotional well-being and can significantly improve relationships.

Support strategies are vital in the journey toward mental health recovery. Men are often taught to be stoic, which can hinder their ability to seek help. By promoting support groups and therapy tailored specifically for men, we can break down these barriers. These resources offer a platform for men to discuss their unique challenges, such as anxiety, depression, and the impact of societal expectations on their mental health. This camaraderie can empower individuals to confront their struggles more openly and effectively.

Coping strategies play a significant role in managing stress and anxiety. Methods such as mindfulness, physical activity, and creative outlets can greatly benefit men experiencing mental health issues. Engaging in regular exercise not only improves physical health but also releases endorphins that elevate mood. Additionally, practices such as meditation or journaling can help men process their emotions and develop emotional intelligence, which is often lacking in traditional masculine roles.

The impact of job loss on mental health is a critical area of concern for many men, particularly those in midlife. Employment often shapes a man's identity and self-worth, making job loss a particularly devastating experience. Open discussions about the emotional fallout of unemployment, along with practical support systems such as career counselling and skills training, can help mitigate feelings of inadequacy and promote resilience during these transitions.

Finally, addressing the mental health challenges faced by fathers is paramount. Fatherhood brings unique pressures that can exacerbate existing mental health issues or trigger new ones. Encouraging fathers to engage in open discussions about their feelings and experiences can strengthen their relationships with their children and partners. Mental health education that includes the challenges of fatherhood can lead to healthier family dynamics and a more supportive environment for men as they navigate the complexities of their roles.

Substance Abuse and Mental Health in Men

The Link Between Substance Abuse and Mental Health

The relationship between substance abuse and mental health is complex and often intertwined, particularly among adult men experiencing andropause. Many men in this phase of life may find themselves grappling with feelings of inadequacy or loss of identity, which can exacerbate underlying mental health challenges. This emotional turmoil often leads individuals to seek solace in substances, creating a dangerous cycle where substance abuse becomes a maladaptive coping mechanism for managing anxiety and depression. Understanding this link is crucial for addressing the mental health needs of men during this transitional period.

As men navigate the challenges of aging, societal expectations of masculinity can further complicate their relationship with mental health. The stigma surrounding mental health issues often discourages men from seeking help, leading them to resort to alcohol or drugs as a means of self-medication. This reluctance to confront emotional struggles can result in a vicious cycle of escalating substance use, ultimately worsening their mental health conditions. Acknowledging and addressing these societal pressures is essential for breaking the cycle of substance abuse and fostering healthier coping strategies.

Moreover, the impact of substance abuse on relationships cannot be overlooked. For men dealing with anxiety and depression, turning to substances can strain familial and social connections. Partners, children, and friends often bear the brunt of the negative consequences, which can lead to further isolation and despair for the individual. Open communication and support from loved ones are vital, yet men often struggle to express their vulnerabilities, perpetuating their sense of isolation.

Coping strategies that promote mental well-being can be beneficial in mitigating the risk of substance abuse. Engaging in physical activities, practicing mindfulness, and seeking therapy can equip men with healthier tools to manage stress and emotional pain. Peer support groups also provide a vital space for men to share their experiences and learn from one another, fostering a sense of community and understanding. These alternative coping mechanisms are crucial in breaking free from the cycle of substance reliance.

Ultimately, addressing the link between substance abuse and mental health is essential for promoting the overall well-being of adult men. By fostering open discussions about mental health and challenging societal norms around masculinity, we can create a supportive environment where men feel empowered to seek help. This proactive approach not only benefits the individual but also enhances their relationships and community, paving the way for a healthier, more fulfilling life during and beyond andropause.

Risk Factors for Substance Abuse

Substance abuse among adult men, particularly those experiencing andropause, is influenced by a variety of risk factors that can exacerbate underlying mental health issues. Many men face increased stress due to job loss, relationship challenges, and the societal expectations of masculinity, which can lead to unhealthy coping mechanisms. The pressure to conform to traditional masculine norms may discourage open discussions about mental health, pushing some men towards substance use to escape their emotional struggles.

Anxiety disorders are prevalent among adult males, often heightening the likelihood of substance abuse as a form of self-medication. Men may turn to alcohol or drugs to alleviate feelings of anxiety, believing that these substances provide temporary relief. However, this cycle can lead to worsening mental health, creating a paradox where the very substance used to cope becomes a source of further distress and dysfunction in their lives.

Depression also plays a critical role in the risk factors for substance abuse in adult men. Feelings of hopelessness and despair can lead to isolation, making it difficult for men to seek help or connect with supportive relationships. In many cases, the impact of depression on their interpersonal relationships can further perpetuate a cycle of substance abuse, as they may seek solace in drugs or alcohol rather than confronting their emotional pain.

The stigma surrounding mental health in men, particularly related to masculinity, adds another layer to the risk factors for substance abuse. Many men are conditioned to believe that expressing vulnerability is a sign of weakness, which can lead to avoidance of mental health services. This stigma not only prevents men from seeking necessary support but also encourages them to resort to substance use as a misguided form of coping.

Lastly, the emotional toll of navigating midlife crises can significantly influence substance abuse behaviours. As men confront aging, career shifts, or changes in family dynamics, they may struggle with feelings of inadequacy or loss. These emotions can drive some to substances, viewing them as a means to regain control or escape from the realities of their changing lives. Understanding these risk factors is essential for addressing substance abuse and promoting healthier coping strategies among adult men.

Recovery and Support

Recovery from mental health challenges is a journey that requires patience, understanding, and support. For adult males, particularly those experiencing andropause, recognizing the signs of anxiety and depression is crucial. These emotional struggles can significantly impact relationships, making it essential to seek help. Whether through professional therapy or support groups, reaching out is the first step towards healing. Men often feel a societal pressure to appear strong, which can hinder their willingness to discuss their mental health openly.

Support systems play a vital role in the recovery process. Friends, family, and peers can provide the encouragement needed to confront mental health issues. Men should be encouraged to share their experiences and feelings, as open communication can foster deeper connections and alleviate the sense of isolation. Engaging in conversations about mental health can also help dismantle the stigma associated with male vulnerability, promoting a culture where seeking help is seen as a strength rather than a weakness.

Coping strategies are essential for managing stress and anxiety. Techniques such as mindfulness, exercise, and healthy lifestyle choices can significantly improve mental health. Additionally, understanding the impact of substance abuse on mental health is crucial for recovery. Many men turn to alcohol or drugs as a coping mechanism during difficult times, but these substances can exacerbate underlying issues and create a cycle of dependency. Finding healthier alternatives to cope with stress can lead to more sustainable recovery.

Navigating life changes, such as job loss or midlife crises, can also affect mental health. These transitions often bring about feelings of inadequacy and fear of the future. Men experiencing such changes should be reminded that it is normal to seek help during these times. Engaging in community activities, pursuing new interests, or even volunteering can provide a sense of purpose and belonging, aiding in recovery.

Lastly, the importance of emotional intelligence cannot be overstated. Developing the ability to recognize and express emotions can lead to healthier relationships and improved mental well-being. For many men, the journey to recovery involves not only addressing mental health issues but also redefining their understanding of masculinity. Embracing vulnerability and seeking support are powerful steps towards overcoming silent struggles and achieving a fulfilling life.

The Role of Masculinity in Mental Health Stigma

Societal Expectations of Masculinity

Societal expectations around masculinity often create a rigid framework that men feel compelled to navigate throughout their lives. These expectations dictate how men should behave, what emotions they can express, and even how they should manage their mental health. This pressure can lead to significant internal conflict, especially for adult males facing the challenges of andropause, where physical and emotional changes may contradict traditional masculine ideals. The stigma surrounding vulnerability and emotional expression can exacerbate feelings of isolation and anxiety, making it difficult for men to seek help when they need it the most.

In many cultures, masculinity is associated with traits such as strength, stoicism, and self-reliance. This can pressure men to suppress emotional pain or distress, leading to untreated anxiety and depression. Adult men often feel that admitting to mental health struggles undermines their masculinity, leaving them trapped in a cycle of silence. As they age and face life transitions like job loss or fatherhood, these societal expectations can weigh heavily on their mental health, influencing their relationships and overall well-being.

The impact of these societal norms extends to relationships, where men may find it challenging to communicate openly about their feelings. This difficulty can strain connections with partners, friends, and family members, often resulting in misunderstandings and conflict. As adult men navigate the complexities of midlife crises, they may feel an intensified need to conform to masculine stereotypes, further isolating themselves from potential support systems. The fear of being perceived as weak can lead to substance abuse as a coping mechanism, further complicating their mental health landscape.

Navigating mental health challenges in the context of societal expectations requires a shift in how masculinity is defined and understood. Encouraging emotional intelligence can empower men to express their feelings and seek help without fear of judgment. Support groups and therapy tailored for men can foster a safe environment where they can discuss their struggles and develop healthier coping strategies. By challenging the stigma surrounding men's mental health, society can create a more inclusive narrative that acknowledges the complexities of masculinity and its impact on emotional well-being.

Ultimately, redefining societal expectations of masculinity is crucial for improving mental health outcomes for adult men. Embracing vulnerability as a strength rather than a weakness can lead to healthier relationships and a greater sense of fulfilment. As men confront the realities of andropause and other life changes, it becomes essential to cultivate a culture that values emotional expression and support. By doing so, men can break free from the constraints of traditional masculinity and find more meaningful ways to engage with their mental health and the world around them.

How Stigma Impacts Help-Seeking Behaviour

Stigma surrounding mental health issues significantly impacts the help-seeking behaviour of adult men, particularly those navigating the complexities of andropause. Many men feel societal pressure to conform to traditional notions of masculinity, which often equate vulnerability with weakness. As a result, the idea of admitting to mental health struggles becomes daunting, leading many to suffer in silence rather than seek the support they desperately need. This reluctance can exacerbate conditions such as anxiety and depression, creating a vicious cycle that is difficult to break.

The fear of being judged or labelled can deter men from discussing their mental health challenges with friends, family, or professionals. When confronted with issues like job loss or relationship difficulties, many men internalize their feelings, believing that they must handle these struggles independently. This perspective not only isolates them but can also lead to increased reliance on unhealthy coping mechanisms, such as substance abuse, as they seek to numb their pain in secrecy. The stigma surrounding mental health makes it difficult for these men to recognize that reaching out for help is a sign of strength, not weakness.

Additionally, the stigma associated with mental health can manifest in the workplace, where men may fear that disclosing their struggles could jeopardize their careers. Such fears can prevent them from accessing necessary support systems, leaving them to deal with their issues alone. The impact of this stigma is particularly pronounced in environments where traditional masculine ideals dominate, making it even more challenging for men to express their vulnerabilities. Therefore, their mental health deteriorates, affecting not only their well-being but also their relationships with loved ones.

In the context of fatherhood, the stigma can be even more pronounced as men grapple with the pressures of being a provider and a role model. Many fathers may feel they cannot admit to struggling with mental health issues for fear of being seen as inadequate or unfit. This can create a barrier to open communication with their children and partners, further isolating them in their struggles. By breaking down these stigmas and encouraging open dialogues about mental health, men can begin to navigate their challenges in a healthier way, fostering stronger familial bonds and personal resilience.

To combat the negative effects of stigma on help-seeking behaviour, it is crucial to promote a culture that values emotional intelligence and mental wellness. Encouraging men to share their experiences and seek professional help can lead to greater understanding and support within their communities. By normalizing conversations about mental health, we can empower men to seek the help they need, ultimately leading to healthier lives and relationships. Addressing stigma is not just about individual change; it is about transforming societal perceptions and creating an environment where men feel safe to talk about their mental health struggles.

Challenging Traditional Masculine Norms

Challenging traditional masculine norms is essential for adult males, especially those experiencing andropause. These norms often dictate that men should be stoic, self-reliant, and emotionally restrained. However, as men navigate this phase of life, they may find that adhering to these outdated expectations can exacerbate mental health challenges, such as anxiety and depression. Acknowledging the need for emotional expression and vulnerability is a crucial step in promoting healthier mental states.

The stigma surrounding mental health in men is deeply rooted in traditional masculinity. Many adult males feel pressured to conform to societal expectations that discourage seeking help or admitting to emotional struggles. This can lead to isolation and an inability to cope effectively with stressors, such as job loss or relationship issues. By challenging these norms, men can begin to redefine what it means to be masculine, allowing for a broader spectrum of emotional experiences and support.

Substance abuse often arises as a coping mechanism for men grappling with their mental health. The pressure to maintain a façade of strength can lead to self-medication, further complicating mental health issues. Addressing the relationship between masculinity and substance use is crucial in creating a supportive environment for men to seek help. Encouraging open discussions about these topics can pave the way for healthier coping strategies and reduce the stigma associated with seeking treatment.

Another significant aspect of challenging traditional masculine norms is the impact on fatherhood. Many men struggle with the expectation to be the primary provider, often neglecting their emotional needs in the process. This can strain relationships with their children and partners, leading to feelings of inadequacy. By embracing a more emotionally intelligent approach to fatherhood, men can foster deeper connections with their families while also prioritizing their mental well-being.

Ultimately, redefining masculinity involves embracing vulnerability and emotional expression. Adult males, especially those facing andropause, must recognize that seeking help is not a sign of weakness but a strength. By challenging traditional norms, men can create a supportive community that addresses mental health challenges, alleviates stigma, and promotes healthier relationships with themselves and others. This shift can lead to a transformative healing process, not only for individual men but for society.

Coping Strategies for Stress in Adult Males

Identifying Sources of Stress

Identifying the sources of stress is a crucial first step in addressing mental health challenges among adult men, particularly those experiencing andropause. This transitional phase can bring about a myriad of physical and emotional changes that often exacerbate underlying stressors. Men may find themselves grappling with feelings of inadequacy or loss, especially in relation to their roles in family and society, which can significantly impact their mental health.

One major source of stress for many adult males is the pressure to conform to traditional masculine norms. This societal expectation can create a significant internal conflict, leading to anxiety and depression. The stigma surrounding mental health often prevents men from seeking help, making it essential to identify and acknowledge these pressures as legitimate sources of stress that need to be addressed.

Job loss is another critical factor that can elevate stress levels in men, particularly those in midlife. The loss of employment not only threatens financial stability but also challenges a man's sense of identity and purpose. This situation can lead to feelings of helplessness and despair, further complicating their mental health landscape during such a vulnerable time in life.

Additionally, the responsibilities of fatherhood can also be a double-edged sword. While being a father can bring immense joy, it can also introduce stressors related to providing for and nurturing children. The balance between work, family obligations, and personal well-being can feel overwhelming and lead to increased anxiety and depressive symptoms if not managed effectively.

Ultimately, recognizing these various sources of stress is essential for developing coping strategies tailored to the unique experiences of adult men. By understanding the factors contributing to their mental health challenges, men can begin to take proactive steps towards improvement, whether through therapy, support groups, or other resources that promote emotional well-being. Taking this first step can help break the cycle of silence surrounding men's mental health issues, fostering a more supportive environment for those in need.

Healthy Coping Mechanisms

Adult men, particularly those experiencing andropause, often face unique mental health challenges. Understanding healthy coping mechanisms can significantly enhance emotional resilience during this transitional phase of life. This transition is often marked by physiological changes that can trigger feelings of anxiety and depression, making it imperative to explore effective strategies for managing these emotions. Implementing healthy coping mechanisms not only aids in personal well-being but also improves relationships with family and friends, fostering a supportive environment.

One effective coping strategy is engaging in regular physical activity. Exercise serves as a powerful tool for alleviating symptoms of anxiety and depression, as it releases endorphins that elevate mood and enhance overall mental health. Men can start with simple activities like walking, jogging, or joining a local sports team. Physical activity also promotes social interaction, which can combat feelings of isolation that often accompany mental health struggles, particularly in men of advancing years.

Mindfulness and meditation are other valuable coping mechanisms that can help men navigate the complexities of their emotions. Practicing mindfulness encourages individuals to focus on the present moment, reducing anxiety and fostering a sense of calm. Techniques such as deep breathing exercises, yoga, or guided meditation can be particularly beneficial. By integrating these practices into daily routines, men can develop greater emotional intelligence, which is crucial for understanding and managing their mental health.

Additionally, establishing a support network is vital for emotional well-being. Men often feel pressured to uphold traditional masculine ideals, which can hinder their willingness to seek help. However, reaching out to friends, family, or support groups can provide a safe space for sharing experiences and emotions. Connecting with others who understand similar struggles can diminish feelings of loneliness and stigma, reinforcing the notion that it is acceptable to seek support during challenging times.

Lastly, engaging in hobbies and interests can serve as an excellent outlet for stress relief. Whether it's woodworking, painting, or playing a musical instrument, these activities offer a creative escape from daily pressures. They not only provide a sense of accomplishment but also allow men to express their emotions in a constructive way. By exploring and investing time in personal interests, adult males can cultivate a fulfilling life that positively impacts their mental health and overall quality of life.

Building Resilience

Building resilience is a crucial skill for adult men, especially those navigating the complexities of andropause. During this phase, men often face heightened emotional challenges such as anxiety and depression, which can impact their relationships and overall well-being. Resilience enables individuals to bounce back from these adversities, allowing them to maintain a sense of stability and purpose in their lives. By developing this strength, men can better manage the stresses associated with job loss, changes in family dynamics, and other midlife transitions.

One vital aspect of building resilience is fostering emotional intelligence. Understanding one's emotions and recognizing their triggers can significantly enhance a man's ability to cope with stress. This awareness paves the way for healthier communication in relationships, reducing the likelihood of misunderstandings and conflicts. Additionally, cultivating emotional intelligence allows men to empathize with others, which can be particularly beneficial in fatherhood and nurturing family bonds.

Another important strategy for resilience is the establishment of a robust support network. Connecting with friends, family, or support groups can provide a sense of belonging and reduce feelings of isolation that often accompany mental health challenges. Sharing experiences and seeking advice from others who have faced similar struggles can offer valuable perspectives and coping mechanisms. This communal approach not only helps in managing anxiety and depression but also reinforces a sense of masculinity that embraces vulnerability rather than shunning it.

Physical well-being also plays a significant role in resilience. Regular exercise, a balanced diet, and adequate sleep can enhance mental health and improve emotional regulation. Engaging in activities that promote physical health can help mitigate the effects of stress and anxiety, making it easier for men to confront their challenges head-on. Additionally, mindfulness practices, such as meditation or yoga, can further strengthen resilience by improving focus and emotional control.

Ultimately, building resilience is an ongoing process that requires commitment and effort. It involves not just managing stressors but also actively seeking personal growth and understanding. By embracing resilience, men can navigate the complexities of their mental health challenges more effectively, fostering stronger relationships and a more fulfilling life. This journey empowers them to redefine masculinity in a way that prioritizes mental health and emotional well-being, breaking down the stigma surrounding these issues.

Mental Health Effects of Job Loss in Men

The Psychological Impact of Unemployment

Unemployment can have a profound psychological impact on men, particularly as they navigate the complexities of andropause. The loss of a job often leads to feelings of inadequacy and diminished self-worth, especially in a society that typically equates employment with identity and success. For many adult males, this can trigger anxiety disorders, as the uncertainty of the future looms large. The pressure to provide, coupled with the shame of being unemployed, can create a perfect storm for mental health challenges.

As men face unemployment, the risk of depression increases significantly. This emotional downturn can strain personal relationships, particularly with partners and children. Men may withdraw from social interactions or become irritable, which can lead to a vicious cycle of isolation. The inability to fulfil traditional roles of provider and protector can exacerbate feelings of guilt and despair, worsening their mental state and affecting those around them.

Substance abuse often becomes a coping mechanism for men dealing with the stresses of unemployment. Alcohol and drugs may provide temporary relief from feelings of hopelessness, but they can also lead to further mental health issues and relationship breakdowns. This cycle can be especially detrimental during andropause, when men may already be grappling with declining physical health and emotional stability. Recognizing the potential for substance abuse as a result of unemployment is crucial for early intervention.

Moreover, the societal stigma surrounding mental health and masculinity can prevent men from seeking help. Many feel that admitting to struggles with anxiety or depression diminishes their masculinity. This internal conflict can lead to avoidance of professional support, further entrenching their mental health issues. It is vital to create an environment where men feel safe discussing their challenges without fear of judgment, thereby fostering a culture of openness and support.

Coping strategies for managing unemployment-related stress are essential for maintaining mental health. Engaging in physical activities, pursuing hobbies, and connecting with supportive communities can significantly alleviate symptoms of depression and anxiety. Men should be encouraged to explore therapy and counselling as viable options for addressing their emotional struggles. By prioritizing mental health and recognizing the impact of unemployment, men can navigate this challenging phase of life with resilience and strength.

Coping with Job Loss

Job loss can be a significant source of distress for adult men, particularly those experiencing andropause. The sudden shift in identity and purpose can trigger feelings of inadequacy and anxiety, leading to a decline in mental health. Men often tie their self-worth to their professional roles, and when that role is stripped away, it can feel like a personal failure. Understanding the emotional impact of losing a job is crucial for navigating this challenging period.

Many men facing job loss may experience anxiety disorders that complicate their ability to cope. The uncertainty of the job market can exacerbate feelings of helplessness, leading to a cycle of negative thoughts and behaviours. It is essential for men to recognize these symptoms as a natural response to a stressful situation rather than a reflection of their character. Seeking professional help can be a vital step in addressing these mental health challenges.

Depression is another common response to job loss, often manifesting in withdrawal from social interactions and strained relationships. Men may find it difficult to communicate their feelings of sadness or frustration, fearing that it will undermine their masculinity. This stigma can prevent them from seeking support from friends and family, leading to isolation. Open conversations about emotions can help alleviate this burden and foster stronger connections.

Coping strategies are essential for managing stress during periods of unemployment. Engaging in physical activity, practicing mindfulness, and maintaining a routine can provide structure and a sense of normalcy. Additionally, exploring new hobbies or volunteering can help men rediscover their passions and purpose, contributing positively to their mental health. Developing emotional intelligence through these activities can also enhance relationships with others, providing a support network during tough times.

Ultimately, navigating the emotional landscape of job loss requires patience and resilience. Men must understand that experiencing such setbacks is a part of life that many share. By fostering open discussions about mental health, embracing vulnerability, and actively seeking support, men can emerge from this experience with a renewed sense of purpose and improved mental well-being. Recognizing the interconnectedness of employment, identity, and mental health is the first step toward recovery and growth.

Seeking Support and Resources

As adult men navigate the complexities of andropause, seeking support and resources becomes crucial in addressing mental health challenges. Many men may feel isolated in their struggles, believing that they must face their issues alone. However, recognizing the importance of community and professional help can significantly alter the course of their mental health journey. Connecting with others who share similar experiences fosters a sense of belonging and reduces feelings of loneliness, ultimately aiding in recovery and personal growth.

Support groups tailored for men can provide a safe space for expressing vulnerabilities and discussing mental health openly. These groups often emphasize the importance of emotional intelligence, helping participants understand their feelings and reactions. Engaging in discussions about anxiety, depression, and other issues can demystify these experiences and reduce the stigma surrounding them. Men are encouraged to share coping strategies and solutions that have worked for them, creating a collaborative environment that empowers all members.

In addition to peer support, professional resources are invaluable for men dealing with mental health challenges. Therapists and counsellors specializing in men's mental health can offer tailored guidance and therapeutic techniques. Engaging with a mental health professional can help men explore underlying issues, such as trauma or substance abuse, that may contribute to their current struggles. This professional help can also assist in developing healthy coping mechanisms and strategies for managing stress, particularly during significant life transitions such as job loss or fatherhood.

Moreover, educational resources, such as workshops and online platforms, provide men with valuable information about mental health. These resources often cover various topics, including the impacts of masculinity on mental health and the importance of emotional expression. By educating themselves, men can better understand their mental health and recognize the signs of distress in themselves and others. This knowledge empowers them to seek help when needed, fostering a proactive rather than reactive approach to mental wellness.

Finally, it is essential for men to prioritize self-care as a foundational aspect of seeking support. Simple practices, such as regular exercise, mindfulness, and maintaining social connections, can significantly enhance mental health. Men should not underestimate the power of small, consistent actions in improving their overall well-being. By actively seeking support and utilizing available resources, men can navigate the challenges of andropause and emerge stronger, more resilient, and more connected to their emotional selves.

Men's Mental Health in the Context of Fatherhood

The Challenges of Parenting

Parenting presents unique challenges, particularly for adult men navigating the complexities of andropause. As physical and emotional changes occur, many men find themselves grappling with feelings of inadequacy and anxiety in their parenting roles. The pressure to conform to traditional masculinity can heighten these feelings, making it difficult to openly discuss fears or seek support. The struggle to balance these internal conflicts while being present for their children can lead to significant stress and emotional turmoil.

Men often experience a societal expectation to be the primary providers and protectors of their families, which can exacerbate feelings of depression and anxiety. The impact of job loss or financial instability further complicates this dynamic, as men may feel they are failing to meet their responsibilities. This can create a vicious cycle, where stress and mental health issues negatively affect parenting, leading to strained relationships with children and partners alike. Understanding how these external pressures influence mental health is essential for men in this stage of life.

Moreover, the stigma surrounding mental health can prevent men from seeking help. Many adult males are conditioned to believe that discussing feelings or vulnerabilities is a sign of weakness, which can lead to isolation. This isolation often manifests in unhealthy coping mechanisms, such as substance abuse, which can further deteriorate family relationships. It is crucial for men to recognize that addressing mental health challenges is not only beneficial for themselves but also for their families.

Navigating the journey of fatherhood during andropause also means developing emotional intelligence. Men are often encouraged to suppress their emotions, but learning to express feelings can enhance parenting skills and improve relationships with their children. Engaging in open dialogue about mental health and emotions can foster a healthier family environment, where children learn the importance of vulnerability and emotional expression.

In conclusion, the challenges of parenting during andropause are multifaceted, involving mental health issues, societal expectations, and emotional growth. Men must prioritize their mental well-being and seek support when needed, not only for their own benefit but also for the sake of their families. By breaking the stigma surrounding mental health and embracing vulnerability, men can become more effective parents and positively influence their children's lives.

Balancing Work and Family Life

Balancing work and family life is a significant challenge for many adult men, especially those undergoing the changes of andropause. The pressures of career obligations can often clash with family responsibilities, leading to heightened stress and anxiety. It's crucial for men to recognize how these competing demands can impact their mental health, relationships, and overall well-being.

Finding equilibrium requires a conscious effort to prioritize both professional commitments and personal life, fostering a more fulfilling existence.

One of the key aspects of achieving this balance is effective time management. Adult men need to develop strategies that allow them to allocate sufficient time for both work and family. This may involve setting boundaries at work, such as limiting overtime or delegating tasks, which can prevent burnout. Additionally, creating dedicated family time, whether through weekly activities or simple daily rituals, can strengthen family bonds and provide emotional support crucial for mental health.

Moreover, the role of masculinity in mental health can't be overlooked. Societal expectations often pressure men to prioritize work over family, perpetuating a cycle of neglect that harms both mental health and relationships. Embracing emotional intelligence and vulnerability can help men to communicate their needs and feelings more openly. This shift not only aids in reducing stigma surrounding mental health issues but also fosters healthier connections with family members.

Coping strategies play an essential role in managing stress associated with balancing work and family life. Engaging in regular physical activity, seeking professional help when necessary, and practicing mindfulness techniques can mitigate anxiety and depression. Furthermore, men should be encouraged to express their feelings and seek support from peers, which can alleviate feelings of isolation often experienced during andropause.

Ultimately, recognizing the importance of balance between work and family can lead to improved mental health outcomes for men. As they navigate the complexities of their roles, it's vital for them to understand that prioritizing family does not equate to failure at work but rather contributes to a more holistic approach to life. Support from loved ones and the cultivation of healthy coping mechanisms can empower men to face the silent struggles of mental health with resilience and strength.

Supporting Mental Health as a father

Fatherhood can be a transformative experience, yet it often brings unique challenges that can impact a father's mental health. Men in midlife, especially those experiencing andropause, may find themselves grappling with feelings of inadequacy or anxiety regarding their parenting abilities. The pressure to provide for their families can exacerbate these feelings, leading to increased stress and potential mental health struggles. Understanding these dynamics is crucial for fathers who wish to support both their own mental health and that of their families.

Communication plays a vital role in supporting mental health as a father. Open and honest conversations with partners and children can foster a supportive environment that acknowledges the emotional struggles fathers may face. Sharing experiences and feelings can reduce feelings of isolation often associated with mental health challenges. Encouraging dialogue not only helps fathers process their experiences but also models emotional intelligence for their children, teaching them the importance of discussing feelings and seeking help.

Coping strategies are essential for fathers to manage stress effectively. Exercise, mindfulness practices, and hobbies can provide necessary outlets for stress relief. Additionally, seeking professional help when needed is a sign of strength, not weakness. Fathers should consider therapy or support groups where they can share their experiences and learn from others facing similar challenges. These strategies not only benefit the fathers themselves but also create a healthier family dynamic.

The stigma surrounding masculinity often discourages men from prioritizing their mental health. Societal expectations can make it difficult for fathers to express vulnerability or seek support, leading to a cycle of silence that can worsen mental health issues. Addressing this stigma is vital, as it allows fathers to embrace their emotional needs openly. By challenging traditional views of masculinity, fathers can foster an environment that values mental health, encouraging their children to do the same.

Ultimately, supporting mental health as a father is a multifaceted endeavor that requires awareness, communication, and a willingness to seek help. Fathers must recognize their own mental health needs and understand how these can affect their relationships with their children and partners. By prioritizing their mental well-being, fathers not only improve their own quality of life but also set a positive example for future generations, ensuring that mental health is openly discussed and valued in their families.

Navigating Midlife Crises and Mental Health

Understanding the Midlife Crisis

The midlife crisis is a complex phenomenon that affects many adult males as they navigate the challenges of aging and shifting life priorities. This period often involves a revaluation of one's achievements, relationships, and overall direction in life. Many men experience heightened feelings of anxiety and depression during this time, as they confront the reality of aging, potential job loss, and the responsibilities associated with fatherhood. Understanding the emotional and psychological impacts of this crisis is vital for men seeking to maintain their mental health and well-being.

Anxiety disorders can frequently emerge or intensify during a midlife crisis. Men may find themselves grappling with a sense of inadequacy and fear of failure, leading to increased stress and emotional turmoil. This anxiety can manifest in various ways, including insomnia, irritability, and a pervasive sense of dread about the future. Recognizing these symptoms as part of the midlife experience is crucial for men, enabling them to seek appropriate support and strategies to cope effectively.

Depression is another significant mental health challenge that can arise during this life stage, often impacting men's relationships with partners, children, and friends. The feelings of sadness and hopelessness can lead to withdrawal and isolation, further exacerbating the crisis. Men often feel societal pressure to maintain a façade of strength, which can hinder their ability to express vulnerability and seek help. Open communication about mental health struggles is essential for fostering healthy relationships and overcoming the stigma associated with seeking treatment.

Substance abuse is also a concern during midlife crises, as men may turn to alcohol or drugs as a means of coping with their emotional pain. This behavior can lead to a vicious cycle, where substance use further deteriorates mental health, intensifying feelings of depression and anxiety. Addressing the root causes of substance abuse, such as unresolved trauma or stress, is essential for effective recovery and long-term well-being.

Coping strategies play a vital role in navigating the midlife crisis and its associated mental health challenges. Men can benefit from practices such as mindfulness, physical activity, and engaging in supportive social networks. Building emotional intelligence is also key, as it enables men to better understand and manage their feelings, ultimately leading to healthier coping mechanisms. By acknowledging the realities of midlife and taking proactive steps to address mental health, men can emerge from this period with renewed strength and purpose.

Common Mental Health Issues During Midlife

Midlife is often a time of significant change and reflection for many men. As they navigate the challenges of andropause, issues such as anxiety and depression often come to the forefront. The pressures of career, family responsibilities, and personal expectations can create a perfect storm for mental health struggles. Men may find themselves feeling more anxious about their future, grappling with a sense of loss regarding their youth, and questioning their identity in a rapidly changing world.

One of the most common mental health issues faced during midlife is anxiety, which can manifest in various forms, including generalized anxiety disorder and panic attacks. Men may experience heightened worries about job security, financial stability, and health concerns as they age. This anxiety can exacerbate feelings of inadequacy and lead to avoidance behaviours, which can further complicate relationships with partners, children, and friends. Understanding the roots of these anxieties is crucial for men to address them effectively.

Depression is another prevalent issue that can significantly impact men during midlife. It often goes unnoticed or unacknowledged due to societal expectations surrounding masculinity, which discourage emotional vulnerability. Men may feel pressured to appear strong and self-reliant, leading them to suppress their feelings. This suppression can strain relationships, as partners may feel shut out or unable to help. Recognizing the signs of depression is essential for men to seek help and foster healthier connections with loved ones.

Substance abuse can also become a coping mechanism for men facing midlife challenges. Alcohol and drug use may temporarily alleviate stress or anxiety, but they can lead to more severe mental health issues and relationship problems. The stigma surrounding men's mental health can discourage them from seeking appropriate treatment, perpetuating a cycle of unhealthy coping strategies. Addressing substance abuse openly and honestly is crucial for recovery and improving overall mental health.

Finally, navigating the complexities of midlife crises can further complicate mental health for men. Many experience a revaluation of their life choices, which can lead to feelings of regret or discontent. The pressure to conform to societal norms of success can intensify these feelings. Developing emotional intelligence and coping strategies to manage stress is vital for men to navigate this challenging period. By fostering self-awareness and seeking support, men can work toward achieving a healthier mental state during these transformative years.

Strategies for Navigating Change

Navigating change can be particularly challenging for adult men, especially those experiencing andropause. As physical and emotional changes occur, many may find themselves grappling with anxiety and depression. Recognizing that these feelings are common is the first step towards managing them effectively. Seeking support from friends, family, or mental health professionals can provide a crucial outlet and help men feel less isolated in their struggles.

Developing coping strategies is essential in the face of change. Techniques such as mindfulness and meditation can help ground men during turbulent times, allowing them to maintain a sense of calm. Regular physical exercise is also beneficial; it not only improves physical health but also releases endorphins, which can boost mood and reduce anxiety. Engaging in hobbies and activities that bring joy can serve as effective distractions from stressors, fostering a more positive mindset.

Addressing the stigma surrounding masculinity and mental health is vital for men navigating these changes. Societal expectations often discourage men from expressing vulnerability, leading to a reluctance to seek help. By challenging these norms and promoting open conversations about mental health, men can create a supportive environment for themselves and others. This shift can empower men to prioritize their mental well-being without fear of judgment.

In addition to personal coping mechanisms, fostering strong relationships is fundamental. Men should strive to communicate openly with their partners, friends, and family about their feelings and experiences. Sharing these struggles not only provides relief but also strengthens bonds and enhances understanding. Building a network of support can be invaluable in navigating the complexities of midlife changes and associated mental health challenges.

Lastly, it's important for men to recognize that change can also bring opportunities for growth. Embracing new experiences, whether it's through learning new skills or engaging in community activities, can create a sense of purpose and fulfillment. By adopting a proactive approach to change, men can transform challenges into stepping stones towards a healthier and more enriching life, ultimately aiding their mental health journey.

PTSD and Trauma Recovery in Male Veterans

Understanding PTSD in Veterans

Post-Traumatic Stress Disorder (PTSD) is a mental health condition that can greatly affect veterans, particularly those who have experienced combat or significant trauma during their service. For adult males and men of advancing years, understanding the symptoms and impacts of PTSD is crucial, as these individuals may be more likely to downplay their struggles due to societal expectations of masculinity. The stigma surrounding mental health can hinder them from seeking help, making it essential to foster an environment where discussing such issues is normalized and encouraged.

Symptoms of PTSD can manifest in various ways, including intrusive memories, avoidance behaviours, negative changes in mood, and heightened arousal responses. Many veterans experience hypervigilance or emotional numbing, which can complicate their ability to form or maintain relationships. This is particularly significant for men navigating the complexities of fatherhood or those facing pressures related to job loss, where emotional availability is critical for fostering healthy connections with family members.

The relationship between PTSD and substance abuse is also a concerning aspect of mental health in veterans. Many individuals may turn to alcohol or drugs as a means to cope with their symptoms, leading to a vicious cycle that exacerbates their mental health challenges. Understanding this connection can aid in developing targeted interventions that address both PTSD and substance use, helping veterans find healthier coping mechanisms and reducing the stigma associated with seeking treatment.

Coping strategies play a vital role in managing PTSD. Techniques such as mindfulness, physical exercise, and engaging in supportive social networks can significantly improve the mental well-being of veterans. Men must recognize the importance of emotional intelligence and vulnerability in their healing journey, as these attributes can foster resilience and provide pathways to recovery. Encouraging open conversations about mental health can empower veterans to take the first step toward seeking help.

Ultimately, understanding PTSD in veterans involves recognizing the unique challenges faced by adult males, particularly in the context of societal expectations of masculinity. By promoting awareness and providing support, we can create a more inclusive conversation around mental health that allows veterans to share their silent struggles. This understanding not only aids in the recovery of those affected but also contributes to a broader cultural shift toward valuing mental health in all men, regardless of age or background.

Symptoms and Diagnosis of PTSD

Post-Traumatic Stress Disorder (PTSD) is a complex mental health condition that can affect adult males, particularly those who have experienced trauma. The symptoms of PTSD can manifest in various forms, including intrusive memories, flashbacks, and severe emotional distress. For men undergoing andropause, the recognition of these symptoms can be particularly challenging as they may be perceived as signs of weakness, conflicting with traditional notions of masculinity. It is essential to understand these symptoms to seek appropriate help and support.

In addition to intrusive thoughts, individuals with PTSD may experience heightened anxiety, irritability, and difficulty concentrating. These symptoms can significantly impact daily functioning, work performance, and personal relationships. Men may find themselves withdrawing from social interactions or feeling detached from loved ones, which can exacerbate feelings of loneliness and depression. Recognizing these signs is crucial for men in acknowledging their mental health struggles without the stigma that often accompanies them.

Diagnosis of PTSD typically involves a comprehensive assessment by a mental health professional. This process includes discussions about the individual's trauma history, current symptoms, and their impact on daily life. For adult males, especially those in midlife or experiencing andropause, discussing emotional and psychological issues can be daunting. However, a professional evaluation is vital for establishing an accurate diagnosis and developing an effective treatment plan tailored to their specific needs.

The relationship between PTSD and other mental health challenges, such as depression and anxiety disorders, is also important to consider. Men may engage in substance abuse as a coping mechanism, using alcohol or drugs to numb their feelings. Understanding this connection helps in addressing not only the symptoms of PTSD but also related issues that may arise from it. Men must recognize that seeking help for PTSD is a step towards reclaiming their emotional well-being and improving their relationships.

Coping strategies for managing PTSD symptoms may include therapy, medication, and self-care practices. Engaging in physical activity, developing emotional intelligence, and building a supportive network can also be effective. Men must learn that it is okay to express vulnerability and seek support, as this can lead to healthier coping mechanisms and improved mental health overall. Breaking the stigma around mental health in men is essential for promoting a culture where seeking help is viewed as a strength rather than a weakness.

Pathways to Recovery

Recovery from mental health challenges requires a multifaceted approach that acknowledges the unique experiences of adult men, particularly those navigating the complexities of andropause. During this phase, men may encounter significant emotional and psychological changes that can exacerbate feelings of anxiety and depression. Understanding these nuances is crucial for implementing effective recovery strategies. This journey often begins with recognizing the signs of distress and seeking help, whether through professional counselling or support groups that foster a sense of community and understanding among peers.

Coping strategies play a vital role in the recovery process. Men can benefit from developing emotional intelligence, which entails recognizing and managing their emotions effectively. This skill not only aids in personal recovery but also enhances relationships with partners, children, and friends. Activities such as mindfulness and physical exercise can serve as powerful tools to alleviate stress, promote emotional well-being, and foster a healthier mindset. Engaging in hobbies or pursuing new interests can also provide a much-needed outlet for expression and a break from negative thought patterns.

Addressing the stigma surrounding mental health is another critical pathway to recovery. The societal pressures on men to embody traditional masculinity often hinder their willingness to seek help. By openly discussing mental health issues, men can challenge these stereotypes, empowering themselves and others to prioritize emotional well-being. Sharing personal experiences can lead to a supportive dialogue that normalizes mental health struggles, ultimately fostering a culture of acceptance and understanding.

For many men, the experience of job loss or significant life changes can trigger mental health challenges. These transitions can evoke feelings of inadequacy and anxiety, making it essential to develop resilience through support networks and coping mechanisms. Establishing routines, pursuing new career opportunities, or engaging in volunteer work can not only provide structure but also enhance self-esteem during recovery. Recognizing that setbacks are a part of life can help men cultivate a more adaptive mindset.

Finally, recovery is often intertwined with the roles men play in their families and communities. As fathers, they may face additional pressures that impact their mental health. Actively participating in their children's lives can foster a sense of purpose and connection, which are fundamental to emotional recovery. By embracing vulnerability and seeking support, men can navigate their mental health challenges more effectively, paving the way for a fulfilling and balanced life.

Emotional Intelligence and Mental Health in Men

The Importance of Emotional Intelligence

Emotional intelligence (EI) is an essential aspect of mental health that plays a critical role in how adult men navigate their emotional landscapes, particularly during challenging life transitions such as andropause. For many men, understanding and managing their emotions can lead to healthier relationships and improved mental well-being. Emotional intelligence encompasses self-awareness, self-regulation, empathy, and social skills, all of which are vital for fostering personal growth and resilience against anxiety and depression that often accompany this phase of life.

As men age, they may find themselves grappling with new emotional challenges, including feelings of inadequacy or loss associated with changing roles in family and society. Developing emotional intelligence allows men to recognize and articulate these feelings rather than suppress them, which can be detrimental to their mental health. By fostering an understanding of their emotional responses, men can better cope with stressors such as job loss, relationship changes, and the pressures of fatherhood, thereby reducing the stigma associated with seeking help.

Furthermore, emotional intelligence can enhance men's ability to engage in supportive relationships, a crucial element in combating isolation and loneliness. By practicing empathy and active listening, men can strengthen their connections with friends and family, creating a supportive network that is essential during times of emotional distress. This support system not only serves as a buffer against anxiety and depression but also promotes healthier coping strategies, reducing the likelihood of substance abuse as a means of escape.

In the context of masculinity, developing emotional intelligence challenges traditional notions of manhood that often discourage emotional expression. Men who embrace their emotional intelligence are better equipped to navigate midlife crises and trauma recovery, particularly for those who have served in the military and may be dealing with PTSD. By redefining what it means to be strong, men can break free from the confines of mental health stigma and create a more supportive environment for themselves and their peers.

Ultimately, the importance of emotional intelligence cannot be overstated for adult men facing mental health challenges. By prioritizing emotional awareness and skills, men can improve their overall mental health, build healthier relationships, and foster resilience. Understanding and cultivating emotional intelligence is not just beneficial; it is a vital component of thriving in the later stages of life, enabling men to embrace their emotional realities and emerge stronger from their silent struggles.

Developing Emotional Awareness

Developing emotional awareness is a crucial step for adult men navigating the complexities of life, particularly during periods of significant transition such as andropause. Recognizing and understanding one's emotions can lead to improved mental health outcomes, helping men address underlying anxiety and depression. Emotional awareness allows individuals to identify triggers and patterns in their feelings, creating a pathway to healthier coping mechanisms and more fulfilling relationships.

As men often face societal pressures to conform to traditional notions of masculinity, they may suppress their emotions, leading to isolation and increased mental health struggles. By embracing emotional awareness, men can break free from these constraints, allowing them to express vulnerability without fear of judgment. This shift not only enhances personal well-being but also fosters deeper connections with friends, partners, and family members, enriching their lives in the process.

Learning to articulate feelings is another important aspect of emotional awareness. Many men are taught to prioritize logic over emotion, which can hinder their ability to communicate effectively in relationships. By practicing emotional literacy, men can better convey their needs and experiences, reducing misunderstandings and conflict. This skill is particularly vital during midlife crises or significant life changes, where emotional turmoil can manifest in various ways, affecting mental health and relationships.

Furthermore, developing emotional awareness can play a significant role in addressing substance abuse issues among men. Understanding the emotions that drive substance use can lead to healthier coping strategies. Men who are aware of their emotional triggers can seek support and find alternative ways to manage stress, ultimately reducing the likelihood of turning to substances as a means of escape.

In conclusion, fostering emotional awareness is not just beneficial; it is essential for adult men, particularly those facing the challenges of andropause. By prioritizing emotional health, men can navigate their struggles more effectively, cultivate resilience, and build stronger, more meaningful connections with those around them. This journey towards emotional intelligence not only enhances individual lives but also contributes to a broader cultural shift in how society views masculinity and mental health.

Improving Relationships Through Emotional Intelligence

Emotional intelligence (EI) plays a crucial role in improving relationships, especially for adult men facing the challenges of andropause. During this stage of life, men often experience shifts in their emotional and psychological well-being, which can lead to increased anxiety and depression. By developing emotional intelligence, men can better understand their emotions and the emotions of those around them, paving the way for healthier interactions and stronger connections with loved ones.

One of the key components of emotional intelligence is self-awareness. This involves recognizing and acknowledging one's feelings, which is often a struggle for men due to societal expectations surrounding masculinity. By fostering self-awareness, men can identify the underlying causes of their emotional responses and address them constructively. This self-reflection can lead to meaningful conversations with partners and friends, enhancing mutual understanding and support.

Empathy is another essential aspect of emotional intelligence that can significantly improve relationships. By learning to put themselves in others' shoes, men can respond more compassionately to the emotions of others. This skill is particularly important for those experiencing anxiety or depression, as it allows men to connect with their loved ones on a deeper level. Empathy can bridge the gap between emotional struggles and relational harmony, creating a safe space for open dialogue about mental health challenges.

Effective communication, a vital skill linked to emotional intelligence, also plays a significant role in relationship improvement. Men often face difficulties expressing their feelings verbally, which can lead to misunderstandings and resentment. By honing their communication skills, men can articulate their emotions more clearly and effectively. This not only reduces the likelihood of conflict but also encourages their partners and friends to share their feelings, fostering a more supportive environment for discussing mental health issues.

Finally, practicing emotional intelligence can help men navigate the complexities of relationships during midlife, especially when dealing with stressors like job loss or changes in family dynamics. By embracing emotional intelligence, men can cultivate resilience and adaptability, essential traits for overcoming challenges. As they learn to manage their emotions better, they can create stronger, healthier relationships that contribute to their overall mental well-being and vitality in this critical stage of life.

Pause for Thought

- As men enter the andropause transitional state, they often encounter emotional and psychological changes that can lead to anxiety and depression. Awareness needs to be promoted through a culture in which mental health is openly discussed, this helps men feel less isolated in their struggle.
- Anxiety disorders in this transitional phase can exacerbate symptoms which can manifest as increased stress, irritability and overwhelming fatigue which can significantly impact daily life. Healthcare practitioners must help men to understand that seeking help for anxiety is not a sign of weakness but an essential step in managing their wellbeing.
- Depression -often leading to withdrawal from social interactions and a decline in communication with loved ones. Men may feel pressured to adhere to traditional masculine norms, which discourage vulnerability and emotional expression. By raising awareness about depression and its

impact, nor can be encouraged to share their feelings and experiences which allows for deeper connections with family and friends.

- Mental health issues may manifest with substance abuse. Many men may turn to alcohol or drugs as a coping mechanism for the mental health challenges, particularly during times of stress an emotional upheaval. Raising awareness about the link between substance abuse and mental health can help men recognise the danger of this behaviour and seek healthier alternatives. Education on the effects of substance abuse or mental health can empower men to make informed choices and pursue recovery options.
- Traditional notions on masculinity often discourage men from expressing vulnerability or seeking help which can perpetuate mental health issues. By challenging these stereotypes and promoting emotional intelligence men can embrace their feelings and seek support without fear of judgement. |Awareness initiatives which facilitate discussions around masculinity, encouraging a more holistic approach to men's mental health embracing vulnerability as a strength rather than a weakness.
- Anxiety disorder in men encompass a range of conditions, including general anxiety disorder, pace disorder and social anxiety disorder, each characterised by excessive fear or worry that can disrupt daily functioning. These anxieties can be triggered by significant life changes, such as job transitions, health concerns, or shift in family dynamics, leading to an increase in stress and emotional turmoil.

- Men often experience societal pressure to embody strength and stoicism which can lead to a reluctance to seek help or express vulnerability. This stigma surrounding mental health can exacerbate feelings of isolation and despair which makes it challenging for men to connect with their partners, friends and family members understanding how anxiety affects communication and emotional intimacy is crucial for fostering healthier relationships during this period of life.
- Navigating midlife crisis can also trigger or amplify anxiety disorder as men confront their mortality, career aspirations and personal achievements, feelings of inadequacy or failure may surface. This introspection can lead to further anxiety and depression, developing emotional intelligence and resilience is vital for managing these challenges, allowing men to address their fears constructively rather than allowing them to spiral into debilitating anxiety.
- Treatment options for mental health challenges in adult men, particularly those experiencing andropause, are diverse and should be personalised. Individuals respond differently to various therapies. Knowledge of this is crucial in crafting an effective treatment plan. Common approaches include physiotherapy, medication and lifestyle changes which can all contribute to improved mental health outcomes. Professional guidance must be sought to identify which combination work best for their unique situation.

- Psychotherapy or talk therapy is one of the most effective treatment modalities for addressing anxiety and depression in adult males. Cognitive behavioural therapy is particularly beneficial as it helps individuals recognise and modify negative thought patterns. This is essential for men who struggle with traditional expression of emotion as it provides them with tools to articulate their feelings and cope with stress engaging in therapy can also dismantle the stigma surrounding mental health encouraging more men to seek help.

Take Home Nuggets

- Treatment options must be approached holistically, considering the various aspects of a man's life, including his responsibilities as a father, his career, and his personal relationships. It is essential for adult males to recognise the importance of seeking help and engaging in conversations about mental health, breaking down the barriers of stigma and isolation.
- Coping strategies tailored to men experiencing depression are essential for recovery. Techniques such as mindfulness, physical activity and establishing a strong support network can provide relief. Encouraging emotional intelligence and vulnerability can help men articulate their feelings and seek help when needed.
- By fostering an environment that normalises discussions around mental health, adult males can navigate their struggles more efficiently,

ultimately enhancing their wellbeing and relationships during challenging times.

- The impact of depression on relationships often manifests in withdrawal and avoidance behaviour. Men might retreat into themselves, avoiding social interactions and isolating themselves from their social network.
- Effective communication is a cornerstone of addressing mental health challenges, especially for adult males navigating the complexities of andropause. Encouraging men to share their experiences not only helps reduce the stigma surrounding mental health but also provides a support network that is crucial during difficult times. Creating a safe space for honest conversations is essential for emotional wellbeing and can significantly improve relationships.
- Coping strategies play a significant role in managing stress and anxiety. Methods such as mindfulness, physical activity and creative outlets can greatly benefit men experiencing mental health issues. Practices such as meditation and journalling can help men process their emotions and develop emotional intelligence, a feature which is often lacking in traditional masculine roles.
- Recovery from mental health challenges is a journey that requires patience, understanding, and support. Emotional struggles can significantly impact relationships, whether professional therapy or support group, reaching out is the first step towards healing.

- Navigating mental health challenges in the context of societal expectations require a shift in how masculinity is defined and understood. Support groups and therapy tailored for men can foster a safe environment where they can discuss their struggles and develop healthier coping strategies.

- Recognising the multiplicity of roles that adult men are expected to perform, coupled with societal pressures of what constitutes manliness present a special challenge to men going through andropause. Additionally, the stigma associated with mental health can manifest in the workplace where men may fear that a disclosure of their struggles can jeopardise their careers. This is further aggravated by the struggles men undergo as they grapple with the pressures of being a provider and a role model.

- Building resilience is a crucial skill for adult men, especially those navigating complexities of andropause. In this phase men often face heightened emotional challenges such as anxiety, and depression, which can impact their relationship and overall wellbeing. Resilience allows individuals to bounce back from these adversities, allowing them to maintain a sense of stability and purpose in their lives. By developing this strength, men can better manage their stresses associated with job loss, changes in family dynamics, and other midlife transitions.

Chapter 7
Andropause, Heart Health and Hormonal Changes

The Link Between Hormones and Cardiovascular Function

Hormones play a crucial role in regulating cardiovascular function, particularly in men experiencing andropause. As testosterone levels decline, various physiological changes occur, which can affect heart health. This decline may lead to increased risks of cardiovascular diseases due to factors such as altered lipid profiles, insulin sensitivity, and changes in vascular function. Understanding the relationship between hormonal changes and cardiovascular health is essential for healthcare personnel and men undergoing this transition, as it lays the groundwork for effective management strategies.

Testosterone influences several aspects of cardiovascular health, including endothelial function and inflammation. Low testosterone levels have been associated with increased arterial stiffness and higher levels of inflammatory markers, which may contribute to the development of atherosclerosis. Furthermore, hormonal imbalances can affect mood and mental health, further complicating cardiovascular well-being during andropause. Identifying these links allows healthcare professionals to provide better support and guidance to men facing these challenges.

Lifestyle modifications are vital in managing heart health during andropause. Regular exercise, a balanced diet, and stress management techniques can help improve cardiovascular function and mitigate the effects of hormonal changes. Engaging in physical activity not only enhances cardiovascular fitness but also positively influences hormone levels, creating a beneficial feedback loop. Men are encouraged to adopt a holistic approach to health, incorporating these lifestyle changes to support their heart function.

Nutritional approaches also play a significant role in supporting heart health for middle-aged men. Diets rich in omega-3 fatty acids, antioxidants, and fibre can help improve cardiovascular health. Foods such as fatty fish, nuts, and whole grains should be emphasised to counteract the effects of hormonal decline. Additionally, certain supplements may provide further benefits, but it is crucial for men to consult with healthcare professionals to ensure safe and effective use.

Finally, the mental health impacts of andropause should not be overlooked, as they can significantly affect cardiovascular wellbeing. Factors such as depression and anxiety can lead to unhealthy lifestyle choices, which may exacerbate heart issues. Addressing mental health through therapy, social support, and lifestyle changes can improve overall health outcomes. By recognising the intricate relationship between hormones and cardiovascular function, healthcare personnel can empower men to make informed decisions about their health during andropause.

How Andropause Affects Heart Health

Andropause, often referred to as male menopause, brings about significant hormonal changes that can adversely affect heart health. As testosterone levels decline, men may experience an increase in body fat, particularly around the abdomen, which is a known risk factor for cardiovascular disease. Furthermore, lower testosterone levels have been associated with reduced muscle mass and strength, further compounding the risks associated with heart health. Understanding these changes is crucial for healthcare professionals and men undergoing andropause to proactively manage heart health.

Lifestyle modifications play a pivotal role in mitigating the heart health risks associated with andropause. Regular exercise is essential, as it not only helps in maintaining a healthy weight but also contributes to improved cardiovascular function. Engaging in aerobic activities, strength training, and flexibility exercises can enhance overall heart health. Health care personnel should encourage men to adopt a balanced exercise regimen tailored to their individual capabilities and preferences to foster long-term adherence.

Nutritional approaches are equally important in supporting heart function during andropause. A diet rich in fruits, vegetables, whole grains, and lean proteins can help manage weight and improve cholesterol levels. Omega-3 fatty acids, found in fish and flaxseeds, have been shown to promote heart health by reducing inflammation and lowering blood pressure. Health professionals should advise men to focus on nutrient-dense foods that support cardiovascular well-being while also considering the effects of hormonal changes on appetite and metabolism.

Mental health impacts are also a significant consideration when discussing cardiovascular wellbeing during andropause. Depression and anxiety are common in men experiencing this transition, potentially leading to neglect of heart health. Addressing mental health through counselling, social support, and stress management techniques is vital. Men should be encouraged to seek help and maintain open communication with their healthcare providers about their mental and emotional health, as these factors are closely linked to heart health.

Finally, the role of testosterone replacement therapy (TRT) in managing cardiovascular risk is an evolving area of study. While TRT may alleviate some symptoms associated with andropause, it is crucial to weigh the potential benefits against the risks for heart health. Regular monitoring and consultation with healthcare professionals are essential to ensure that any treatment plan is safe and effective. Preventative measures, including sleep hygiene and regular health screenings, can further aid in maintaining cardiovascular health during this critical period of life.

Recognising Symptoms of Cardiovascular Issues

Recognising the symptoms of cardiovascular issues is crucial for men undergoing andropause. This phase of life can bring about significant hormonal changes that may affect heart health. It is essential for healthcare personnel to educate men about these signs, as early recognition can lead to timely intervention and better outcomes. Common symptoms include chest pain, shortness of breath, and increased fatigue, which can often be mistaken for normal ageing or stress. Understanding these indicators is the first step towards managing cardiovascular health effectively during andropause.

Men experiencing andropause may also report symptoms such as palpitations or irregular heartbeats, which should not be ignored. These symptoms can signal underlying cardiovascular problems that require further evaluation. Healthcare professionals should be vigilant in assessing these symptoms, especially given the increased risk of heart disease associated with hormonal fluctuations in middle-aged men. Regular check-ups and monitoring can help in identifying any potential heart-related issues early.

Lifestyle modifications play a pivotal role in managing heart health during andropause. Encouraging men to adopt a heart-healthy diet rich in fruits, vegetables, whole grains, and lean proteins can significantly improve their cardiovascular wellbeing. Additionally, reducing saturated fats, sugars, and sodium intake can help mitigate the risk of developing heart disease. Healthcare personnel should provide practical guidance on making these dietary changes, making it easier for men to incorporate them into their daily lives.

Exercise regimens tailored to the needs of men experiencing andropause-related heart issues are equally important. Regular physical activity not only strengthens the heart but also aids in managing stress and improving mental health. Healthcare providers should recommend activities that are both enjoyable and beneficial, such as walking, swimming, or cycling, while also considering individual fitness levels and any existing health concerns. This holistic approach can lead to better cardiovascular outcomes and enhance overall quality of life.

Lastly, understanding the mental health impacts of andropause on cardiovascular wellbeing cannot be overlooked. Men may experience anxiety or depression during this transition, which can adversely affect heart health. It is essential for healthcare personnel to address these concerns, providing support and resources to manage mental health effectively. By recognising the interconnectedness of hormonal changes, mental health, and cardiovascular health, healthcare professionals can offer comprehensive care that supports men through this challenging life stage.

Lifestyle Modifications for Heart Health

Importance of a Healthy Lifestyle

The importance of a healthy lifestyle cannot be overstated, particularly for men experiencing andropause. This transitional phase often brings about significant hormonal changes that can adversely affect cardiovascular health. A proactive approach to lifestyle modifications can make a substantial difference in managing these changes, offering men a pathway to improved heart function and overall well-being. Adopting a holistic view of health allows for a better understanding of how various factors interconnect and impact cardiovascular wellness during andropause.

Nutrition plays a vital role in supporting heart health, particularly in middle-aged men. A diet rich in fruits, vegetables, whole grains, and lean proteins can provide essential nutrients that foster cardiovascular function. Moreover, specific dietary choices can help mitigate the risks associated with hormonal fluctuations.

For instance, incorporating omega-3 fatty acids, found in fish and nuts, has been linked to improved heart health and may counteract some of the negative impacts of andropause.

Regular exercise is another critical component of a healthy lifestyle, especially for men facing heart issues related to andropause. Engaging in a well-rounded exercise regimen can enhance cardiovascular fitness, boost mood, and alleviate some mental health impacts associated with this life stage. Activities such as walking, swimming, and strength training not only improve heart function but also help in maintaining a healthy weight, which is essential for reducing cardiovascular risk.

In addition to diet and exercise, mental health must also be addressed when considering cardiovascular wellness during andropause. Sleep disorders, anxiety, and depression can significantly impact heart health. Men should be encouraged to seek support and engage in stress-relieving activities, such as mindfulness and yoga, which can enhance their mental well-being and, in turn, benefit their cardiovascular health.

Lastly, exploring supplements and natural remedies can provide additional support for heart health during andropause. Vitamins and minerals, such as magnesium and vitamin D, play crucial roles in maintaining cardiovascular function. Furthermore, discussions regarding testosterone replacement therapy should not be overlooked, as they may influence cardiovascular risk factors. By integrating these elements into a comprehensive lifestyle strategy, men can take significant strides towards better heart health during andropause.

Dietary Changes for Cardiovascular Wellness

Dietary changes play a crucial role in promoting cardiovascular wellness, especially for men undergoing andropause. During this transitional phase, hormonal fluctuations can significantly impact heart health, making it essential to adopt a heart-healthy diet. Emphasising whole foods, such as fruits, vegetables, whole grains, and lean proteins, can help mitigate the risks associated with these hormonal changes. Moreover, reducing the intake of saturated fats, trans fats, and high-sugar foods can contribute positively to cardiovascular health.

Incorporating omega-3 fatty acids into the diet is particularly beneficial for men experiencing andropause. These healthy fats, found in fish such as salmon and mackerel, have been shown to lower triglyceride levels and reduce the risk of heart disease. Additionally, plant-based sources like flaxseeds and walnuts can provide similar benefits. By prioritising these foods, men can support their heart function while navigating the challenges of hormonal changes.

Another vital aspect of dietary changes is the inclusion of fibre-rich foods. A diet high in fibre not only aids digestion but also helps maintain healthy cholesterol levels. Foods like legumes, oats, and fresh produce can be easily incorporated into daily meals. This shift towards a fibre-rich diet can play a significant role in preventing cardiovascular diseases, which are more prevalent during andropause due to increased weight and metabolic changes.

Hydration also deserves attention when discussing dietary changes for cardiovascular wellness. Adequate water intake supports overall body functions and can enhance heart health. Moreover, limiting alcohol consumption is crucial, as excessive intake can exacerbate heart issues and negatively influence hormonal balance. By maintaining proper hydration and moderating alcohol, men can further improve their cardiovascular health during this pivotal stage of life.

Finally, it is important to consider the psychological aspects of dietary changes. The mental health impacts of andropause can affect motivation and adherence to dietary modifications. Health care personnel should encourage men to establish a supportive environment and incorporate social aspects into meal planning, such as cooking with family or friends. This holistic approach can not only make healthy eating more enjoyable but also reinforce positive lifestyle changes for better heart health.

Nutritional Approaches to Support Heart Function

Essential Nutrients for Heart Health

Heart health is a critical concern for men undergoing andropause, as hormonal changes can significantly impact cardiovascular function. Essential nutrients play a pivotal role in supporting heart health, and understanding these can empower healthcare professionals and patients alike. Key nutrients such as omega-3 fatty acids, fibre, and antioxidants are vital in reducing inflammation and improving heart function. Adequate intake of these nutrients can help mitigate the risks of heart disease, which tends to increase during andropause due to declining testosterone levels and other hormonal shifts.

Omega-3 fatty acids, found in fatty fish like salmon, walnuts, and flaxseeds, are renowned for their heart-protective properties. They have been shown to lower triglyceride levels, reduce blood pressure, and combat inflammation. For men experiencing andropause, incorporating omega-3-rich foods into their diet can be a crucial step towards maintaining cardiovascular health. Additionally, supplements such as fish oil may be beneficial for those who struggle to meet their omega-3 needs through diet alone.

Fibre is another essential nutrient that plays a significant role in heart health. A diet high in soluble fibre, found in oats, beans, and fruits, can help lower cholesterol levels and improve overall heart function. As men age, their digestion may slow down, making it even more important to ensure a fibre-rich diet to support not only heart health but also digestive wellbeing. Healthcare personnel should encourage patients to include a variety of fibre sources in their meals to reap the benefits.

Antioxidants, particularly vitamins C and E, are crucial in combating oxidative stress, which can lead to cardiovascular problems. Foods rich in these vitamins, such as berries, nuts, and green leafy vegetables, should be staples in the diet of men facing andropause. These nutrients help protect the heart by neutralising free radicals and supporting endothelial function, which is vital for maintaining healthy blood vessels. Encouraging a colourful plate filled with fruits and vegetables can make a significant difference in overall heart health.

Finally, it is essential to recognise the interplay between nutrition and mental health during andropause. Nutrient deficiencies can lead to mood changes and increased stress, which can negatively affect heart health. Therefore, healthcare providers should consider not only the physical but also the emotional wellbeing of their patients. By promoting a balanced diet rich in essential nutrients, they can help men manage the cardiovascular risks associated with andropause effectively, fostering a holistic approach to health and wellness.

Dietary Patterns for Men in Andropause

As men enter andropause, they experience various hormonal changes that can significantly impact their cardiovascular health. It is essential to understand the dietary patterns that can support heart function during this transition. A diet rich in whole foods, including fruits, vegetables, whole grains, lean proteins, and healthy fats, can help mitigate some of the negative effects associated with andropause. These foods provide vital nutrients that support overall health and specifically benefit heart function, making them crucial for men in this stage of life.

Incorporating antioxidant-rich foods into the diet is particularly important for men undergoing andropause. Foods such as berries, nuts, and green leafy vegetables can combat oxidative stress, which is a significant factor in cardiovascular disease. Additionally, omega-3 fatty acids found in fatty fish, flaxseeds, and walnuts can reduce inflammation and improve heart health. By focusing on these nutrient-dense foods, men can enhance their heart function and overall wellbeing during andropause.

Limitations on processed foods, added sugars, and excessive sodium are equally important in establishing a heart-healthy diet. These foods can contribute to weight gain, hypertension, and elevated cholesterol levels, all of which pose risks for cardiovascular health. Men should aim to minimise their intake of these harmful substances while increasing their consumption of fibre-rich foods, which can help in managing cholesterol levels and maintaining a healthy weight.

Furthermore, hydration plays a crucial role in cardiovascular health. Men should ensure they are drinking sufficient water throughout the day, as dehydration can negatively impact heart function. Herbal teas and natural juices can also be beneficial, but it is essential to avoid sugary beverages that can lead to increased blood sugar levels. Maintaining proper hydration supports overall bodily functions, including those of the heart.

Finally, it is vital for men to consider their mental health during andropause, as psychological wellbeing is closely linked to cardiovascular health. Stress management techniques, along with a balanced diet, can aid in maintaining a healthy heart. The integration of mindfulness practices, such as yoga or meditation, alongside dietary modifications can create a holistic approach to managing heart health during this challenging phase of life. By adopting these dietary patterns and lifestyle changes, men can significantly improve their cardiovascular wellness as they navigate andropause.

Foods to Include and Avoid

When addressing the dietary needs of men undergoing andropause, it is essential to focus on foods that promote cardiovascular health. Incorporating fruits and vegetables rich in antioxidants can help combat oxidative stress, which is crucial as men experience hormonal changes. Whole grains, such as oats and brown rice, provide necessary fibre that supports heart function and helps maintain healthy cholesterol levels. Additionally, including sources of lean protein like fish, chicken, and legumes is important for muscle maintenance and overall wellbeing during this transitional phase.

Conversely, certain foods should be avoided to mitigate cardiovascular risks. Trans fats, often found in processed foods and fried items, can elevate cholesterol levels and increase the likelihood of heart disease. High sodium intake, commonly present in processed and packaged foods, can lead to hypertension, which is a significant concern for older men. It is also advisable to limit added sugars, as these can contribute to weight gain and metabolic issues, further exacerbating heart health problems associated with andropause.

Incorporating healthy fats into the diet is vital for supporting cardiovascular function. Foods high in omega-3 fatty acids, such as fatty fish, walnuts, and flaxseeds, can lower inflammation and improve heart health. Additionally, avocados and olive oil provide monounsaturated fats that are beneficial for heart health. Balancing these healthy fats with a reduction in saturated fats found in red meats and full-fat dairy products can help manage cholesterol levels effectively during andropause.

Hydration plays a crucial role in maintaining heart health as well. Encouraging adequate water intake helps to regulate blood pressure and supports overall bodily functions. Herbal teas and beverages rich in polyphenols, like green tea, can also offer cardiovascular benefits. Men should be advised to limit alcohol consumption, as excessive intake can have detrimental effects on both cardiovascular health and hormonal balance during andropause.

Lastly, a holistic approach to nutrition should include consideration of mental health, as emotional wellbeing can significantly impact heart health. Encouraging the intake of foods that support mood, such as those rich in omega-3s and antioxidants, can help manage stress and anxiety during andropause. Engaging in regular physical activity, alongside a balanced diet, will further enhance cardiovascular wellbeing and alleviate some of the mental health challenges faced during this stage of life.

Mental Health and Cardiovascular Wellbeing

The Psychological Impact of Andropause

Andropause, often referred to as male menopause, can have profound psychological effects on men, particularly as they navigate the complexities of hormonal changes. These hormonal fluctuations can lead to feelings of depression, anxiety, and a general sense of malaise, which can significantly impact cardiovascular health. It is essential for healthcare personnel to recognise these symptoms in men undergoing andropause, as mental wellbeing is intricately linked to physical health, particularly heart health. Understanding the mind-body connection during this transitional phase can aid in developing comprehensive treatment plans that address both psychological and physiological concerns.

The emotional turmoil associated with andropause can manifest as stress, which is a well-known risk factor for cardiovascular diseases. Elevated stress levels can lead to unhealthy lifestyle choices, including poor dietary habits and lack of physical activity, further exacerbating heart health issues. Healthcare providers should encourage men to engage in lifestyle modifications, such as stress management techniques and mindfulness practices, which can improve mental health and thus support cardiovascular function. This holistic approach can empower men to take control of their health amidst the challenges posed by andropause.

Nutrition plays a pivotal role in managing both psychological and cardiovascular health. Men experiencing andropause should focus on a balanced diet rich in nutrients that support heart function, such as omega-3 fatty acids, antioxidants, and vitamins. These dietary choices not only help in maintaining heart health but also contribute to improved mood and cognitive function. Healthcare professionals should provide guidance on nutritional approaches that can alleviate symptoms of andropause while promoting overall wellness, reinforcing the importance of food as medicine in this context.

Physical activity is equally crucial in mitigating the psychological impacts of andropause. Regular exercise has been shown to enhance mood, reduce anxiety, and improve overall cardiovascular health. Tailored exercise regimens that take into account the unique challenges faced by men in this life stage can be particularly beneficial. Healthcare providers should advocate for physical activity as a primary strategy to combat the negative effects of andropause, encouraging men to participate in activities that they enjoy and that fit their lifestyle, thus making exercise a sustainable part of their routine.

Finally, it is essential to address the role of testosterone replacement therapy (TRT) in managing both psychological and cardiovascular health during andropause. While some men may benefit from TRT, it is crucial to weigh the potential risks and benefits, especially concerning cardiovascular risk factors. Open discussions about TRT, alongside alternative supplements and natural remedies, can empower men to make informed decisions regarding their health. Preventative measures, including monitoring sleep patterns which are often disrupted during andropause, can also play a significant role in maintaining heart health and overall wellbeing in older men.

Mental Health Disorders and Heart Health

Mental health disorders and heart health are intricately linked, particularly during andropause, a phase marked by significant hormonal changes in men. These changes can lead to various mental health issues, including depression and anxiety, which have been shown to adversely affect cardiovascular health. The stress associated with these mental health disorders can elevate blood pressure and contribute to the development of heart disease. Therefore, understanding this connection is essential for healthcare personnel working with men undergoing andropause.

To effectively manage heart health during andropause, lifestyle modifications play a crucial role. Incorporating regular physical activity can alleviate symptoms of depression and anxiety, while simultaneously improving cardiovascular function. Exercise regimens tailored for men experiencing andropause-related heart issues can help in reducing stress levels and enhancing overall mental resilience. It is vital for healthcare professionals to encourage patients to engage in consistent physical activity as part of a holistic approach to health.

Nutritional approaches also significantly influence both mental and heart health. A diet rich in omega-3 fatty acids, fruits, and vegetables can support heart function and improve mood. Specific nutrients, such as magnesium and B vitamins, are particularly beneficial in managing stress and anxiety, which are common during andropause. Healthcare personnel should advocate for dietary changes that not only promote cardiovascular wellness but also enhance mental wellbeing.

In addition to lifestyle modifications, the role of supplements and natural remedies cannot be overlooked. Certain supplements, such as fish oil and vitamin D, have been associated with improved heart health and mood enhancement. Healthcare providers should be knowledgeable about these options and discuss them with patients as potential adjuncts to traditional treatments. Moreover, testosterone replacement therapy may also be a consideration, as it can alleviate symptoms of andropause while potentially lowering cardiovascular risks.

Lastly, recognising the connection between sleep disorders and heart health is essential. Poor sleep can exacerbate mental health issues and lead to a decline in cardiovascular function. Encouraging good sleep hygiene practices and addressing sleep disorders can significantly improve both mental health and heart health in older men. In conclusion, a comprehensive approach that encompasses mental health, lifestyle modifications, nutrition, and sleep management is vital for promoting cardiovascular wellness in men undergoing andropause.

Strategies for Maintaining Mental Wellbeing

Mental wellbeing is a crucial aspect of overall health, particularly for men undergoing andropause. This life stage often brings about various hormonal changes that can significantly impact emotional and psychological states. It is essential for health care personnel to understand these dynamics and provide support to men navigating this transition. Strategies for maintaining mental wellbeing can include fostering a strong support network, engaging in open discussions about feelings, and encouraging men to seek professional help if needed.

Regular physical activity is a fundamental strategy in promoting mental wellbeing. Exercise not only helps to manage cardiovascular health but also releases endorphins, which can enhance mood and reduce feelings of anxiety and depression. Health care professionals should encourage men experiencing andropause to adopt tailored exercise regimens that suit their individual capabilities. Activities such as walking, swimming, or joining a fitness class can provide both physical and psychological benefits.

Nutrition plays a pivotal role in mental health and can be used as a tool to combat the emotional effects of andropause. A balanced diet rich in omega-3 fatty acids, whole grains, and antioxidants can support brain function and mood regulation. Health care personnel can guide men towards nutritional approaches that not only enhance heart health but also promote mental clarity and emotional stability. This includes recommending foods that are known to reduce inflammation and improve cognitive function.

Mindfulness and stress reduction techniques have gained recognition as effective strategies for maintaining mental wellbeing. Practices such as meditation, yoga, or deep-breathing exercises can help men manage stress and improve their emotional resilience. Health care professionals should advocate for these practices as part of a holistic approach to health during andropause, emphasising their benefits for both mental and cardiovascular health.

Finally, sleep quality is often overlooked but is a vital component of mental wellbeing. Andropause can lead to sleep disturbances, which in turn can exacerbate mood disorders and impact heart health. Encouraging good sleep hygiene, such as establishing a regular sleep schedule and creating a restful environment, can help men improve their sleep quality. Addressing sleep issues can significantly contribute to overall wellbeing and provide a foundation for healthier lifestyle choices during this transitional phase.

Exercise Regimens for Andropause-Related Heart Issues

Importance of Physical Activity

Physical activity plays a crucial role in maintaining cardiovascular health, particularly for men experiencing andropause. As hormonal changes occur during this phase, the risk of heart-related issues increases significantly. Regular exercise not only helps mitigate these risks but also promotes overall well-being. Engaging in physical activity can lead to improved heart function, better circulation, and a strengthened cardiovascular system, making it an essential component of a heart-healthy lifestyle for middle-aged men.

Moreover, exercise serves as a powerful tool for managing weight, which is particularly important during andropause. Weight gain can lead to a range of complications, including increased blood pressure and elevated cholesterol levels. By incorporating regular physical activity into their routines, men can effectively manage their weight, thereby reducing the likelihood of developing heart disease. This lifestyle modification is vital for those looking to maintain their cardiovascular health amid hormonal fluctuations.

The mental health benefits of physical activity cannot be overstated, especially for men undergoing andropause. Exercise has been shown to alleviate symptoms of anxiety and depression, which can be exacerbated by hormonal changes. A regular workout regimen can boost mood, enhance cognitive function, and improve sleep quality, all of which contribute positively to heart health. As mental well-being is closely linked to physical health, prioritising exercise becomes even more critical during this transitional phase.

In addition to traditional exercises, incorporating specific regimens tailored to the needs of men experiencing andropause-related heart issues can yield significant benefits. Activities such as strength training, aerobic exercises, and flexibility workouts can help improve cardiovascular endurance and muscular strength. Furthermore, consulting with healthcare professionals to create a personalised exercise plan can ensure that men engage in safe and effective physical activity that addresses their unique health concerns.

Finally, it is essential to recognise that supplements and nutritional approaches can complement physical activity in supporting heart function. A balanced diet rich in omega-3 fatty acids, antioxidants, and fibre can enhance the effects of exercise. Moreover, the role of testosterone replacement therapy should also be considered, as it may influence cardiovascular risk factors. By integrating physical activity with proper nutrition and medical guidance, men can take proactive steps towards maintaining their heart health during andropause, ultimately leading to a better quality of life.

Recommended Types of Exercise

Exercise plays a pivotal role in managing the health of men undergoing andropause, particularly concerning cardiovascular wellness. Engaging in regular physical activity helps to mitigate the hormonal changes associated with this life stage, which can lead to increased cardiovascular risk. A well-rounded exercise regimen that includes aerobic, strength training, and flexibility exercises can significantly contribute to improved heart health. Health care personnel should encourage men to incorporate such activities into their daily routines to foster a proactive approach to their well-being.

Aerobic exercises, such as walking, cycling, and swimming, are essential for cardiovascular health. These activities elevate the heart rate, improve circulation, and enhance overall cardiovascular function. For men experiencing andropause-related heart issues, starting with moderate-intensity aerobic exercises can lead to significant improvements in heart health without overwhelming the body. Gradually increasing the intensity and duration of these activities can further optimise cardiovascular benefits.

Strength training is equally important, as it helps to combat muscle loss associated with andropause and hormonal changes. Incorporating weightlifting or resistance bands into an exercise regimen can improve muscle mass, which in turn supports metabolic health and cardiovascular function. Health care professionals should advise men to engage in strength training exercises at least twice a week, targeting all major muscle groups to maximise the benefits.

Flexibility and balance exercises, such as yoga or tai chi, should not be overlooked, as they contribute to overall physical health and can mitigate stress. Stress management is crucial during andropause, given its potential negative impact on cardiovascular health. By promoting flexibility and balance, these exercises also reduce the risk of injuries, making it easier for men to remain active and engaged in their exercise routines.

In summary, a comprehensive exercise programme tailored to the needs of men undergoing andropause can significantly enhance cardiovascular health. Health care personnel should advocate for a balanced approach that includes aerobic, strength, and flexibility exercises, catering to the unique challenges posed by andropause. By making these lifestyle modifications, men can improve their overall health and reduce their risk of heart disease during this transitional phase of life.

Creating an Effective Exercise Plan

Creating an effective exercise plan is crucial for men experiencing andropause, particularly in relation to cardiovascular health. As hormonal changes occur, physical activity can help mitigate some of the negative effects on heart function. A well-structured exercise regimen should incorporate a mix of aerobic, strength training, and flexibility exercises to ensure comprehensive health benefits. Understanding the balance of these components can empower men to take charge of their cardiovascular wellness during this transitional phase in their lives.

Aerobic exercises, such as brisk walking, cycling, and swimming, play a vital role in improving heart health. These activities increase heart rate and promote better circulation, which is essential in combating the risks associated with andropause. Men should aim for at least 150 minutes of moderate-intensity aerobic exercise weekly, as recommended by health authorities. Gradually increasing the intensity and duration of these workouts can lead to significant improvements in cardiovascular function and overall stamina.

Strength training is equally important, as it helps to maintain muscle mass and metabolic rate, both of which can decline with age and hormonal changes. Engaging in resistance exercises two to three times a week can enhance muscle strength and bone density, reducing the risk of osteoporosis and other related issues. Furthermore, strength training has been shown to improve insulin sensitivity, which is crucial for managing weight and overall cardiovascular health.

Flexibility and balance exercises should not be overlooked in an effective exercise plan. Activities such as yoga or tai chi can help improve flexibility, reduce stress levels, and enhance mental well-being. These practices are particularly beneficial for men undergoing andropause, as they not only contribute to physical health but also support emotional resilience. Integrating these elements into a weekly routine can lead to a holistic approach to managing health during andropause.

Finally, it is essential to consult with a healthcare professional before starting any new exercise programme, especially for those with pre-existing heart conditions. A tailored approach, considering individual fitness levels and health concerns, will yield the best outcomes. By committing to a balanced and well-rounded exercise plan, men can significantly improve their cardiovascular health and quality of life during andropause.

Supplements and Natural Remedies

Overview of Useful Supplements

In the context of andropause, understanding the role of supplements can be crucial for maintaining cardiovascular health. As men experience hormonal changes during this phase, the body may require additional nutritional support to manage heart function effectively. Various supplements have been researched for their potential benefits, including omega-3 fatty acids, Coenzyme Q10, and magnesium, which are known to contribute positively to heart health. This overview explores how these supplements can be integrated into the lifestyle of men undergoing andropause, enhancing their overall wellbeing and supporting cardiovascular function.

Omega-3 fatty acids, found in fish oil and certain plant oils, have been extensively studied for their cardioprotective properties. These essential fats are known to lower triglyceride levels, reduce inflammation, and improve endothelial function. For men facing the challenges of andropause, incorporating omega-3 supplements may help mitigate some of the heart-related risks associated with declining testosterone levels. The anti-inflammatory effects of omega-3s also support mental health, which can be significantly impacted during this transition, further contributing to cardiovascular wellbeing.

Coenzyme Q10 (CoQ10) is another supplement that holds promise for heart health, especially in older men. This naturally occurring antioxidant plays a vital role in energy production within cells, particularly in heart tissue. As men age, CoQ10 levels decline, which can affect cardiac function. Supplementation may enhance energy levels and support heart muscle health, making it a valuable addition to the regimen of men experiencing andropause. Furthermore, CoQ10 has been linked to improved exercise tolerance, which is essential for maintaining an active lifestyle.

Magnesium is often overlooked but is crucial for cardiovascular health, particularly in the context of hormonal changes during andropause. It aids in regulating blood pressure, maintaining heart rhythm, and preventing arterial calcification. Many men may not receive adequate magnesium from their diet, making supplementation a practical approach to support heart function. Additionally, magnesium has been shown to have positive effects on mood and sleep quality, tackling two significant concerns for men undergoing this transitional period.

While supplements can play a vital role in supporting cardiovascular health during andropause, it is essential to approach their use thoughtfully. Men should consult healthcare professionals before starting any supplementation regimen, ensuring that their overall health and specific needs are considered. A holistic approach that includes dietary modifications, exercise, and mental health support, alongside appropriate supplementation, can lead to improved outcomes for men navigating the complexities of andropause and its impact on heart health.

Natural Remedies for Heart Health

Heart health is crucial for men experiencing andropause, a phase marked by significant hormonal changes. Natural remedies can play a vital role in supporting cardiovascular function during this transition. These remedies often include dietary adjustments, lifestyle changes, and supplementation that align with the unique needs of middle-aged men. By focusing on heart-healthy habits, individuals can mitigate risks associated with cardiovascular disease and enhance their overall well-being.

Nutritional approaches to heart health are foundational. Incorporating omega-3 fatty acids, found in fish and flaxseeds, can help reduce inflammation and promote healthy blood circulation. Antioxidant-rich foods, such as berries, leafy greens, and nuts, support heart function by combating oxidative stress. Additionally, limiting saturated fats and sugars can help manage weight and lower cholesterol levels, which are crucial factors in maintaining cardiovascular health during andropause.

Exercise regimens tailored for men undergoing andropause-related heart issues are equally important. Regular physical activity can improve heart efficiency, regulate blood pressure, and enhance mood. Activities such as brisk walking, cycling, and swimming not only build cardiovascular endurance but also help in managing stress and anxiety, which are often heightened during andropause. A consistent routine encourages the release of endorphins, promoting mental health and overall vitality.

Supplements can also provide an additional layer of support for heart health. Coenzyme Q10, vitamin D, and magnesium are frequently recommended due to their roles in energy production and muscle function, including the heart muscle. Herbal remedies like hawthorn and garlic have been traditionally used to support cardiovascular health. However, it's essential for healthcare personnel to advise patients to consult with their doctors before starting any supplementation, ensuring safety and efficacy.

Finally, understanding the interplay between sleep disorders and heart health is vital for men in this demographic. Poor sleep can exacerbate hormonal imbalances and increase cardiovascular risk. Encouraging sleep hygiene practices, such as maintaining a regular sleep schedule and creating a restful environment, can significantly improve sleep quality. This holistic approach, combining natural remedies, exercise, nutrition, and mental health support, is essential for managing heart health during andropause.

Consulting with Healthcare Professionals

Consulting with healthcare professionals is a crucial step for men undergoing andropause, particularly when addressing cardiovascular health. Many men experience hormonal changes that can significantly impact their heart function. It is essential for healthcare personnel to understand these changes and guide patients in recognising symptoms that may arise during this transitional phase. A comprehensive approach to assessing heart health can help in formulating effective management strategies tailored to individual needs.

During consultations, discussing lifestyle modifications is vital. Healthcare professionals should emphasise the importance of a balanced diet, regular exercise, and stress management techniques. Men in andropause may find it beneficial to learn about nutritional approaches that specifically support heart function. Encouraging the inclusion of heart-healthy foods, such as omega-3 fatty acids, fruits, and vegetables, can play a significant role in improving overall cardiovascular wellness.

Mental health impacts are another crucial aspect to address when consulting with patients. The emotional and psychological effects of andropause can lead to increased stress, anxiety, and depressive symptoms, all of which can adversely affect heart health. Healthcare professionals should be prepared to discuss these concerns openly and offer resources for mental health support, ensuring that patients understand the importance of addressing both physical and emotional wellbeing.

Exercise regimens tailored to men experiencing andropause-related heart issues should also be a focal point in consultations. Physical activity is not only beneficial for maintaining cardiovascular health but also plays a role in improving mood and energy levels. Healthcare professionals can guide patients in developing customised exercise plans that take into account their current fitness levels and any limitations they may have due to age or medical conditions.

Finally, discussions regarding supplements and natural remedies are pertinent when consulting with men undergoing andropause. The role of testosterone replacement therapy in managing cardiovascular risk should also be carefully evaluated. Healthcare personnel must stay informed about preventative measures for heart disease and the connection between sleep disorders and heart health, providing patients with comprehensive advice that enhances their quality of life during this challenging period.

Testosterone Replacement Therapy and Cardiovascular Risk

Understanding Testosterone Replacement

Testosterone replacement therapy (TRT) is a significant consideration for men experiencing andropause, particularly regarding its impact on cardiovascular health. As testosterone levels decline with age, many men face various symptoms, including fatigue, reduced libido, and mood disturbances. These changes can also correlate with an increased risk of cardiovascular issues. Understanding the role of testosterone in heart health is crucial for healthcare personnel and men undergoing andropause to make informed decisions about treatment options.

Research indicates that low testosterone levels may contribute to the development of metabolic syndrome, characterised by obesity, insulin resistance, and increased blood pressure, all of which are risk factors for cardiovascular disease. TRT has been shown to improve these metabolic parameters, potentially reducing cardiovascular risk. However, the relationship between testosterone and heart health is complex, necessitating careful assessment before initiating therapy. Healthcare professionals must evaluate individual patient needs, considering both benefits and potential risks associated with TRT.

Lifestyle modifications play a vital role in managing heart health during andropause. Nutritional approaches, regular exercise, and mental health support are all essential components of a comprehensive strategy. A diet rich in whole foods, including fruits, vegetables, lean proteins, and healthy fats, can help support heart function. Additionally, exercise regimens tailored for men experiencing andropause-related heart issues can improve overall cardiovascular fitness, enhance mood, and promote a healthier body composition.

Moreover, mental health impacts cannot be overlooked, as depression and anxiety are common during andropause and can adversely affect cardiovascular wellbeing. Addressing these issues through counselling, support groups, or mindfulness practices can lead to improved heart health outcomes. Supplements and natural remedies may also aid in supporting heart function, but they should be approached with caution and discussed with a healthcare provider to ensure safety and efficacy.

Finally, a thorough understanding of the connection between sleep disorders and heart health in older men is essential. Poor sleep quality can exacerbate hormonal imbalances and increase cardiovascular risk. Therefore, integrating strategies to improve sleep hygiene should be part of any treatment plan for men undergoing TRT. Ultimately, a holistic approach that combines testosterone replacement when appropriate with lifestyle modifications, mental health support, and sleep improvement can lead to better cardiovascular health in men experiencing andropause.

Benefits and Risks of Therapy

Therapy can offer numerous benefits to men undergoing andropause, particularly in the context of cardiovascular health. Psychological support through therapy can help address the emotional and mental health challenges that often accompany hormonal changes. This support can lead to improved coping strategies, which in turn can positively impact lifestyle choices, including diet and exercise. By fostering a greater sense of well-being, therapy can play a crucial role in enhancing overall heart health during this transitional phase of life.

However, the decision to engage in therapy is not without its risks. Some individuals may find that discussing personal issues brings up uncomfortable emotions or memories, leading to increased anxiety or stress. Additionally, therapy may require a significant time commitment, which could be a challenge for men with busy lifestyles. It is essential for healthcare personnel to evaluate the readiness and willingness of their patients to engage in therapeutic processes, ensuring that the potential benefits outweigh any possible drawbacks.

Lifestyle modifications are vital for managing heart health during andropause, and therapy can facilitate this change. Through therapeutic interventions, men can learn to set realistic health goals, such as adopting a heart-healthy diet or establishing a regular exercise routine. These lifestyle changes not only support cardiovascular wellness but also help mitigate the mental health impacts of andropause, creating a holistic approach to treatment. Therefore, the integration of therapy into a comprehensive health plan can significantly enhance the effectiveness of lifestyle modifications.

Furthermore, nutritional approaches to support heart function can also be reinforced through therapy. A therapist can aid in addressing emotional eating habits and provide guidance on making healthier food choices. This support can be crucial as men navigate the complexities of hormonal changes that may affect their appetite and cravings. By fostering a healthier relationship with food, therapy can contribute to better nutritional outcomes and, consequently, improved heart health.

In conclusion, while therapy presents both benefits and risks for men undergoing andropause, its positive impact on cardiovascular health cannot be overlooked. The potential for therapy to improve mental well-being and encourage lifestyle changes makes it a valuable tool in the management of andropause-related heart issues. Healthcare personnel should consider incorporating therapeutic options into their treatment plans, ensuring that men receive comprehensive support during this critical phase of life.

Monitoring Cardiovascular Health During Treatment

Monitoring cardiovascular health during treatment for andropause is crucial for men experiencing hormonal changes that can impact their heart function. Regular assessments, including blood pressure checks, cholesterol levels, and cardiac function tests, are essential to identify any emerging risks. Health care personnel should be vigilant in evaluating these parameters, as they can provide critical insights into a patient's cardiovascular status and guide appropriate interventions.

Lifestyle modifications play a significant role in managing heart health during andropause. Encouraging patients to adopt a heart-healthy diet, rich in fruits, vegetables, whole grains, and lean proteins, can help mitigate the risks associated with hormonal fluctuations. Additionally, promoting regular physical activity is vital; tailored exercise regimens can enhance cardiovascular fitness and improve overall wellbeing, addressing both physical and mental health aspects.

Nutritional approaches are also paramount for supporting heart function in middle-aged men. Incorporating omega-3 fatty acids, found in fish and flaxseed, can be beneficial for cardiovascular health. Furthermore, educating patients on the importance of micronutrients, such as magnesium and potassium, can help prevent complications related to heart disease, especially in those undergoing testosterone replacement therapy, which may influence cardiovascular risk.

Mental health impacts should not be overlooked, as psychological wellbeing is intrinsically linked to cardiovascular health. Men going through andropause often experience mood swings, anxiety, and depression, which can adversely affect heart health. Health care personnel must address these issues through counselling, stress management techniques, and possibly medication, to ensure a holistic approach to treatment.

Lastly, sleep disorders are common in older men and can significantly affect heart health. Encouraging good sleep hygiene practices and addressing sleep apnoea can play a critical role in improving cardiovascular outcomes. Preventative measures, including regular monitoring and addressing sleep issues, are imperative in managing heart disease risks in men undergoing andropause, ultimately contributing to their overall health and quality of life.

Preventative Measures for Heart Disease

Identifying Risk Factors

Identifying risk factors associated with andropause is crucial for understanding how hormonal changes can impact cardiovascular health in men. As testosterone levels decline, various physiological changes occur that may predispose men to heart-related issues. These changes can include an increase in body fat, a decrease in muscle mass, and alterations in lipid profiles, which can all contribute to a heightened risk of cardiovascular disease. Therefore, health care personnel must be vigilant in recognising these risk factors to provide appropriate interventions.

One of the primary risk factors to consider is the impact of lifestyle modifications on heart health during andropause. Poor dietary choices, lack of physical activity, and stress can exacerbate the cardiovascular risks associated with hormonal changes. Health professionals should advocate for healthier lifestyle choices, including balanced nutrition and regular exercise, as these can significantly mitigate the risks of heart disease. Effective communication about these changes can empower men to take control of their heart health during this transitional phase of life.

Nutritional approaches also play a vital role in supporting heart function for middle-aged men. Diets rich in omega-3 fatty acids, antioxidants, and fibre can help counteract some of the negative impacts of andropause on cardiovascular health. Furthermore, educating patients on the importance of maintaining a healthy weight and managing blood pressure through dietary choices is essential. Incorporating heart-healthy foods can lead to improved outcomes and enhance overall well-being during andropause.

Mental health impacts are another critical aspect to consider when discussing cardiovascular wellbeing. Men experiencing andropause may face emotional challenges such as depression and anxiety, which can further contribute to heart health issues. Recognising the connection between mental health and cardiovascular risk allows healthcare providers to offer comprehensive care that addresses both physical and psychological factors. Encouraging men to seek support for mental health can lead to improved heart health outcomes.

Finally, the role of testosterone replacement therapy (TRT) in managing cardiovascular risk is a topic of significant debate. While TRT may alleviate some symptoms of andropause, its effects on heart health require careful consideration. It is essential for healthcare professionals to evaluate the potential benefits and risks associated with TRT, guiding men through informed decisions. Preventative measures, including monitoring for sleep disorders that can affect heart health, should also be integrated into the overall management plan for men undergoing andropause.

Strategies for Prevention

Preventing cardiovascular issues during andropause requires a multifaceted approach that includes lifestyle modifications, nutritional strategies, and regular exercise. Health care personnel should emphasise the importance of a balanced diet rich in heart-healthy nutrients. Foods high in omega-3 fatty acids, such as fish, nuts, and seeds, can help reduce inflammation and improve overall heart function. Moreover, incorporating a variety of fruits and vegetables can provide essential vitamins and antioxidants that support cardiovascular health.

Regular physical activity is paramount for men experiencing andropause-related heart issues. Exercise regimens should focus on both aerobic and resistance training to enhance cardiovascular fitness and build muscle mass. Activities such as brisk walking, swimming, or cycling can increase heart rate and improve circulation. Additionally, strength training can counteract the muscle loss associated with hormonal changes, thereby supporting better heart health.

Mental health also plays a significant role in cardiovascular wellbeing during andropause. Stress management techniques, including mindfulness and relaxation exercises, can mitigate the adverse effects of hormonal fluctuations on mental health. Encouraging men to engage in social activities and seek support from peers or mental health professionals can help reduce feelings of isolation, which can adversely affect heart health.

Nutritional approaches are equally vital, with certain supplements and natural remedies showing promise in supporting heart function. Omega-3 fatty acids, Coenzyme Q10, and magnesium supplements may offer benefits for cardiovascular health. Health care personnel should guide men in choosing the right supplements based on their individual health profiles and needs, ensuring that they complement a healthy diet rather than replace it.

Finally, the role of testosterone replacement therapy should be carefully considered in the context of cardiovascular risk. While it may alleviate some symptoms of andropause, evaluation of the potential benefits and risks is crucial. Preventative measures, including regular check-ups and screenings for heart disease, should be a priority for men undergoing andropause, as early detection and intervention can significantly influence outcomes in cardiovascular health.

Importance of Regular Health Check-ups

Regular health check-ups are essential for men undergoing andropause, as they serve as a proactive approach to managing cardiovascular health. During andropause, hormonal fluctuations can significantly impact heart function, making it crucial for healthcare personnel to encourage routine screenings. These check-ups can help identify potential risks early, allowing for timely interventions that may prevent serious heart conditions. By prioritising regular assessments, men can take control of their health, especially during this transitional phase.

In addition to monitoring cardiovascular health, regular check-ups provide an opportunity to assess overall wellbeing, including mental health. The psychological impacts of andropause, such as anxiety and depression, can affect cardiovascular health. By integrating mental health evaluations into routine check-ups, healthcare providers can offer comprehensive care, ensuring that both physical and mental health are addressed. This holistic approach is vital for promoting heart health in middle-aged men.

Lifestyle modifications are another key component of maintaining cardiovascular wellness during andropause. Health check-ups can serve as a platform for educating men about the importance of exercise, nutrition, and supplements tailored to support heart function. Healthcare professionals can provide personalised recommendations based on individual health assessments, empowering men to make informed choices that positively impact their heart health.

Furthermore, check-ups can facilitate discussions regarding testosterone replacement therapy and its implications for cardiovascular risk. Understanding the balance between hormonal treatment and heart health is critical for men experiencing andropause. Regular consultations allow for the monitoring of therapy effects, ensuring that any potential risks are managed effectively.

Lastly, addressing the connection between sleep disorders and heart health is vital during health check-ups. Many men undergoing andropause experience sleep disturbances, which can exacerbate cardiovascular issues. By incorporating sleep assessments into regular check-ups, healthcare providers can identify and address these concerns, further enhancing the overall health and wellbeing of men during this life stage. Regular check-ups, therefore, play a fundamental role in fostering a proactive approach to cardiovascular health during andropause.

The Connection Between Sleep Disorders and Heart Health

Impact of Sleep on Cardiovascular Health

The relationship between sleep and cardiovascular health is a critical area of study, especially for men undergoing andropause. Adequate sleep is essential for the body's recovery and maintenance functions, including heart health. Research indicates that sleep deprivation can lead to increased risks of hypertension, heart attacks, and other cardiovascular issues. This is particularly concerning for men experiencing hormonal changes associated with andropause, where the body's ability to manage stress and repair itself may already be compromised.

Hormonal fluctuations during andropause can significantly impact sleep patterns, leading to insomnia or disrupted sleep. Poor sleep quality not only affects mood and cognitive function but also has a direct correlation with cardiovascular health. Men may find themselves in a cycle where hormonal changes affect sleep, and inadequate sleep further exacerbates cardiovascular risks. Understanding this connection is vital for healthcare personnel as they support men in implementing effective lifestyle modifications.

Lifestyle modifications, including establishing a regular sleep routine, can play a pivotal role in enhancing sleep quality and, consequently, heart function. Encouraging men to adopt practices such as winding down before bed, limiting screen time, and creating a restful sleeping environment can improve overall sleep quality. Additionally, these adjustments can have a beneficial effect on hormonal balance, thereby supporting cardiovascular health during andropause.

Nutrition also plays a significant role in this context. A diet rich in antioxidants, omega-3 fatty acids, and essential vitamins can not only promote better sleep but also support heart health. Healthcare professionals should guide men towards nutritional strategies that incorporate foods known for their heart-protective qualities, such as leafy greens, nuts, and fatty fish. This dual approach addresses both sleep and cardiovascular health, allowing for a holistic strategy to manage the challenges of andropause.

Finally, addressing mental health is crucial as stress and anxiety can further disrupt sleep and negatively affect heart health. Encouraging mindfulness practices, regular physical activity, and possibly discussing the role of testosterone replacement therapy may provide comprehensive support for men experiencing these changes. Integrating these elements creates a multi-faceted approach to improving sleep and cardiovascular outcomes, ultimately enhancing the quality of life for men during andropause.

Common Sleep Disorders in Older Men

As men age, especially during the andropause phase, they may experience various sleep disorders that can significantly impact their overall health and well-being. Common sleep disorders in older men include insomnia, sleep apnoea, restless leg syndrome, and circadian rhythm disturbances. These conditions can lead to poor sleep quality, which is closely linked to cardiovascular health, putting older men at higher risk for heart-related issues.

Insomnia is one of the most prevalent sleep disorders among older men undergoing andropause. It can manifest as difficulty falling asleep, staying asleep, or waking up too early. The hormonal changes associated with andropause, particularly the decline in testosterone, can exacerbate insomnia symptoms. This lack of restorative sleep can lead to increased stress levels and negatively affect heart health, further complicating cardiovascular conditions.

Sleep apnoea is another common concern, characterised by interruptions in breathing during sleep. This disorder is often unnoticed but can have severe implications for cardiovascular health, including elevated blood pressure and increased risk of heart failure. Older men may be particularly susceptible to this condition due to factors such as obesity and the relaxation of throat muscles, which can occur with age.

Restless leg syndrome (RLS) can also be prevalent among older men, causing uncomfortable sensations in the legs that lead to an irresistible urge to move them, especially at night. RLS can disrupt sleep patterns, leading to chronic fatigue and a host of mental health issues, which are intertwined with cardiovascular well-being. Addressing RLS through lifestyle modifications, such as dietary changes and appropriate exercise, can improve sleep quality and subsequently heart health.

Finally, circadian rhythm disturbances, often exacerbated by lifestyle factors, can affect sleep quality in older men. Irregular sleep patterns can lead to a misalignment between the body's internal clock and external environment, which can adversely impact metabolic processes related to heart health. Understanding and managing these disorders through lifestyle interventions and, when necessary, medical treatments, is crucial for maintaining cardiovascular wellness in men undergoing andropause.

Improving Sleep Quality for Better Heart Health

Sleep quality plays a critical role in maintaining heart health, particularly for men undergoing andropause. As hormonal changes occur during this life stage, they can lead to sleep disturbances such as insomnia or sleep apnoea, which negatively impact cardiovascular wellness. Adequate sleep is essential for the body to repair itself, regulate hormones, and manage stress levels, all of which are crucial for a healthy heart. By addressing sleep quality, men can significantly enhance their overall cardiovascular health and well-being during andropause.

Implementing lifestyle modifications can profoundly influence sleep quality. Simple practices like establishing a regular sleep schedule, creating a calming bedtime routine, and optimising the sleep environment can help improve restfulness. Reducing exposure to screens before bedtime and avoiding stimulants like caffeine and nicotine in the evening are also effective strategies. Health care personnel should encourage men to adopt these habits, as they can lead to better sleep and, consequently, better heart health.

Nutrition also plays a vital role in sleep quality and cardiovascular health. A balanced diet rich in whole foods, such as fruits, vegetables, whole grains, and lean proteins, can support both restful sleep and heart function. Specific nutrients, such as magnesium and omega-3 fatty acids, are known to promote better sleep and reduce inflammation in the body. Health care providers should emphasise the importance of dietary choices that not only aid sleep but also contribute to overall heart health.

Mental health is another critical factor influencing sleep quality and heart health during andropause. Many men experience anxiety or depression as they navigate hormonal changes, which can further exacerbate sleep disorders. Addressing mental health through therapy, stress management techniques, and social support can improve sleep quality and ultimately benefit cardiovascular health. Encouraging open discussions about mental well-being can empower men to seek help and make positive changes.

Finally, incorporating regular exercise into daily routines is essential for both improving sleep quality and promoting heart health. Physical activity helps regulate sleep patterns and reduces stress, which can positively impact cardiovascular function. Health care professionals should recommend tailored exercise regimens suitable for men experiencing heart issues related to andropause. By focusing on holistic approaches that include sleep, nutrition, mental health, and exercise, men can enhance their cardiovascular wellness during this challenging life stage.

Pause for Thought

- As testosterone levels decline, various physiological changes occur which can affect heart health. This decline may lead to increased risk of cardiovascular disease due to factors such as altered lipid profiles, insulin sensitivity and changes in vascular function, understanding this relationship lays the basis for effective management strategies.
- Testosterone influences several aspects of cardiovascular health including endothelial function and inflammation. Low testosterone levels have been associated with increased arterial stiffness and higher levels of inflammatory markers, which may contribute to the development of atherosclerosis. Furthermore, hormonal imbalances can affect mood and

mental health, further complicating cardiovascular wellbeing during andropause.

- Lifestyle modifications are vital in managing heart health during andropause. Regular exercise, a balanced diet, and stress management techniques can help improve cardiovascular function and mitigate the effects of hormonal changes engaging in physical activity not only enhances cardiovascular fitness but also positively influences hormone levels, creating a beneficial feedback loop.
- Nutritional approaches also play a significant role in supporting heart health for middle aged men. Diets rich in omega -3 fatty acids, antioxidants and fibre can help improve cardio-vascular health. Foods such as fatty fish, nuts and whole grains should be emphasised to counteract the effects of hormonal decline.
- Factors such as depression and anxiety can lead to unhealthy lifestyle choices, which may exacerbate heart issues. Addressing mental health through therapy, social support and lifestyle changes can improve overall health outcomes.
- It is essential that healthcare providers recognize the interconnectedness of hormonal changes, mental health and cardiovascular health so that more comprehensive care plan can be extended to men through this challenging life stage.
- Heart health is a critical concern for men during andropause, as hormonal changes can significantly impact cardiovascular function.

Essential nutrients play a pivotal role in supporting heart health. Key nutrients such as omega-3 fatty acids, fibre and antioxidants are vital in reducing inflammation and improving heart function. Adequate intake of these nutrients can help mitigate the risks of heart disease which tends to increase during andropause.

- Fibre is an essential nutrient that plays a significant role in heart health. A diet rich in soluble fibre, found in oats, beans and fruits, can help lower cholesterol levels and improve overall heart function. As men age their digestion may slow down which makes it important to ensure a fibre rich diet to support not only heart health but also digestive wellbeing.
- Antioxidants, specifically vitamins C and E are crucial in combatting oxidative stress, which can lead to cardiovascular problems. Foods rich in these vitamins, such as berries, nuts and green leafy vegetables should be staples in the diet of men facing andropause. These nutrients help protect the heart by neutralising free radical and supporting endothelial function, which is vital for maintaining healthy blood vessels.
- Limitations on the use of processed foods, added sugars and excessive sodium are equally important in establishing a heart healthy diet. These foods can contribute to weight gain, hypertension, and elevated cholesterol levels, all of which pose risks for cardiovascular health. Men should therefore aim to minimise their intake of these harmful substances while increasing their intake of fibre rich foods which can help in

managing cholesterol levels and maintaining a healthy weight. Hydration also plays a crucial role in cardiovascular health.

Take Home Nuggets

- When addressing the dietary needs of men undergoing andropause, it is essential to focus on foods that promote cardiovascular health. Incorporating fruits and vegetable rich in antioxidants can help combat oxidative stress, which is crucial as men experience hormonal changes. Whole grains such as oats and brown rice, provide necessary that supports heart function and helps maintain healthy cholesterol levels. Additionally, sources of lean protein like fish, chicken and legumes are important for muscle maintenance and overall wellbeing during this transitional phase.
- Foods like trans fats, often found in processed foods and fried items, can elevate cholesterol levels and increase the likelihood of heart disease. High sodium intake, commonly present in processed and packaged foods can lead to hypertension though its ability to cause the body to retain water, thus increasing blood volume and pressure , it can cause nerve activation, inflammation and vascular changes that stiffen arteries, all contributing to higher resistance and causing the heart to work harder. A holistic approach to nutrition should include consideration of mental health, as emotional wellbeing can significantly impact heart health. Encouraging the intake of foods that support mood, such as those rich in omega-3 s and antioxidants can help manage stress and anxiety during

andropause. Engaging in regular physical activity alongside a balanced diet, will further enhance cardiovascular wellbeing and alleviate some of the mental health challenges faced during this stage of life.

- The hormonal fluctuations seen in andropause can lead to feelings of depression, anxiety and a general sense of malaise, which can significantly impact cardiovascular health. Hence it is important to understand the mind-body connection which can aid in the development of comprehensive care plans that address both the psychological and physiological concerns.
- The emotional turmoil associated with andropause can manifest as stress, which is a well-known factor for cardiovascular disease. Elevated stress levels can lead to unhealthy lifestyle choices, including poor dietary habits and lack of physical activity further exacerbating heart health issues.
- Engaging in physical activity can lead to improved heart function, better circulation, and a strengthened cardiovascular system, making it an essential component of a heart-healthy lifestyle for middle aged men.
- A well-rounded exercise regime that includes aerobic, strength training and flexibility exercise can significantly contribute to improved heart health. Aerobic exercise such as walking, cycling, and swimming are essential exercise components for heart health, strength training help to combat muscle loss associated with andropause. Incorporating weightlifting or resistance bands into an exercise regime can improve

muscle mass which in turn supports metabolic health and cardiovascular function.

- Flexibility and balance exercises such as yoga or tai chi should not be overlooked. By promoting flexibility and balance, these exercises also reduce the risk of falls and consequent injuries, making it easier for men to remain active.
- Understanding the role of supplements can be crucial for maintaining cardiovascular health as men experience hormonal changes during this phase, the body may require additional nutritional support to effectively manage heart function. Omega-3 fatty acids, coenzyme Q-10 and magnesium are known supplements which contribute positively to cardio-vascular health.
- Men should consult with their health care providers before starting any supplementation regime ensuring that their specific needs and overall health are considered. A holistic approach that includes dietary modifications, exercise and mental health support with appropriate use of supplements can lead to an improved outcome for men.

Chapter 8
Erectile Dysfunction

Understanding Erectile Dysfunction

Definition and Overview

Erectile dysfunction (ED) is defined as the persistent inability to achieve or maintain an erection sufficient for satisfactory sexual performance. This condition affects millions of men worldwide and can stem from a myriad of causes, including physical, psychological, and lifestyle factors. Understanding the complexities of ED requires a comprehensive approach that encompasses not only the physiological aspects but also psychological, relational, and cultural dimensions. As the medical landscape evolves, modern management strategies focus on a holistic view that addresses the multifaceted nature of erectile dysfunction.

Modern management of ED has witnessed significant advancements, particularly in the realms of psychological approaches and nutritional interventions. Psychological factors, such as anxiety and depression, can play a crucial role in the manifestation of ED. Cognitive-behavioural therapy and other psychological interventions have shown promise in alleviating these issues, thereby improving sexual function. Concurrently, nutritional interventions, including dietary changes and supplements, are gaining recognition for their potential benefits in enhancing erectile function and overall health. This intersection of mental and physical health underscores the importance of a comprehensive treatment plan.

The impact of technology on ED treatment cannot be overstated. Telemedicine has emerged as a pivotal tool, enabling patients to access care and support from the comfort of their homes. This is particularly beneficial for those who may feel uncomfortable discussing their condition in person. Furthermore, advances in medical devices, such as vacuum erection devices and penile implants, offer innovative solutions for men with ED. These technological advancements not only improve accessibility but also enhance the efficacy of treatment options available today.

Exercise and physical activity are integral components of managing erectile dysfunction. Regular physical activity has been associated with improved cardiovascular health, which is crucial since many ED cases are linked to vascular issues. Exercise helps to enhance blood flow, reduce stress, and improve overall well-being, all of which can contribute to better erectile function. Encouraging men to adopt a more active lifestyle can be a key strategy in both prevention and treatment of ED, emphasizing the interconnectedness of physical health and sexual performance.

Lastly, the dynamics of relationships and cultural perspectives play a significant role in how ED is perceived and managed. The stigma surrounding erectile dysfunction can create barriers to seeking help, affecting not only the individual but also their partner. Open communication within relationships is essential for addressing the emotional and psychological ramifications of ED.

Furthermore, cultural attitudes toward masculinity and sexuality can influence treatment-seeking behaviour and acceptance of various management strategies. Understanding these dynamics is crucial for healthcare providers and researchers alike, as they work toward developing effective, culturally sensitive interventions for erectile dysfunction.

Causes of Erectile Dysfunction

Erectile dysfunction (ED) can stem from a myriad of causes that intertwine physiological, psychological, and lifestyle factors. On a physiological level, vascular health plays a crucial role in erectile function. Conditions such as atherosclerosis, hypertension, and diabetes can impede blood flow, making it difficult to achieve or maintain an erection. Neurological disorders, including Parkinson's disease and multiple sclerosis, can also disrupt the nerve signals essential for an erection. Hormonal imbalances, particularly involving testosterone, can further exacerbate these issues, leading to diminished sexual desire and erectile difficulties.

Psychological factors are equally significant contributors to erectile dysfunction. Anxiety, depression, and stress can create a cycle where the fear of failure in sexual performance leads to increased anxiety, further hindering the ability to achieve an erection. Relationship dynamics can amplify these psychological impacts; conflicts or unresolved issues between partners may create an environment that is less conducive to intimacy, thereby affecting sexual performance. Understanding these psychological underpinnings is vital for developing effective treatment strategies that address not only the physical but also emotional and relational aspects of ED.

Lifestyle choices are another integral component influencing erectile function. Poor nutrition, lack of physical activity, and substance abuse can negatively impact overall health and, by extension, sexual health. Diets high in saturated fats and sugars can contribute to obesity and cardiovascular issues, which are known risk factors for erectile dysfunction. Conversely, regular exercise has been shown to improve circulation and boost testosterone levels, thereby enhancing erectile function. By adopting healthier lifestyle habits, men can often mitigate some of the risk factors associated with ED.

Advancements in technology and medicine have introduced new avenues for the management of erectile dysfunction. Telemedicine solutions allow for greater accessibility to healthcare providers, enabling men to seek advice and treatment options from the comfort of their homes. Additionally, innovative medical devices, such as vacuum erection devices and penile implants, have provided alternatives for those who may not respond to traditional treatments. These developments reflect a growing recognition of the importance of personalized care in dealing with erectile dysfunction, where each patient's unique circumstances dictate the most effective approach.

Cultural perspectives also play a crucial role in shaping attitudes toward erectile dysfunction and its treatment. In some cultures, discussing sexual health openly is stigmatized, leading men to suffer in silence rather than seek help. This cultural reluctance can perpetuate feelings of inadequacy and shame, further worsening the psychological aspects of ED. Education and awareness are essential in breaking down these barriers, promoting a more open discourse around sexual health, and ensuring that men feel empowered to seek assistance. By understanding the multifaceted causes of erectile dysfunction, individuals and healthcare providers can work together to create comprehensive management plans that address the needs of men and their partners effectively.

Prevalence and Demographics

Erectile dysfunction (ED) is a prevalent condition that affects a significant portion of the male population worldwide. Research indicates that approximately 30 million men in the United States alone experience ED, with prevalence rates increasing with age. It is estimated that about 40% of men in their 40s and nearly 70% of men in their 70s encounter some degree of erectile dysfunction. These statistics underscore the importance of understanding the demographics and factors contributing to ED, as they can inform both treatment strategies and the development of effective management programs.

Demographically, erectile dysfunction does not discriminate, affecting men across various age groups, ethnicities, and socioeconomic backgrounds. However, certain populations are more susceptible to the condition. Studies suggest that men with chronic health issues such as diabetes, hypertension, and cardiovascular disease are at a higher risk for developing ED. Additionally, lifestyle factors such as smoking, obesity, and sedentary behaviour contribute significantly to the incidence of erectile dysfunction, emphasizing the need for targeted interventions that consider these risk factors.

Psychological influences also play a crucial role in the prevalence of erectile dysfunction. Conditions such as anxiety, depression, and stress are commonly associated with ED, creating a complex interplay between psychological well-being and sexual health. Research shows that men experiencing psychological distress are more likely to report difficulties with erectile function. This highlights the importance of addressing mental health as part of a comprehensive approach to managing erectile dysfunction, particularly in younger men who may face unique pressures related to performance and self-esteem.

Cultural perspectives on erectile dysfunction significantly shape how the condition is perceived and treated. In some cultures, societal stigma surrounding ED can deter men from seeking help, leading to underreporting and untreated cases. Conversely, in more open societies, there is a growing acceptance of discussing sexual health issues, resulting in increased demand for modern treatments and interventions. Understanding these cultural nuances is vital for healthcare providers and researchers aiming to improve access to care and tailor educational resources that resonate with diverse populations.

Finally, advances in technology have transformed the landscape of erectile dysfunction management. The rise of telemedicine, for instance, has made it easier for men to access care without the embarrassment often associated with discussing sexual health issues in person. Additionally, innovations in medical devices and nutritional interventions are providing new avenues for treatment, catering to the varied needs of individuals seeking relief from erectile dysfunction. As research continues to evolve, it is essential to stay informed about these developments to ensure effective and comprehensive care for men dealing with this common condition.

Modern Management of Erectile Dysfunction

Traditional Treatments

Traditional treatments for erectile dysfunction (ED) have long been the cornerstone of management strategies, offering a range of options that have stood the test of time. Commonly, these treatments include oral medications, injections, vacuum erection devices, and penile implants. Oral phosphodiesterase type 5 inhibitors, such as sildenafil, tadalafil, and vardenafil, are among the most recognized and widely used. These medications work by enhancing blood flow to the penis, thereby facilitating an erection in response to sexual stimulation. Their effectiveness has made them a first-line treatment for many men experiencing ED.

In addition to oral medications, intracavernosal injections have gained popularity as an alternative for those who may not respond to oral therapies. This method involves injecting medication directly into the corpora cavernosa of the penis, resulting in an erection within minutes. The most used agents for injection include alprostadil, papaverine, and phentolamine. While this treatment can be effective, it requires careful patient education to ensure proper technique and minimize discomfort or complications. For some men, the idea of self-injection can be daunting, but with appropriate support and guidance, many find it a viable option.

Vacuum erection devices (VEDs) are another traditional approach to managing ED, particularly for men who prefer a non-invasive method. These devices create a vacuum around the penis, drawing blood into the organ and facilitating an erection. Once achieved, a constriction ring is placed at the base of the penis to maintain the erection during intercourse. VEDs are often recommended for men with certain medical conditions, such as diabetes or cardiovascular disease, where other treatments may pose risks. While VEDs can be effective, they require practice and can be less spontaneous than other methods.

Penile implants represent a more invasive yet permanent solution for men with severe ED who have not found success with other treatments. These devices are surgically placed inside the penis and can be inflated or deflated as needed, allowing for greater control over the timing of sexual activity. Despite the surgical risks, penile implants have high satisfaction rates among patients, offering a reliable option for restoring sexual function. Men considering this option should engage in thorough discussions with their healthcare providers to understand the benefits and potential complications.

While traditional treatments remain integral to managing erectile dysfunction, their effectiveness can be influenced by psychological, relational, and lifestyle factors. Many men may benefit from complementary approaches, such as counselling, lifestyle modifications, and nutritional interventions, which address underlying causes or contributing factors to ED. As research continues to evolve, combining traditional methods with modern solutions may provide a more holistic approach to managing erectile dysfunction, improving not only sexual function but overall quality of life for men and their partners.

Emerging Therapies

Emerging therapies for erectile dysfunction (ED) represent a significant frontier in the management of this condition, addressing not only physiological aspects but also encompassing psychological, nutritional, and technological interventions. Traditional treatments, such as oral medications and injections, have paved the way for innovative approaches that seek to enhance effectiveness and improve patient outcomes. These emerging therapies are increasingly personalized, considering the diverse factors contributing to ED, which may include hormonal imbalances, psychological distress, and lifestyle choices.

One notable advancement in the realm of psychological approaches involves cognitive-behavioural therapy (CBT), which aims to address the mental health aspects associated with ED. Research indicates that psychological factors, such as anxiety and depression, can significantly hinder erectile function. By utilizing CBT techniques, men can learn to reframe negative thoughts, reduce performance anxiety, and ultimately improve their sexual health. Additionally, couples therapy has gained traction, emphasizing the importance of communication and emotional intimacy in overcoming the challenges posed by ED.

Nutritional interventions have also emerged as a vital component in the management of erectile dysfunction. A growing body of evidence suggests that diets rich in fruits, vegetables, whole grains, and lean proteins can enhance erectile function by improving cardiovascular health and reducing inflammation. Specific dietary patterns, such as the Mediterranean diet, have shown promise in promoting healthy blood flow and hormone regulation. Furthermore, supplements like L-arginine and ginseng are being explored for their potential benefits in enhancing nitric oxide production, which is crucial for achieving and maintaining an erection.

Integrative Approaches

Integrative approaches to managing erectile dysfunction (ED) are gaining traction as they combine multiple therapeutic modalities to address the complex nature of this condition. Traditional treatments often focus on pharmacological solutions, but integrative strategies recognize that ED can stem from various factors, including psychological, physiological, and relational dimensions. By understanding and addressing these interrelated components, men, couples, and healthcare professionals can create a more holistic treatment plan that enhances overall well-being and sexual health.

Psychological interventions play a crucial role in the integrative management of ED. Cognitive-behavioural therapy (CBT), mindfulness practices, and counselling can help address underlying anxiety, depression, or relationship issues that may contribute to erectile difficulties. By fostering better communication between partners and reducing performance anxiety, these psychological approaches can significantly improve sexual function. Couples therapy can also be beneficial, as it encourages partners to work together to overcome challenges, thus reinforcing emotional intimacy and support.

Nutritional interventions are another essential aspect of an integrative approach. Diet plays a significant role in sexual health, and certain foods have been shown to enhance blood flow, hormone levels, and overall vitality. Diets rich in fruits, vegetables, whole grains, and healthy fats can support vascular health and hormonal balance, which are crucial for erectile function. Additionally, specific nutrients, such as zinc, L-arginine, and omega-3 fatty acids, have been linked to improved sexual health. Educating men and couples about making informed dietary choices can empower them to take charge of their sexual health.

Exercise and physical activity represent vital components of an integrative strategy for managing ED. Regular physical activity helps to improve cardiovascular health, reduce stress, and enhance overall physical fitness, all of which can positively impact erectile function. Exercise increases blood flow and can improve self-esteem and body image, which are often closely connected to sexual performance. Tailored exercise programs that include both aerobic and strength-training elements can be particularly effective in promoting sexual health.

Finally, the role of technology in managing erectile dysfunction cannot be overlooked. Advances in medical devices, telemedicine solutions, and digital health applications provide new avenues for treatment and support. These tools can facilitate remote consultations with healthcare providers, making it easier for men to access care and receive personalized recommendations. The convenience of technology can help reduce stigma and encourage more individuals to seek help, ultimately leading to better outcomes. By integrating these various approaches, men and their partners can create a comprehensive and personalized plan to address erectile dysfunction effectively.

Psychological Approaches to Erectile Dysfunction Management

Cognitive Behavioural Therapy

Cognitive Behavioural Therapy (CBT) has emerged as a vital psychological approach in addressing erectile dysfunction (ED), particularly when the condition has psychological underpinnings. CBT focuses on the interplay between thoughts, feelings, and behaviours, and aims to modify negative thought patterns that can contribute to sexual dysfunction. For many men, anxiety, depression, and low self-esteem can create a cycle of fear and avoidance that exacerbates ED. By employing CBT techniques, individuals can learn to identify and challenge these detrimental thoughts, ultimately fostering a healthier mindset towards sexual performance and intimacy.

The structured nature of CBT often includes specific techniques such as cognitive restructuring, where patients are guided to replace irrational beliefs with more rational and positive thoughts. This process not only alleviates the psychological burdens associated with ED but also empowers men to regain confidence in their sexual health. Moreover, CBT sessions typically involve behavioural interventions, including gradual exposure to sexual situations that may have previously been anxiety-inducing. This gradual approach helps in reducing performance anxiety, which is a significant barrier for many men facing ED.

Couples experiencing ED can also benefit from CBT as it encourages open communication and shared problem-solving. Relationship dynamics play a crucial role in sexual health, and when one partner struggles with ED, it can create tension and misunderstanding. Through CBT, couples can engage in joint sessions that focus on enhancing intimacy and reducing the stigma often associated with erectile issues. This collaborative approach not only improves the individual's experience but also strengthens the relationship, fostering a supportive environment that can lead to improved sexual satisfaction.

Research has shown that CBT can be as effective as pharmacological treatments for ED, particularly in cases where psychological factors are predominant. By integrating CBT into a comprehensive treatment plan, individuals and couples can explore not just the symptoms but also the underlying issues that contribute to erectile dysfunction. Furthermore, the accessibility of teletherapy solutions has made CBT more convenient for those seeking help, allowing men to engage in therapy from the comfort of their own homes, thus reducing the stigma and anxiety associated with seeking treatment.

In conclusion, Cognitive Behavioural Therapy offers a modern and effective psychological approach to managing erectile dysfunction. By addressing the cognitive and emotional aspects of ED, CBT not only enhances individual well-being but also improves relationship dynamics. As men, couples, and researchers continue to explore the multifaceted nature of erectile dysfunction, the integration of CBT into treatment protocols represents a promising avenue for holistic management, encouraging both psychological resilience and enhanced sexual health.

Mindfulness and Relaxation Techniques

Mindfulness and relaxation techniques have gained recognition as valuable tools in managing erectile dysfunction (ED). These practices focus on enhancing mental clarity, reducing stress, and promoting emotional well-being—all of which are essential for a healthy sexual function. Research has shown that psychological factors such as anxiety, stress, and negative self-image can significantly influence erectile performance. By integrating mindfulness and relaxation techniques into daily routines, men can cultivate a more positive mindset, which may contribute to improved sexual health and intimacy.

Mindfulness involves being fully present in the moment without judgment. This practice encourages individuals to focus on their thoughts, feelings, and bodily sensations, allowing them to recognize and manage stressors that may impact their sexual performance. Techniques such as deep breathing, meditation, and guided imagery can be beneficial in creating a relaxed state of mind. For men experiencing ED, these practices can alleviate performance anxiety, foster a sense of control and reduce the fear of failure during intimate moments.

Relaxation techniques, including progressive muscle relaxation and yoga, can also play a critical role in managing erectile dysfunction. These methods work to release physical tension and promote a state of calm. Engaging in regular physical activity, such as yoga, not only enhances flexibility and strength but also serves as a means to connect with one's body. This connection can diminish feelings of disconnection or inadequacy that often accompany ED. Furthermore, yoga and similar practices are known to improve circulation, which can be beneficial for erectile function.

Couples can also benefit from practicing mindfulness and relaxation techniques together. Engaging in shared experiences such as meditation or yoga can strengthen emotional bonds and improve communication. This shared focus can foster intimacy and reduce the pressure associated with sexual performance. By creating a supportive environment, couples can navigate the challenges of ED collaboratively, reinforcing the idea that they are in this journey together rather than facing it in isolation.

Incorporating mindfulness and relaxation techniques into one's lifestyle can be a significant step toward addressing the psychological and emotional aspects of erectile dysfunction. As men and their partners work to enhance their connection and manage stress, they may find that these practices not only improve their sexual health but also enrich their overall quality of life. As research continues to explore the intersection of mental health and sexual function, mindfulness and relaxation techniques stand out as promising avenues for holistic ED management.

Addressing Anxiety and Depression

Addressing anxiety and depression is a critical component in the comprehensive management of erectile dysfunction (ED). The interrelationship between psychological health and sexual function is well documented, with anxiety and depression frequently cited as underlying causes of ED. Men experiencing these emotional challenges may find it difficult to achieve or maintain an erection, creating a vicious cycle of fear and performance anxiety. Understanding how these psychological factors contribute to ED is essential for developing effective treatment strategies that encompass both mental and physical health.

Psychological approaches to managing ED often begin with therapeutic interventions aimed at alleviating anxiety and depression. Cognitive-behavioural therapy (CBT) has been shown to be particularly effective in addressing maladaptive thoughts and behaviours that contribute to sexual dysfunction. By working with a qualified therapist, men can learn to reframe negative thought patterns and develop coping strategies for managing anxiety in sexual situations. Additionally, couples therapy can be beneficial, as it fosters open communication between partners and helps to address relational dynamics that may exacerbate feelings of inadequacy and distress.

Nutritional interventions also play a role in addressing the psychological aspects of ED. A well-balanced diet rich in fruits, vegetables, whole grains, and healthy fats can positively influence mood and overall mental health. Certain nutrients, such as omega-3 fatty acids and antioxidants, have been linked to reduced symptoms of anxiety and depression. By incorporating these nutritional strategies, men can not only improve their physical health but also bolster their psychological resilience, creating a solid foundation for sexual wellness.

Exercise and physical activity are crucial for managing both erectile dysfunction and mental health issues like anxiety and depression. Regular physical activity has been shown to reduce symptoms of anxiety and depression through the release of endorphins and improved self-esteem. Furthermore, exercise can enhance blood flow and overall cardiovascular health, which are vital for erectile function. A tailored exercise regimen that includes both aerobic and strength training can provide significant benefits, helping men feel more empowered and in control of their bodies and their sexual health.

Finally, the impact of technology on ED treatment cannot be overlooked. Telemedicine offers an accessible platform for men to seek help for anxiety and depression without the stigma often associated with seeking mental health support. Online therapy services and mental health apps can provide immediate resources and support, bridging the gap between psychological care and sexual health management. By leveraging modern technology, men can access comprehensive care that addresses both their mental and sexual health needs, fostering a holistic approach to overcoming erectile dysfunction.

Nutritional Interventions for Erectile Dysfunction

Dietary Modifications

Dietary modifications play a crucial role in managing erectile dysfunction (ED), as nutrition directly influences overall health, blood circulation, and hormonal balance. A diet rich in fruits, vegetables, whole grains, and healthy fats can enhance vascular health, which is essential for erectile function. Specific nutrients, such as antioxidants and amino acids, are vital for improving blood flow and reducing oxidative stress within the body. For men experiencing ED, it is beneficial to adopt a diet that supports cardiovascular health, as heart-related issues are often linked to erectile problems. Foods high in nitrates, such as leafy greens and beets, can help improve blood flow by dilating blood vessels, thereby potentially alleviating some symptoms of ED.

Incorporating specific dietary patterns, like the Mediterranean diet, has shown promise in studies focusing on ED management. This diet emphasizes whole foods, healthy fats from sources like olive oil, and lean proteins, which contribute to improved heart health and circulation. The inclusion of fish, nuts, and legumes provides essential fatty acids and nutrients that support hormonal balance and overall vitality. Moreover, reducing the intake of processed foods, sugars, and unhealthy fats can mitigate the risk factors associated with ED, such as obesity and diabetes. By prioritizing nutrient-dense foods, men can create a foundation for not only improved erectile function but also enhanced overall well-being.

Hydration is another often overlooked aspect of dietary modifications that can impact erectile function. Adequate hydration is essential for maintaining optimal blood volume and circulation. Dehydration can lead to decreased blood flow and increased fatigue, both of which can contribute to ED. Men should aim to drink sufficient water throughout the day, along with incorporating hydrating foods such as cucumbers, oranges, and watermelons into their diet. Additionally, limiting alcohol and caffeine intake is essential, as excessive consumption can negatively affect libido and erectile function.

Beyond specific foods and hydration, it is also important to consider the timing and frequency of meals. Eating smaller, more frequent meals can help maintain energy levels and prevent the blood from diverting away from the genitals during digestion. On the other hand, heavy meals can lead to sluggishness and decreased sexual desire. Men should aim for balanced meals that include a combination of protein, healthy fats, and complex carbohydrates to sustain energy and maximize performance. Additionally, incorporating foods that are rich in zinc and vitamin D, such as shellfish and fortified dairy products, can support testosterone production, further benefiting erectile function.

Lastly, dietary modifications should be viewed as part of a comprehensive approach to managing erectile dysfunction. While nutrition plays a significant role, it should be complemented by other lifestyle changes such as regular exercise, stress management, and open communication within relationships. Addressing psychological factors through counselling or therapy is equally important, as mental health can significantly impact sexual health. By combining dietary adjustments with holistic approaches, men can take significant steps toward improving their erectile function and enhancing their quality of life.

Supplements and Natural Remedies

Supplements and natural remedies have gained popularity as complementary approaches in the management of erectile dysfunction (ED). Many men seeking alternatives to pharmaceutical interventions often turn to these options, hoping to improve their sexual health without the side effects associated with conventional medications. Commonly used supplements include L-arginine, ginseng, and ginkgo biloba, each of which has been studied for its potential to enhance blood flow and improve erectile function. These natural agents may work by increasing nitric oxide levels, promoting vasodilation, and improving overall cardiovascular health, which is crucial for achieving and maintaining an erection.

L-arginine, an amino acid, is frequently cited in discussions about supplements for ED. It plays a vital role in the production of nitric oxide, a compound that relaxes blood vessels and facilitates increased blood flow to the penis. Research has shown that men with ED may have lower levels of nitric oxide, leading to impaired erectile function. Supplementing with L-arginine could potentially address this deficiency, although results can vary among individuals. It's essential for users to consult healthcare professionals before starting any supplementation, as the efficacy and safety of L-arginine can depend on underlying health conditions and concurrent medications.

Ginseng, particularly Korean red ginseng, has also been linked to improved sexual function. Traditionally used in herbal medicine, ginseng is believed to enhance energy levels and reduce fatigue, factors that can significantly impact sexual performance. Some studies have indicated that ginseng might help with erection quality and overall sexual satisfaction. However, like other supplements, the outcomes may not be universal, and more rigorous clinical trials are needed to establish definitive guidelines regarding its use in ED treatment.

Another natural remedy, ginkgo biloba, is often discussed for its potential benefits in improving blood circulation. While ginkgo is primarily known for its cognitive enhancement properties, its role in increasing blood flow could have implications for erectile function. Some men report positive experiences with ginkgo supplementation, yet scientific evidence remains inconclusive, underscoring the need for further research to determine its effectiveness and safety. Men considering ginkgo as a treatment option should be aware of potential interactions with other medications, particularly anticoagulants.

In conclusion, while supplements and natural remedies for erectile dysfunction present a promising avenue for some individuals, they should not be viewed as a replacement for comprehensive medical evaluation and treatment. The integration of these alternatives into a broader management plan—encompassing psychological support, lifestyle modifications, and medical interventions—can provide a more holistic approach to addressing ED. Men, couples, and researchers must continue to explore the efficacy and safety of these natural options, ensuring that any approach taken is well-informed and tailored to the individual's specific health needs.

The Role of Hydration

The role of hydration in managing erectile dysfunction (ED) is often overlooked, yet it plays a crucial part in overall sexual health and function. Proper hydration is essential for maintaining optimal blood circulation, which is vital for achieving and sustaining an erection. Blood vessels need to be adequately hydrated to function efficiently, as dehydration can lead to a reduction in blood volume and, consequently, blood flow. This diminished blood flow can directly impact erectile function, making it more difficult for men to achieve the hardness necessary for sexual activity. Therefore, understanding the significance of hydration is paramount for men seeking to improve their sexual health.

In addition to its effects on blood circulation, hydration influences hormonal balance, which is critical in managing erectile dysfunction. Hormones such as testosterone play a significant role in sexual desire and performance. Dehydration can lead to an imbalance in the body's hormone levels, potentially diminishing libido and sexual function. Ensuring adequate fluid intake supports the body's natural processes, including hormone regulation. For men experiencing ED, maintaining proper hydration can be a simple yet effective strategy to support hormonal health and enhance sexual performance.

Moreover, hydration has implications for overall physical performance, which can indirectly affect erectile dysfunction. Regular physical activity is an important factor in managing ED, and staying hydrated is key to maintaining stamina and endurance during exercise. When men are well-hydrated, they are more likely to engage in regular physical activity, which has been shown to improve erectile function. Exercise not only promotes cardiovascular health but also helps in weight management and reduces stress levels, all of which are beneficial for sexual health. Therefore, hydration can be seen as a foundational element that supports a more active lifestyle, ultimately contributing to improved erectile function.

The impact of hydration extends beyond physical health; it also plays a role in psychological well-being. Dehydration can lead to fatigue, irritability, and decreased cognitive function, all of which can negatively affect mental health and, by extension, sexual performance. Psychological factors are often intertwined with erectile dysfunction, as anxiety and stress can create a cycle that exacerbates the condition. By ensuring adequate hydration, individuals may find themselves in a better mental state, which can help alleviate the psychological barriers associated with ED. This highlights the importance of viewing hydration not just as a physical necessity but as a holistic approach to managing erectile dysfunction.

In conclusion, hydration is a vital yet sometimes underestimated aspect of managing erectile dysfunction. Its effects on blood circulation, hormonal balance, physical performance, and psychological well-being underscore its importance in the overall approach to sexual health. For men, couples, and researchers alike, recognizing the role of hydration in the context of erectile dysfunction can lead to more effective strategies for management. By integrating proper hydration practices into daily life, individuals may experience significant improvements in their sexual health and overall quality of life.

Impact of Technology on Erectile Dysfunction Treatment

Digital Health Innovations

Digital health innovations have revolutionized the landscape of erectile dysfunction (ED management), offering new avenues for diagnosis, treatment, and ongoing care. These technological advancements encompass a wide range of applications, from mobile health apps that track symptoms and treatment efficacy to telemedicine platforms that facilitate remote consultations with healthcare professionals. By harnessing the power of technology, individuals can access information, resources, and support systems that were previously limited to in-person visits and traditional healthcare models.

One significant aspect of digital health innovations is the development of mobile applications designed specifically for men experiencing ED. These apps provide users with tailored exercise programs, nutritional advice, and psychological support, creating a holistic approach to managing their condition. By allowing users to monitor their symptoms and progress, these tools empower men to take an active role in their health. Additionally, many apps include educational resources that help demystify erectile dysfunction, encouraging users to engage in open conversations about their experiences and reducing the stigma often associated with the condition.

Telemedicine has emerged as a vital component in the management of erectile dysfunction, especially in response to the growing demand for accessible healthcare options. Through virtual consultations, patients can connect with specialists from the comfort of their own homes, ensuring that even those in remote areas or with mobility challenges receive the care they need. This approach not only increases the reach of healthcare providers but also offers a level of privacy and convenience that can be particularly beneficial for individuals hesitant to seek in-person treatment for ED.

Moreover, wearable technology has begun to play a role in monitoring and managing erectile dysfunction. Devices such as smartwatches and fitness trackers can collect data on physical activity, sleep patterns, and heart health, all of which are critical factors influencing erectile function. By integrating these insights into a comprehensive health management plan, men can make informed lifestyle changes that contribute to improved sexual health. Additionally, some devices are designed to aid in the treatment of ED by providing biofeedback or other therapeutic interventions, further enhancing their utility in a modern treatment regimen.

As the field of digital health continues to evolve, it is essential for men, couples, and researchers to remain informed about these innovations. Understanding the potential benefits and limitations of digital tools can facilitate better decision-making regarding treatment options. As technology becomes increasingly integrated into healthcare, the future of erectile dysfunction management looks promising, with the potential for enhanced outcomes and greater patient engagement.

Mobile Applications for Monitoring

Mobile applications for monitoring erectile dysfunction (ED) represent a significant advancement in the management of this condition, leveraging technology to provide users with tools for self-assessment, tracking, and improving their sexual health. These applications offer features that allow men to log their symptoms, track their medication usage, and even note lifestyle factors that may impact their erectile function. By facilitating regular self-monitoring, these applications empower users to take an active role in their health, leading to better communication with healthcare providers and improved outcomes.

Many mobile applications incorporate questionnaires and surveys to assess the severity of ED, helping users understand their condition better and identify patterns over time. This data can be invaluable not only for personal insight but also for discussions with healthcare providers. By sharing this information during medical consultations, men can receive tailored advice and treatment options based on their specific needs and experiences, making the management of ED more personalized and effective.

In addition to tracking symptoms, some applications provide educational resources to inform users about the psychological, nutritional, and lifestyle factors that can influence erectile function. By raising awareness of these factors, users can make informed decisions regarding their health. For instance, they might receive reminders to engage in physical activity or suggestions for dietary changes that could enhance their sexual health. This holistic approach aligns well with modern management strategies that emphasize the integration of psychological and physical health.

The impact of technology on erectile dysfunction treatment extends beyond individual monitoring. Many applications now offer features for telemedicine, allowing users to connect with healthcare providers remotely. This can be especially beneficial for men who may feel embarrassed or reluctant to discuss their condition in person. By providing a discreet and convenient way to access care, mobile applications help to reduce the stigma surrounding ED and increase the likelihood that individuals will seek the help they need.

As mobile applications for monitoring erectile dysfunction continue to evolve, they are likely to incorporate more advanced features such as artificial intelligence and data analytics. These innovations could provide users with predictive insights and tailored recommendations based on their specific health profiles. As technology advances, the potential for these applications to enhance the management of ED becomes increasingly promising, offering users a modern solution that reflects the complexities of erectile dysfunction and its treatment.

Online Support Communities

Online support communities have emerged as a vital resource for men experiencing erectile dysfunction (ED), offering a platform for sharing experiences, information, and emotional support. These communities vary in format, ranging from forums and social media groups to dedicated websites and mobile applications. Their primary appeal lies in providing anonymity, which can be crucial for men who may feel embarrassed or stigmatized by their condition. In these spaces, individuals can connect with others facing similar challenges, fostering a sense of camaraderie and understanding that can be profoundly beneficial for mental health.

Participation in online support communities can enhance psychological approaches to ED management. Often, men encounter emotional distress linked to their condition, which can exacerbate the problem. Through interaction with peers, members can discuss coping strategies, share success stories, and receive encouragement. This communal support can help mitigate feelings of isolation and shame, allowing men to approach their condition with a more positive mindset. Additionally, these forums often provide access to expert opinions and evidence-based information, empowering members to make informed decisions regarding their treatment options.

Nutrition plays a critical role in the management of erectile dysfunction, and online communities often serve as platforms for sharing dietary advice and insights. Members frequently exchange tips on nutritional interventions that may improve blood flow and overall health, such as the Mediterranean diet or the incorporation of specific superfoods. By learning from one another's experiences, men can adopt healthier eating habits that contribute to better erectile function. Furthermore, these communities may host discussions about the latest research in nutritional science, helping individuals stay informed about innovations and trends in dietary management.

The impact of technology on ED treatment is another significant topic within online support communities. Many men explore various telemedicine solutions and medical devices designed to address erectile dysfunction. Through discussions, users can share reviews and experiences with different products and services, ranging from prescription medications to vacuum erection devices and innovative apps. This exchange of information facilitates a more comprehensive understanding of available options and encourages men to consider treatments that they may not have previously known about or felt comfortable discussing with healthcare providers.

Finally, online support communities can address the relationship dynamics affected by erectile dysfunction. The emotional toll of ED often extends beyond the individual to their partner, which can lead to communication breakdowns and increased tension in relationships. Within these online spaces, men and their partners can find resources and support aimed at improving their relational health. Discussions on how to foster open communication, rebuild intimacy, and navigate the psychological challenges associated with ED can empower couples to work together towards effective solutions, ultimately strengthening their bond in the face of adversity.

Role of Exercise and Physical Activity in Managing Erectile Dysfunction

Types of Beneficial Exercises

Exercise plays a crucial role in managing erectile dysfunction (ED) by enhancing physical health, boosting mood, and improving circulation. Among the various types of exercises beneficial for ED, cardiovascular activities, strength training, flexibility exercises, pelvic floor exercises, and mind-body practices stand out. Each category contributes uniquely to overall well-being and can have a direct impact on erectile function.

Cardiovascular exercises, such as running, cycling, and swimming, are essential for improving heart health and blood flow. Enhanced cardiovascular fitness can lead to better circulation, which is vital for achieving and maintaining an erection. Engaging in regular aerobic activity helps lower blood pressure and reduces body fat, both of which are linked to improved erectile function. Studies have shown that men who participate in consistent cardiovascular exercise report fewer instances of ED.

Strength training, involving resistance exercises like weightlifting and bodyweight workouts, also plays a critical role in ED management. Building muscle mass not only contributes to physical strength but also boosts testosterone levels, which can be beneficial for sexual health. Incorporating strength training into a weekly exercise routine can improve body composition and increase metabolism, further supporting erectile function. This approach is particularly effective when combined with cardiovascular activities.

Flexibility exercises, including yoga and stretching routines, enhance physical health by improving range of motion and reducing muscle tension. These exercises can help alleviate stress and anxiety, which are often psychological contributors to erectile dysfunction. By promoting relaxation and mindfulness, flexibility training can foster a healthier mental state and improve confidence in sexual performance. The practice of yoga has been linked to improved erectile function through its focus on breath control and stress reduction.

Pelvic floor exercises, commonly known as Kegel exercises, specifically target the muscles involved in erectile function. Strengthening these muscles can enhance control over erections and improve sexual performance. Research indicates that men who regularly perform pelvic floor exercises may experience improved erectile function and greater satisfaction in sexual activities. This type of exercise is discreet, can be done anywhere, and requires no special equipment, making it an accessible option for many men seeking to manage ED.

Mind-body practices, such as tai chi and meditation, can also contribute positively to erectile function by promoting mental well-being. These exercises help reduce stress, anxiety, and depression, which can all play significant roles in erectile dysfunction. By fostering a greater connection between the mind and body, these practices can enhance overall sexual health and improve intimate relationships. Integrating these exercises into a comprehensive approach to managing ED can lead to significant improvements in both physical and psychological aspects of sexual health.

Exercise Guidelines for Men

Exercise plays a crucial role in managing erectile dysfunction (ED), as it contributes to overall health and well-being. For men experiencing ED, regular physical activity can enhance blood circulation, boost testosterone levels, and improve psychological health, all of which are vital for sexual function. The American Heart Association recommends at least 150 minutes of moderate-intensity aerobic exercise or 75 minutes of vigorous-intensity exercise each week. Activities such as brisk walking, cycling, swimming, or jogging can elevate heart rate and improve cardiovascular health, which is essential for erectile function.

Strength training is another important component of an exercise regimen for men dealing with ED. Engaging in resistance training at least two days a week can help increase muscle mass and strength, which in turn can elevate testosterone levels. Exercises such as weightlifting, bodyweight exercises, and resistance band workouts should be incorporated into a balanced fitness plan. These activities not only enhance physical strength but also contribute to improved body image and confidence, which are often affected in men with erectile dysfunction.

Flexibility and balance exercises, such as yoga or tai chi, can also be beneficial. These practices not only promote physical flexibility but also reduce stress and anxiety, which are common psychological factors associated with ED. Stress management through these activities can lead to improved mental health, thus enhancing sexual function. Incorporating mindfulness and relaxation techniques into an exercise routine can foster a more holistic approach to managing erectile dysfunction.

When developing an exercise program, it is essential for men to consider their individual health status and any pre-existing conditions. Consulting with a healthcare professional before starting a new exercise routine is advisable, especially for those with cardiovascular issues or other health concerns. A tailored exercise plan can ensure that the activities chosen are safe and effective, maximizing the potential benefits for erectile function and overall health.

Incorporating exercise into daily life can be a sustainable and empowering approach to managing erectile dysfunction. Setting realistic goals, finding enjoyable activities, and establishing a consistent routine can make a significant difference. Whether it's joining a local sports team, participating in group classes, or simply walking daily, the key is to stay active. As men engage in regular physical activity, they may find not only improvements in erectile function but also in their overall quality of life, relationships, and self-esteem.

Long-term Benefits of Physical Activity

Engaging in regular physical activity offers a multitude of long-term benefits that extend beyond general health, particularly for men experiencing erectile dysfunction (ED). Exercise has been shown to improve cardiovascular health, enhance circulation, and promote hormonal balance, all of which are crucial factors in achieving and maintaining erectile function. The physiological mechanisms underlying these benefits include the improved flow of blood to the pelvic area and the release of endorphins, which can alleviate stress and anxiety—common psychological barriers to sexual performance.

Moreover, physical activity is known to positively influence body composition, reducing the risks associated with obesity, which is a significant risk factor for erectile dysfunction. By maintaining a healthy weight through regular exercise, men can lower their chances of developing diabetes and hypertension, both of which can impair erectile function. Studies have demonstrated that even moderate exercise can lead to significant improvements in these risk factors, thereby enhancing overall sexual health and performance.

In addition to the physical benefits, regular participation in exercise can also serve as a powerful tool for improving mental well-being. Physical activity has been linked to reductions in anxiety and depression, conditions that can severely impact sexual desire and performance. The psychological benefits of exercise can create a more positive self-image and increase confidence, both of which are essential for a healthy sexual life. As men feel better about themselves, they are more likely to engage in intimate relationships, fostering emotional connections that can further alleviate symptoms of erectile dysfunction.

Social interactions that occur through group exercise or sports can also provide psychological benefits. Engaging with others in physical activities can mitigate feelings of isolation and foster a sense of community, further improving mental health. This social support is particularly vital for men experiencing ED, as it encourages open discussions about sexual health and can lead to shared experiences and coping strategies among peers.

Finally, establishing a routine of physical activity can lead to long-lasting lifestyle changes that promote overall health. The commitment to regular exercise can serve as a catalyst for adopting healthier dietary choices and improving sleep patterns, both of which are integral to managing erectile dysfunction. As men incorporate physical activity into their daily lives, they not only improve their sexual health but also enhance their quality of life, fostering a holistic approach to managing erectile dysfunction that encompasses physical, psychological, and social dimensions.

Advances in Medical Devices for Erectile Dysfunction

Vacuum Erection Devices

Vacuum erection devices (VEDs) represent a non-invasive treatment option for men experiencing erectile dysfunction (ED). These devices work by creating a vacuum around the penis, which enhances blood flow and facilitates an erection. VEDs typically consist of a cylindrical chamber, a pump, and a constriction band. When the pump is activated, air is removed from the chamber, resulting in a pressure differential that draws blood into the penis. Once an adequate erection is achieved, the constriction band can be placed at the base of the penis to maintain the erection by preventing blood from flowing back out.

The effectiveness of VEDs has been supported by numerous studies, which indicate that they can successfully produce an erection in a significant percentage of men with ED. They are particularly beneficial for men who may not be suitable candidates for pharmacological treatments due to contraindications or those who prefer non-drug options. Furthermore, VEDs can be used in conjunction with other therapies, offering a holistic approach to managing erectile dysfunction, especially in cases where psychological or relational factors are involved.

While VEDs have proven effective, patient education is crucial for optimal use. Men may initially find the idea of using a mechanical device for sexual function daunting or embarrassing. However, with proper instruction and practice, many users report positive outcomes. It is essential for healthcare providers to address any misconceptions and provide clear guidance on how to operate the device safely and effectively. Additionally, discussing the device with partners can enhance comfort and intimacy, fostering a supportive environment for both parties.

Technological advancements have also played a role in the evolution of VEDs, with newer models offering enhanced features such as automatic pumps, digital pressure gauges, and customizable settings. These innovations aim to improve user experience and outcomes. As men become more comfortable with technology in their healthcare, VEDs can be integrated into a broader telemedicine framework, allowing for virtual consultations and follow-ups that enhance adherence to treatment plans and provide ongoing support.

In conclusion, vacuum erection devices represent a valuable tool in the modern management of erectile dysfunction. They offer a viable alternative for men seeking non-invasive solutions, particularly when psychological factors are at play. The incorporation of technology into VEDs and the potential for telemedicine solutions underscore the importance of adapting to the needs of patients in a rapidly evolving healthcare landscape. As men, couples, and researchers continue to explore the diverse approaches to ED management, VEDs remain a crucial component of a comprehensive treatment strategy.

Penile Implants

Penile implants represent a significant advancement in the management of erectile dysfunction (ED), especially for men who find little relief from oral medications or other non-invasive treatments. These devices are surgically placed within the penis and can provide a reliable solution for achieving an erection. There are two primary types of implants: inflatable and malleable. Inflatable implants consist of fluid-filled cylinders that can be expanded and contracted, allowing for a more natural erection and aesthetic appearance. Malleable implants, on the other hand, are firm rods that can be bent into position when needed, offering simplicity and ease of use.

The decision to pursue a penile implant often comes after a thorough evaluation of the underlying causes of ED, which may include psychological factors, hormonal imbalances, or vascular issues. For many men, the psychological burden of ED can exacerbate the condition, leading to a cycle of anxiety and performance pressure. Therefore, it is essential for healthcare providers to assess not only the physical but also the emotional and relational aspects of a man's health. The process usually involves consultations with urologists, mental health professionals, and possibly partners, ensuring a comprehensive approach to treatment.

Once a man chooses to undergo penile implant surgery, the procedure is typically performed in a hospital setting and may take one to two hours. Recovery times vary, but most men can return to normal activities within a few weeks. The success rates for penile implants are high, with studies indicating that over 90% of men report satisfaction with the results. Moreover, these devices can significantly improve quality of life and relationship dynamics, as they restore the ability to engage in sexual activity without the fear of failure associated with other treatment options.

While penile implants are highly effective, it is crucial to consider the potential risks and complications, which include infection, mechanical failure, and dissatisfaction with the results. Men must engage in an informed discussion with their healthcare provider about the potential benefits and drawbacks of the procedure. Additionally, cultural perspectives on erectile dysfunction may influence a man's decision to pursue surgical options. In some cultures, seeking help for ED can carry stigma, impacting the willingness to consider surgical interventions.

Advances in technology continue to enhance the design and functionality of penile implants. Newer models are more durable and easier to use, while innovations in materials have reduced the risk of complications. As telemedicine becomes more prevalent, consultations for surgical options can be conducted remotely, allowing for broader access to this treatment. For men and couples navigating the complexities of erectile dysfunction, understanding the role of penile implants as a viable treatment option is essential in making informed decisions that align with their health needs and relationship goals.

Emerging Technologies

Emerging technologies are playing a pivotal role in the management of erectile dysfunction (ED), offering innovative solutions that enhance traditional treatment methods. One of the most significant advancements is the development of medical devices such as vacuum erection devices (VEDs) and penile implants, which provide physical solutions to address erectile issues. These devices have evolved to incorporate user-friendly designs and enhanced functionality, making them more accessible and effective for men experiencing ED. As a result, men are increasingly turning to these devices not only for immediate relief but also as a long-term management strategy.

Telemedicine has also transformed the landscape of ED treatment, allowing patients to seek professional help from the comfort of their homes. Virtual consultations have become a viable option, enabling men to discuss sensitive topics related to erectile dysfunction without the stigma often associated with in-person visits. This approach has significantly increased accessibility to specialists and has made it easier for men to receive timely advice and treatment. The integration of telehealth platforms into ED care is particularly beneficial for those living in remote areas, where access to healthcare facilities may be limited.

Another notable advancement in the management of ED comes from the field of pharmacology, with the introduction of oral medications and novel compounds that target erectile function more effectively. Research into new pharmacological agents aims to provide alternatives for patients who do not respond to traditional treatments like phosphodiesterase type 5 inhibitors. These emerging drugs are designed to work through different mechanisms, potentially offering solutions for those with varying underlying causes of erectile dysfunction including psychological factors, hormonal imbalances, or vascular issues.

Wearable technology is also making waves in the realm of ED management. Devices such as smartwatches and fitness trackers can monitor health metrics that are closely linked to erectile function, including heart rate, physical activity levels, and even sleep patterns. By providing real-time data and analytics, these devices empower men to take proactive steps toward improving their overall health, which is intrinsically connected to erectile function. Furthermore, some emerging technologies are exploring biofeedback mechanisms that help users understand their physiological responses, potentially reducing anxiety associated with sexual performance.

The intersection of psychology and technology is another area where innovative solutions are emerging. Virtual reality (VR) therapy is being explored as a means to address the psychological barriers that contribute to ED. By immersing individuals in controlled environments that simulate intimate scenarios, VR therapy may help reduce performance anxiety and enhance sexual confidence. As mental health plays a crucial role in erectile dysfunction, these technological advances may provide effective tools for couples seeking to improve their sexual relationships while addressing the underlying psychological components of ED.

Telemedicine Solutions for Erectile Dysfunction Care

Virtual Consultations

Virtual consultations have emerged as a transformative approach in the management of erectile dysfunction (ED), providing patients with convenient access to healthcare professionals. This method allows men to seek advice and treatment from the comfort of their homes, reducing the stigma often associated with discussing sexual health issues. Through telemedicine platforms, individuals can engage in private, one-on-one sessions with qualified specialists, facilitating a more open dialogue about their concerns without the anxiety of an in-person visit. This accessibility is particularly beneficial for those living in remote areas where specialized care may be limited.

The psychological aspects of erectile dysfunction are significant, and virtual consultations play a crucial role in addressing these issues. Many men experience anxiety and embarrassment when discussing ED, which can exacerbate the condition. Online consultations create a safe environment where patients can express their feelings and thoughts candidly. Healthcare providers can employ psychological approaches to help address these concerns, utilizing techniques such as cognitive behavioural therapy (CBT) to help patients manage anxiety related to sexual performance. The ability to connect with professionals who understand the psychological dimensions of ED can lead to more effective treatment outcomes.

Nutrition also plays a vital role in managing erectile dysfunction, and virtual consultations can incorporate dietary guidance tailored to individual needs. During these sessions, healthcare providers can assess a patient's current dietary habits and recommend nutritional interventions that may enhance sexual health. For instance, a diet rich in fruits, vegetables, whole grains, and healthy fats can improve blood circulation and overall health, which are essential for erectile function. By utilizing technology, men can receive personalized meal plans and ongoing support, ensuring they stay accountable to their health goals while managing ED.

The impact of technology on ED treatment cannot be overstated, as virtual consultations have streamlined the process of obtaining medical advice and prescriptions. Patients can easily follow up with their healthcare providers regarding medication adjustments or new treatment options without the need for physical appointments. This flexibility not only saves time but also encourages adherence to treatment plans. Moreover, the integration of wearable devices and mobile applications can enhance the monitoring of health metrics, facilitating more informed discussions during virtual consultations and allowing for tailored adjustments to treatment strategies.

Finally, the dynamics of relationships are often affected by erectile dysfunction, and virtual consultations provide a platform for couples to address these challenges together. Many providers offer joint sessions, allowing both partners to participate in the discussion. This inclusive approach fosters understanding and support, which are critical for navigating the emotional complexities surrounding ED. By encouraging open communication, these consultations can help couples develop strategies to strengthen their relationship while managing the impact of erectile dysfunction, ultimately improving both emotional intimacy and sexual health.

Online Prescription Services

Online prescription services have emerged as a pivotal resource in the management of erectile dysfunction (ED), providing a convenient and discreet option for men seeking treatment. These services allow individuals to consult with licensed healthcare professionals through telemedicine platforms, eliminating the need for in-person visits. This accessibility is particularly beneficial for men who may feel embarrassed about discussing ED face-to-face, thus reducing the stigma associated with the condition. By utilizing online prescription services, patients can receive tailored treatment plans that address their unique needs while maintaining privacy and comfort.

The process typically begins with an online consultation, where patients complete a detailed questionnaire about their medical history, symptoms, and lifestyle factors that may contribute to their ED. This information is crucial for healthcare providers to assess the underlying causes of the condition accurately. After the evaluation, prescriptions for medications such as PDE5 inhibitors can be issued electronically, allowing for timely access to treatment. This streamlined approach not only saves time but also ensures that men receive appropriate care without the lengthy delays often associated with traditional healthcare settings.

Moreover, the integration of technology in ED management through online prescription services represents a significant advancement in patient care. With the ability to monitor treatment efficacy and make adjustments based on feedback, healthcare providers can offer a more personalized approach. Many platforms also provide educational resources about ED, empowering patients with knowledge about their condition and the options available for management. This educational component is essential, as it helps demystify ED and encourages men to take an active role in their health.

In addition to pharmaceutical interventions, online prescription services can also facilitate access to complementary therapies, such as nutritional guidance and exercise regimens. Many platforms collaborate with health professionals who specialize in holistic approaches to ED, ensuring that patients receive comprehensive care. By addressing lifestyle factors alongside medical treatments, these services promote a more integrated management strategy that can improve overall sexual health and wellbeing. This multifaceted approach is particularly beneficial for men whose ED may be influenced by psychological or relational dynamics.

Finally, the growing acceptance of online prescription services marks a shift in cultural attitudes toward ED treatment. As more men utilize these platforms, the conversation surrounding erectile dysfunction is becoming more normalized, helping to break down barriers to seeking help. By fostering an environment where men feel comfortable discussing their experiences and challenges, these services contribute to a broader understanding of ED and its impact on relationships. As technology continues to evolve, the potential for online prescription services to enhance ED management and promote healthier attitudes toward sexual health remains promising.

Benefits and Limitations of Telemedicine

Telemedicine has emerged as a transformative approach to healthcare, providing a range of benefits particularly in the management of erectile dysfunction (ED). One of the primary advantages of telemedicine is its ability to increase accessibility to care for men facing ED. Geographic barriers and stigma associated with seeking help can deter many from pursuing treatment. Telemedicine effectively eliminates these hurdles, allowing patients to consult with healthcare professionals from the comfort of their homes. This convenience not only encourages men to seek help but also fosters a more open dialogue about sexual health, which is crucial for effective management.

Another significant benefit is the flexibility telemedicine offers in terms of appointment scheduling. Traditional office visits often require time off work and long waiting periods, which can be particularly challenging for those juggling professional and personal commitments. Telemedicine allows for greater flexibility, enabling patients to schedule consultations at times that suit their lifestyles. This ease of access can lead to more consistent follow-up appointments, essential for monitoring progress and making necessary adjustments to treatment plans.

However, while telemedicine presents numerous advantages, it also has limitations. A significant concern is the lack of physical examination during virtual consultations. Certain aspects of ED management, such as physical assessments and lab tests, are essential for accurate diagnosis and treatment. Although telehealth can effectively handle many aspects of care, it may not replace the need for in-person visits in cases where a thorough physical evaluation is necessary. This limitation can hinder the comprehensive understanding of a patient's condition, potentially impacting treatment outcomes.

Privacy and technology-related challenges also pose limitations to telemedicine. While many patients appreciate the discretion offered by virtual visits, concerns about data security and privacy can deter some individuals from engaging with telehealth services. Additionally, not all patients are comfortable with technology or possess reliable internet access, which can create disparities in who can benefit from telemedicine. These barriers can lead to unequal access to care, particularly among older populations or those in underserved areas.

In conclusion, telemedicine represents a modern solution with significant potential for the management of erectile dysfunction, offering accessibility and convenience that traditional healthcare models may lack. However, it is essential to acknowledge its limitations, particularly regarding the need for physical assessments and the challenges of technology use. As telemedicine continues to evolve, it will be crucial for healthcare providers to find ways to integrate these services with traditional care to ensure comprehensive, equitable, and effective treatment for all men experiencing ED.

Erectile Dysfunction and Relationship Dynamics

Communication Strategies

Effective communication strategies are essential for addressing erectile dysfunction (ED), as they can significantly influence treatment outcomes and relationship dynamics. Open and honest dialogue between men and their partners can foster a supportive environment, facilitating a deeper understanding of the condition. This communication is not only crucial for the individuals directly affected but also for couples navigating the emotional and psychological impacts of ED. Encouraging discussions about feelings, concerns, and expectations can help demystify the condition and reduce associated stigma, enabling both partners to participate actively in the management process.

Incorporating psychological approaches to ED management necessitates a multifaceted communication strategy. Men may feel vulnerable discussing their experiences with ED, leading to feelings of shame or inadequacy. Mental health professionals can aid in developing communication techniques that encourage expression of emotions and thoughts. Cognitive-behavioural therapy (CBT), for instance, can provide tools to help individuals articulate their feelings about ED, thereby reducing anxiety and improving overall mental health. This therapeutic dialogue can also extend to couples, helping partners understand each other's perspectives and emotional responses related to ED.

Nutritional interventions play a significant role in managing erectile dysfunction, and effective communication is vital in this context as well. Men seeking dietary changes to enhance their sexual health must be able to discuss their nutritional needs and preferences openly. Healthcare providers should foster an atmosphere where patients feel comfortable discussing their diets, lifestyle choices, and any barriers to implementing recommended changes. By empowering men to communicate their challenges and successes, practitioners can tailor nutritional advice more effectively, leading to better adherence and outcomes.

As technology increasingly impacts ED treatment, communication strategies must evolve to accommodate new modalities of interaction. Telemedicine solutions, for instance, allow patients to consult with healthcare professionals remotely, which can be particularly beneficial for those hesitant to seek in-person help. Clear and consistent communication through digital platforms ensures that men receive timely support and information. It is important for practitioners to educate their patients on how to use these technologies effectively, ensuring they understand how to communicate their symptoms and treatment responses during virtual visits.

Lastly, the cultural perspectives surrounding ED treatment are critical in shaping communication strategies. Different cultures may have varying levels of acceptance and openness regarding sexual health issues, influencing how men and their partners discuss ED. Understanding these cultural contexts can help healthcare providers tailor their communication approaches, ensuring that they are respectful and sensitive to the beliefs and values of their patients. By fostering an inclusive dialogue that acknowledges cultural differences, practitioners can enhance patient engagement and adherence to treatment plans, ultimately improving outcomes for men experiencing erectile dysfunction.

Partner Support and Involvement

Partner support plays a crucial role in the management of erectile dysfunction (ED), as the condition often affects not only the individual but also the dynamics of the relationship. Open communication between partners can foster a supportive environment where feelings of anxiety, shame, or embarrassment can be addressed. This dialogue is essential in reducing the emotional burden associated with ED. Couples who engage in discussions about their experiences and share their feelings can enhance their emotional intimacy, which is often impacted by sexual health issues. Understanding that ED is a medical condition rather than a personal failing can help both partners approach the situation with empathy and a collaborative mindset.

Involving partners in treatment decisions can significantly improve outcomes for men experiencing ED. Couples may benefit from joint consultations with healthcare providers, allowing both partners to voice concerns and preferences regarding treatment options. Such involvement ensures that both individuals feel invested in the process, fostering a sense of teamwork. Many couples find that participating together in therapy sessions, whether they focus on psychological approaches or relationship dynamics, can further enhance their bond and create a shared understanding of the challenges and potential solutions related to ED.

Psychological support from a partner can be a powerful tool in overcoming the stress and anxiety that often accompany erectile dysfunction. Cognitive-behavioral therapy (CBT) techniques can be adapted for couples to help them navigate the emotional challenges presented by the condition. By learning how to manage stress and anxiety together, couples can mitigate the negative impacts of ED on their relationship. This psychological support can also enhance partners' abilities to provide encouragement and reassurance, which can be vital for men struggling with self-esteem issues related to their sexual performance.

Nutritional interventions and lifestyle changes can be more effective when partners are involved in the process. Encouraging a healthier diet and exercise regimen can become a shared goal, promoting not only better sexual health but also overall well-being. Engaging in physical activities together can strengthen the relationship while also addressing some of the physiological factors contributing to ED. This collaborative approach can make lifestyle changes feel less daunting and more achievable, as partners can motivate each other and celebrate progress along the way.

As technology continues to advance, telemedicine solutions have emerged as a valuable resource for couples dealing with erectile dysfunction. Remote consultations can facilitate access to specialists and provide couples with educational resources without the pressure of an in-person visit. Involving partners in these virtual appointments can enhance understanding and commitment to treatment plans. Additionally, digital platforms often offer tools for tracking progress, which can foster accountability and provide a sense of achievement for both partners. By embracing modern solutions and maintaining open lines of communication, couples can effectively navigate the challenges of erectile dysfunction together, strengthening their relationship in the process.

Navigating Intimacy Issues

Navigating intimacy issues related to erectile dysfunction (ED) is a complex and sensitive task that can significantly affect relationships. For many men, the psychological implications of ED can lead to feelings of inadequacy, embarrassment, and anxiety, which can further exacerbate the condition. Couples often find themselves in a challenging dynamic, where communication about sexual health becomes strained. Understanding these intimacy issues is crucial for both partners, as it allows them to approach the situation collaboratively rather than allowing it to create distance in their relationship.

One of the first steps in addressing intimacy issues is fostering open communication. Couples should create a safe space where both partners feel comfortable discussing their feelings about ED. This dialogue can help demystify the condition and reduce the stigma associated with it. Sharing concerns, fears, and desires can strengthen the emotional connection between partners, making it easier to navigate the physical challenges posed by ED. Engaging in honest discussions about sexual expectations can also prevent misunderstandings and resentment from developing.

Psychological approaches to managing intimacy issues play a pivotal role in addressing the emotional aspects of ED. Cognitive-behavioural therapy (CBT) and couples therapy can be effective in helping both partners cope with the psychological burdens of ED. These therapies focus on changing negative thought patterns and improving communication skills, which can lead to a more supportive environment for both individuals. Additionally, mindfulness practices can help reduce anxiety related to sexual performance, allowing couples to reconnect on a deeper level without the pressure of expectations.

Nutritional interventions and lifestyle changes can also influence intimacy and sexual health. A balanced diet rich in fruits, vegetables, whole grains, and lean proteins can improve overall health and potentially enhance sexual function.

Exercise is another critical component; regular physical activity not only boosts blood flow but also improves mood and reduces stress, which can positively impact intimacy. Couples can benefit from engaging in physical activities together, reinforcing their bond while also addressing the underlying health issues that may contribute to ED.

Finally, the role of technology cannot be overlooked in navigating intimacy issues. Telemedicine solutions have made it easier for couples to seek help discreetly and conveniently. Online counselling options can provide couples with access to professionals who specialize in sexual health, allowing them to address their intimacy challenges from the comfort of their homes. Furthermore, advances in medical devices and treatments offer new hope for managing ED, which can, in turn, enhance intimacy. By embracing these modern solutions, couples can work together to overcome the barriers posed by erectile dysfunction, fostering a more fulfilling and connected relationship.

Cultural Perspectives on Erectile Dysfunction Treatment

Global Attitudes Toward Erectile Dysfunction

Global attitudes toward erectile dysfunction (ED) have evolved significantly over the years, influenced by cultural, social, and medical advancements. In many regions, ED was once shrouded in stigma, often viewed as a taboo subject that men were reluctant to discuss openly. However, increased awareness and education about sexual health have contributed to a gradual shift in perceptions. More men are now recognizing ED as a common condition rather than an embarrassing failure, leading to greater acceptance of seeking help and exploring treatment options. This change is essential for improving the quality of life for those affected and fostering healthier communication within relationships.

Cultural perspectives play a crucial role in shaping attitudes toward erectile dysfunction. In some cultures, traditional masculinity ideals place immense pressure on men to maintain sexual prowess, leading to feelings of shame and inadequacy when faced with ED. Conversely, other cultures may approach the topic with more openness, allowing for discussions about sexual health without fear of judgment. Understanding these cultural differences is vital for healthcare providers who aim to offer personalized care that respects and addresses the unique beliefs and practices of their patients. In this context, the interplay between cultural attitudes and the willingness to seek treatment significantly influences the effectiveness of interventions.

The psychological dimension of erectile dysfunction is also critical in shaping global attitudes. Many men experience anxiety, depression, and diminished self-esteem as a result of ED, which can create a cycle of avoidance and further exacerbation of the condition. Modern management strategies increasingly emphasize psychological support as a key component in treatment. Therapeutic approaches, including cognitive-behavioural therapy and counselling, are being integrated into ED management, helping men address the emotional and psychological factors contributing to their condition. This holistic view is gradually gaining traction worldwide, encouraging men to view ED as a treatable health issue rather than a personal failing.

The advent of technology has transformed how men access information and treatment for erectile dysfunction. The rise of telemedicine has made it easier for individuals to consult healthcare professionals from the comfort of their homes, reducing the stigma associated with in-person visits. Online platforms and mobile applications have emerged, providing educational resources and connecting men with specialists who understand their concerns. This technological shift not only enhances accessibility but also encourages proactive engagement in sexual health, fostering a more informed and empowered patient population.

As global attitudes toward erectile dysfunction continue to evolve, the importance of supportive partnerships cannot be overstated. Couples are increasingly recognizing the impact of ED on their relationships and are seeking solutions together. This collaborative approach emphasizes communication, understanding, and shared responsibility in managing the condition. By fostering an environment where partners can openly discuss their feelings and experiences related to ED, couples can strengthen their emotional connection and resilience. As societal attitudes shift toward greater acceptance and understanding, the potential for improved outcomes in both individual and relational health becomes increasingly promising.

Cultural Barriers to Treatment

Cultural barriers to treatment can significantly impede the management of erectile dysfunction (ED), affecting not just individual men but also their partners and families. Many cultures harbour stigmas surrounding sexual health issues, leading to feelings of shame and embarrassment that prevent open discussions about ED. This reluctance can result in delayed diagnosis and treatment, causing unnecessary suffering for those affected. Understanding these cultural nuances is essential for healthcare professionals, partners, and research students who seek to address ED comprehensively.

In many societies, traditional notions of masculinity dictate that men should be strong and sexually potent. This cultural expectation places immense pressure on men, making it difficult for them to acknowledge or seek help for ED. The fear of being perceived as less masculine can lead to avoidance of medical consultations, even when symptoms are apparent. This cultural context not only exacerbates the condition but also affects relationship dynamics, as partners may feel confused or rejected when sexual issues arise. Therefore, addressing these cultural perceptions is crucial for encouraging men to pursue treatment without fear of judgment.

Cultural attitudes also influence the types of treatment that are acceptable or preferred. In some communities, there may be a strong preference for traditional remedies or herbal treatments over modern medical interventions. While these alternatives may provide some benefits, they can also delay the implementation of evidence-based treatments that are more effective. Understanding these preferences allows healthcare providers to tailor their approach, integrating culturally relevant practices with contemporary medical solutions to enhance patient receptivity and compliance.

The role of technology in breaking down cultural barriers cannot be overstated. Telemedicine solutions have emerged as a vital tool for providing discreet access to healthcare providers, allowing men to seek help for ED from the privacy of their homes. This technology not only circumvents the embarrassment associated with face-to-face consultations but also reaches those in remote areas where traditional medical options may be limited. By leveraging technology, healthcare systems can improve access to information and treatment, ultimately contributing to better outcomes for men suffering from ED.

Ultimately, addressing cultural barriers to treatment requires a multifaceted approach involving education, community engagement, and sensitivity to diverse perspectives. Research students and professionals in the field must be equipped to navigate these complexities, ensuring that interventions are culturally competent and tailored to individual needs. By fostering an environment where men feel safe to discuss their concerns about erectile dysfunction, we can promote more effective treatment strategies and improve the overall quality of life for those affected by this common condition.

Case Studies from Different Cultures

Case studies from various cultures provide valuable insights into the multifaceted approaches to managing erectile dysfunction (ED) across the globe. Each culture brings its unique beliefs, practices, and preferences that influence how individuals perceive and address ED. By exploring these case studies, we can better understand the intersection of cultural norms, health practices, and treatment outcomes, ultimately leading to more effective and culturally sensitive solutions for men experiencing this condition.

In many Asian cultures, traditional medicine plays a significant role in the management of erectile dysfunction. For instance, a case study from China highlights the use of acupuncture and herbal remedies as a preferred treatment method. Patients often report significant improvements in sexual function after undergoing a series of acupuncture sessions combined with the application of specific herbal formulas. This approach underscores the importance of considering traditional practices alongside modern medical interventions, demonstrating that integrative strategies can enhance overall treatment efficacy and patient satisfaction.

Conversely, a case study from a Western context, particularly the United States, illustrates the growing trend of using technology in ED management. Telemedicine has emerged as a powerful tool, allowing men to consult with healthcare professionals from the comfort and privacy of their homes. This case study showcases a patient who benefited from online consultations and the subsequent prescription of oral medications. The convenience of telehealth services not only improved access to care but also encouraged open discussions about sexual health, which can often be stigmatized. This highlights the impact of technology in reshaping the landscape of ED treatment, making it more accessible and less intimidating for patients.

In contrast, cultures that emphasize community and familial support, such as some African societies, often rely on collective wisdom and shared experiences to address erectile dysfunction. A case study from Nigeria illustrates this communal approach, where men gather in support groups to discuss their experiences and share coping strategies. These gatherings foster a sense of solidarity and reduce the stigma associated with ED. Participants reported feeling empowered by their shared experiences, which enhanced their willingness to seek medical treatment and improved their overall psychological well-being. This communal perspective can serve as a model for integrating social support into ED management strategies.

Finally, a study from a Latin American culture emphasizes the importance of nutritional interventions in managing erectile dysfunction. In this case, a patient adopted a Mediterranean diet rich in fruits, vegetables, whole grains, and healthy fats, which led to significant improvements in erectile function. This case underscores the role of diet as not only a lifestyle choice but also as a viable intervention for ED. Emphasizing nutritional education within the context of cultural dietary preferences can pave the way for more personalized and effective treatment plans, enhancing both physical health and sexual performance.

These diverse case studies illustrate the importance of cultural context in understanding and treating erectile dysfunction. By recognizing the varying beliefs and practices that shape men's experiences with ED, healthcare providers can develop more effective, culturally attuned management strategies. Ultimately, this approach will not only improve individual outcomes but also contribute to breaking down the stigma surrounding erectile dysfunction, fostering a more open dialogue about this common yet often overlooked issue.

Hormonal Treatments and Erectile Dysfunction Management

Understanding Hormonal Imbalances

Hormonal imbalances can significantly influence erectile function and contribute to the development of erectile dysfunction (ED). Hormones such as testosterone, oestrogen, and thyroid hormones play crucial roles in sexual health. Testosterone is vital for libido, erectile function, and overall sexual satisfaction in men. Low levels of testosterone, a condition known as hypogonadism, can lead to reduced sexual desire, difficulty achieving or maintaining an erection, and even impact mood and energy levels. Understanding the hormonal underpinnings of erectile dysfunction is essential for both men experiencing these issues and healthcare providers aiming to offer effective solutions.

The relationship between testosterone levels and erectile dysfunction is complex. Research indicates that men with lower testosterone levels often report higher instances of ED. This connection is not solely due to the direct effects of testosterone on erectile function but also involves other physiological processes. For instance, testosterone influences vascular health, which is critical for achieving an erection. Impaired blood flow, often associated with cardiovascular disease, is a common cause of ED. Therefore, addressing hormonal imbalances can be a pivotal step in restoring sexual health and improving erectile function.

In addition to testosterone, oestrogen and thyroid hormones also play important roles in male sexual health. Elevated oestrogen levels can disrupt the balance of testosterone, leading to further complications in sexual function.

Moreover, thyroid dysfunction, whether hypothyroidism or hyperthyroidism, can manifest as changes in libido and erectile performance. Thus, a comprehensive evaluation of hormone levels is essential for understanding the broader context of erectile dysfunction. Men experiencing ED should consider hormone testing as a part of their diagnostic process to identify any underlying hormonal issues that could be addressed.

Management of hormonal imbalances often involves a multifaceted approach, including lifestyle modifications, nutritional interventions, and medical treatments. Lifestyle changes such as regular exercise, a balanced diet, and weight management can positively impact hormone levels. For instance, physical activity has been shown to increase testosterone levels and improve overall health, which can mitigate some of the factors contributing to erectile dysfunction. Nutritional interventions, such as increasing intake of zinc and vitamin D, can also support healthy hormone levels. In some cases, hormone replacement therapy may be warranted, but this should always be carefully managed by healthcare professionals to avoid potential side effects.

Understanding hormonal imbalances is crucial not only for individual men but also for their partners and healthcare providers. Addressing these issues can lead to significant improvements in sexual health and intimacy within relationships. As research continues to evolve, integrating hormonal assessments into the broader management of erectile dysfunction can enhance treatment outcomes. This holistic approach acknowledges the complex interplay of hormones, physical health, and psychological well-being, ultimately fostering a more comprehensive understanding of erectile dysfunction in modern healthcare.

Testosterone Replacement Therapy

Testosterone Replacement Therapy (TRT) has emerged as a significant intervention for men experiencing erectile dysfunction (ED) linked to low testosterone levels. Testosterone plays a crucial role in various bodily functions, including libido, erectile function, and overall sexual health. For men whose ED is associated with hypogonadism, or insufficient testosterone production, TRT can help restore hormonal balance and improve sexual performance. Understanding the mechanisms of TRT is essential for men, couples, and research students exploring modern solutions to ED, as it offers a pathway to enhance quality of life and intimate relationships.

The process of TRT typically begins with thorough testing to establish testosterone levels, which can vary widely among individuals. Blood tests are conducted to measure total and free testosterone levels, often complemented by assessments of luteinizing hormone and follicle-stimulating hormone to rule out other underlying conditions. Once a diagnosis of low testosterone is confirmed, various treatment options are available, including injections, transdermal patches, gels, and pellets. Each method has its unique advantages and potential side effects, making it vital for patients to discuss their preferences and medical history with healthcare providers to determine the most appropriate form of therapy.

While TRT can significantly improve erectile function in men with low testosterone, it is not a one-size-fits-all solution. Psychological factors may also contribute to ED, necessitating a comprehensive approach that includes mental health support. Therapy or counselling can address issues such as anxiety, depression, or relationship dynamics that may exacerbate erectile challenges. Combining TRT with psychological interventions can lead to more sustainable improvements in sexual health and overall well-being, emphasizing the importance of an integrated treatment strategy for managing ED.

Nutritional interventions and lifestyle changes also play a vital role in conjunction with TRT. A balanced diet rich in vitamins and minerals, particularly those supporting testosterone production such as zinc and vitamin D, can enhance the effectiveness of hormone therapy. Regular physical activity is equally important, as exercise has been shown to increase testosterone levels naturally and improve cardiovascular health, which is closely linked to erectile function. Men undergoing TRT should consider adopting a holistic approach that incorporates nutrition, exercise, and psychological well-being alongside hormonal treatment.

As technology evolves, telemedicine solutions have become an invaluable resource for men seeking TRT. Remote consultations allow patients to access expert advice and medication management without the barriers of traditional in-person visits. This is particularly beneficial for those who may feel uncomfortable discussing their ED face-to-face. Additionally, advances in medical devices, such as low-intensity shockwave therapy, are being explored as adjuncts to TRT. These innovations offer promising avenues for enhancing sexual function and underscore the dynamic landscape of ED management. As research in this field continues to expand, individuals and couples can look forward to more effective and personalized treatment options.

Monitoring and Safety Considerations

Monitoring and safety considerations are critical components in managing erectile dysfunction (ED), particularly given the diverse approaches available today. As men and couples navigate treatment options, it is essential to understand the importance of ongoing assessment and the potential risks associated with different interventions. Personalized care plans, which may include psychological support, nutritional guidance, and physical activity recommendations, should incorporate regular monitoring to evaluate efficacy and safety. This proactive approach not only ensures that treatments remain appropriate but also fosters open communication between patients and healthcare providers.

Psychological approaches to ED management often require careful monitoring of both mental health and relationship dynamics. Cognitive-behavioural therapy and other psychological interventions may be beneficial, yet they necessitate regular check-ins to assess progress and adjust strategies. Practitioners should be vigilant for signs of anxiety or depression that may exacerbate erectile difficulties. Furthermore, addressing relationship dynamics openly can enhance treatment outcomes, making it essential for couples to maintain an ongoing dialogue about their experiences and feelings during the management process.

Nutritional interventions play a significant role in managing ED, and monitoring dietary changes can lead to improved outcomes. Additionally, the role played by microplastics which are often inadvertently ingested needs to be more fully understood. Men are encouraged to adopt a heart-healthy diet rich in fruits, vegetables, whole grains, and lean proteins. Regular follow-up appointments can help track progress, ensuring that dietary modifications are effectively implemented and that patients are aware of their impact on erectile function. Safety considerations also include monitoring for potential side effects of supplements or herbal remedies, which may interact with other medications and pose health risks.

The integration of technology in ED treatment has revolutionized care but also necessitates cautious monitoring. Telemedicine solutions, for instance, provide convenient access to care but require robust security measures to protect patient data. Additionally, men using medical devices such as vacuum pumps or penile implants must be educated about proper usage and potential complications. Continuous monitoring of device performance and patient satisfaction is vital to ensure safety and effectiveness. Healthcare providers should offer clear guidelines and follow-up assessments to address any concerns that may arise.

Exercise and physical activity are also pivotal in managing erectile dysfunction, with safety considerations surrounding the type and intensity of exercise being paramount. Men should engage in regular physical activity tailored to their individual health status and fitness levels. Monitoring progress through fitness assessments can help ensure that exercise regimens are effective and safe. An emphasis on gradual increases in activity can prevent injury and enhance cardiovascular health, which is closely linked to erectile function. By prioritizing monitoring and safety across all facets of ED management, men and couples can achieve a more holistic and effective approach to treatment.

Pause for thought

- Erectile dysfunction is the persistent inability to achieve or maintain an erection sufficient for satisfactory sexual performance. This condition which affects millions of men worldwide has a plethora of causes which include physical causes, psychological causes and lifestyle causes.
- Understanding the complexities of erectile dysfunction requires a comprehensive approach that involves physiological, psychological, relational and cultural dimensions. Modern management therefore has a holistic approach which seeks to address the multifaceted nature of erectile dysfunction.
- Psychological factors such as anxiety and depression can play a crucial role in the manifestation of erectile dysfunction. Cognitive behavioural therapy and other psychological interventions have shown some permission in alleviating these issues thereby improving sexual function, so too are nutritional interventions including dietary changes and the addition of supplements. This combination of mental and physical health underscores the importance of a comprehensive treatment plan.
- Technological approaches such as telemedicine have emerged as a pivotal tool, this enables patients to access care and support from the comfort of their homes. Advances in vacuum erection devices and penile implants, offer a solution and may enhance the efficacy of the available treatment options.

- Exercise and physical activity also have an integral role to play. Regular physical activity leads to improved cardiovascular health, a crucial need, since many erectile dysfunction cases are linked to vascular issues. Erectile dysfunction can be improved with exercise, since exercise helps to enhance blood flow, reduce stress and improve overall wellbeing. Hence encouraging men to adopt a more active lifestyle can be strategic in terms of both prevention and treatment of erectile dysfunction.

- Physiologically, there may be vascular causes of erectile dysfunction, conditions such as atherosclerosis, hypertension, and diabetes can impede blood flow, which would make it difficult to achieve or maintain an erection. So too, can neurological disorders including Parkinson's disease and multiple sclerosis, can also disrupt nerve signals essential for an erection. Hormonal imbalances such as reduced testosterone levels can both disrupt sexual desire as well as cause erectile difficulties.

- Psychologically, anxiety, depression and stress can create a cycle where the fear of failure in sexual performance leads to increased anxiety, further hindering the ability to achieve an erection an erection. Relationship dynamics can amplify this psychological impact; conflicts or unresolved issues between partners may create an environment that is less conducive to intimacy, which adversely affects sexual performance. Treatment strategies that address the physical, emotional and relational aspects must be effective.

- Lifestyle choices also play an integral role in influencing erectile function. Poor nutrition, Lack of physical activity and substance abuse can negatively impact overall health and by extension, sexual health. Diets high in saturated fats and sugars can contribute to obesity and cardiovascular disease which are also known risks factors for erectile dysfunction. Conversely regular exercise has been shown to improve circulation and boost testosterone levels thereby enhancing erectile function. By adopting healthier lifestyle habits, therefore, men can often mitigate some of the risk factors associated with erectile dysfunction. The multifaceted causation for erectile dysfunction argues for personalised care to effect best results.
- Cultural perspective also plays a crucial role in shaping attitude towards erectile dysfunction and its treatment. In some cultures, discussing sexual health openly is stigmatised leaving men to suffer in silence rather than seek help. This cultural reluctance can perpetuate feelings of inadequacy and shame which further worsens the psychological aspect of erectile dysfunction.

Take Home Nuggets

- Research suggests that approximately 30 million men in the USA experience Erectile Dysfunction. It is estimated that about 40% of men in their forty's and nearly 70% of men in their 70's encounter some degree of erectile dysfunction.

- Demographically, erectile dysfunction affects men across various age groups, ethnicities and socioeconomic backgrounds. Some populations are more susceptible example men with chronic health issues such as diabetes, hypertension and cardiovascular disease are at a higher risk. Lifestyle factors such as smoking, obesity and sedentary behaviour contribute significantly to the incidence of erectile dysfunction.
- Traditional treatments of erectile dysfunction employ oral medications and injectables. A notable advancement in the realm of psychological approaches involves cognitive behavioural therapy which aims to address the mental health aspects associated with erectile dysfunction. Through cognitive behavioural therapy men can learn to reframe negative thoughts, reduce performance anxiety and ultimately improve their sexual health. Couples therapy has also gained traction, thus emphasising the importance of communication and emotional intimacy in overcoming the challenges posed by erectile dysfunction.
- A growing body of evidence suggest that diets rich in fruits, vegetables, whole grains, and lean proteins can enhance erectile dysfunction by improving cardiovascular health and reducing inflammation. Specific dietary patterns such as the Mediterranean diet have shown promise in promoting healthy blood flow and hormone regulation. Supplements such as ginseng and L-arginine are being explored for their potential benefits in enhancing nitric oxide production, a crucial requirement for achieving and maintaining an erection.

- Integrative approaches to the management of erectile dysfunction recognises that erectile dysfunction can stem from various factors including psychological, physiological, and relational dimensions, thus arguing for the explanation of developing holistic treatment plans that enhance overall wellbeing and sexual health.
- Specific nutrients such as zinc, L-arginine and omega -3 fatty acid have been linked to improve sexual health informed dietary choices can empower men and couples to take charge of their sexual health.
- Cognitive behavioural therapy has emerged as a vital psychological approach in addressing erectile dysfunction. Cognitive behavioural therapy focuses on the interplay between thoughts, feeling, and behaviour, and aims to modify negative thought patterns that can contribute to sexual dysfunction. For many men, anxiety, depression and how self-esteem can create a cycle of fear and avoidance that exacerbate erectile dysfunction. By employing cognitive behavioural therapy techniques, individuals can learn to identify and challenge these detrimental thoughts, ultimately fostering a healthier mindset towards sexual performance and intimacy.
- Cognitive behavioural therapy offers a structural approach which includes a cognitive restructuring where patients are guided replace irrational beliefs with more rational and positive thoughts. This process has the capacity to replace the psychological burdens associated with erectile dysfunction and empower men to regain confidence in their sexual

health. Cognitive behavioural therapy sessions typically involve behavioural interventions including gradual exposure to sexual situations that may have previously been anxiety-inducing. This gradual approach helps in reducing performance anxiety, which is a significant barrier for many men facing erectile dysfunction.

- Couples experiencing erectile dysfunction can also benefit from cognitive behavioural therapy as it encourages open communication and shared problem-solving relationship dynamics play a crucial role in sexual health through cognitive behavioural therapy couples can engage in joint sessions that focus on enhancing intimacy and reducing the stigma often associated with erectile issues. This collaborative approach not only improves the individual's experience but also strengthens the relationship, fostering a supportive environment that can lead to improved sexual satisfaction.
- Mindfulness and relaxation techniques are valuable tools in managing erectile dysfunction. These practices focus on enhancing mental clarity, reducing stress, and promoting emotional wellbeing.

Chapter 9
Modern Therapeutic Options for Erectile Dysfunction

Modern erectile dysfunction (ED) treatment has moved far beyond just tablets. Today's options range from lifestyle optimisation and oral medications to regenerative therapies like shockwave, PRP, stem cells, and neuromuscular stimulation. These approaches target the underlying vascular, neurological, hormonal, and muscular causes of ED, not just the symptoms.

How Each One Works

1. Lifestyle & Foundational Interventions

These are first-line because they directly improve vascular and metabolic health — the root of most ED.

What they include

- Regular aerobic exercise
- Weight reduction
- Smoking cessation
- Reduced alcohol intake
- Better sleep and stress management

How they work

- Improve endothelial function and nitric oxide availability
- Reduce inflammation and insulin resistance
- Enhance testosterone levels naturally

Evidence: Lifestyle changes are recommended as first-line therapy and improve vascular health and erectile function.

2. Oral Medications (PDE5 Inhibitors)

Still the most used treatment.

Examples

- Sildenafil (Viagra)
- Tadalafil (Cialis)
- Vardenafil (Levitra)

How they work

They block the enzyme PDE5, allowing nitric oxide to work more effectively. This increases blood flow to the penis during sexual stimulation.

Evidence: PDE5 inhibitors enhance penile blood flow and are effective for most men.

3. Low-Intensity Shockwave Therapy (LiSWT)

One of the most important modern advances.

How it works

- Uses low-intensity acoustic waves
- Stimulates **angiogenesis** (new blood vessel growth)
- Activates stem cells and growth factors
- Repairs microvascular damage

Benefits

- Non-invasive
- Long-lasting improvements (up to 2+ years)
- Particularly effective for vascular ED

Evidence: Shockwave therapy improves blood flow and promotes tissue regeneration.

4. Platelet-Rich Plasma (PRP) Therapy

A regenerative, injection-based treatment.

How it works

- Patient's own blood is processed to concentrate platelets
- Growth factors are injected into penile tissue
- Stimulates tissue repair and nerve regeneration

Benefits

- Improves erectile function for 12–18 months
- Useful for men with nerve or tissue damage

Evidence: PRP improves erectile function and repairs damaged tissue.

5. Stem Cell Therapy

Still emerging but highly promising.

How it works

- Uses mesenchymal stem cells (fat-derived or bone marrow)
- Regenerates smooth muscle, nerves, and blood vessels
- Reduces fibrosis in penile tissue

Benefits

- Long-lasting improvements (1–2+ years)
- Addresses root causes rather than symptoms

Evidence: Stem cells repair penile tissue at the cellular level.

6. Botox (Botulinum Toxin) Injections

A newer option gaining traction.

How it works

- Relaxes smooth muscle in penile arteries
- Improves blood flow
- May also help premature ejaculation

Benefits

- Effects last 6–9 months

Evidence: Botox can improve blood flow and erectile function.

7. Electromagnetic / Neuromuscular Stimulation

Often used in multi-modal ED clinics.

How it works

- Uses focused electromagnetic pulses
- Strengthens pelvic floor muscles
- Improves nerve signalling and venous occlusion

Benefits

- Non-invasive
- Useful for men with pelvic floor weakness

Evidence: Neuromuscular stimulation is part of modern multi-technology ED protocols.

8. Testosterone Replacement Therapy (TRT)

Only for men with clinically low testosterone.

How it works

- Restores normal testosterone levels
- Improves libido, energy, and erectile function

Forms

- Gels
- Injections

- Patches

Evidence: TRT improves libido and erectile function in men with low testosterone.

9. Vacuum Erection Devices (VEDs)

A mechanical, non-invasive option.

How it works

- Creates negative pressure to draw blood into the penis
- A constriction ring maintains the erection

Benefits

- Safe for men who cannot take medications

Evidence: VEDs are effective non-invasive tools for ED management.

10. Penile Implants (Surgical Option)

Reserved for severe or treatment-resistant ED.

Types

- Inflatable implants
- Malleable rods

How they work

Provide a mechanically induced erection on demand.

Comparison Table: Modern ED Treatments

How to Choose the Right Treatment

A clinician typically evaluates:

- Vascular health
- Hormone levels
- Pelvic floor strength
- Psychological factors
- Medication tolerance
- Severity and duration of ED

Modern clinics increasingly use **multi-technology protocols**, combining shockwave, electromagnetic therapy, PRP, and lifestyle optimisation for superior outcomes.

Personalised Erectile Dysfunction Treatment Pathway

Built around vascular health, pelvic neuromuscular function, hormones, and tissue integrity

Foundational Assessment Layer

A modern pathway always begins with identifying *which system is failing*.

Key domains a clinician evaluates

- **Vascular health**: blood pressure, lipids, diabetes risk
- **Hormonal profile:** testosterone, SHBG, LH/FSH, prolactin
- **Pelvic floor function:** strength, coordination, hypertonicity

- **Neurological integrity:** pudendal nerve, post-surgical changes
- **Lifestyle factors:** sleep, stress, alcohol, smoking
- **Medication review:** SSRIs, antihypertensives, etc.

This determines which branch of therapy is most appropriate.

If vascular insufficiency is the primary issue

(Most common cause of ED)

Phase 1 — Optimise vascular health

- Aerobic exercise programme
- Weight optimisation
- Smoking/alcohol reduction
- Mediterranean-style diet

Phase 2 — Pharmacological support

- PDE5 inhibitors (sildenafil (Viagra)/tadalafil)
- Consider daily low-dose tadalafil for endothelial support

Phase 3 — Regenerative vascular therapies

- **Shockwave therapy (LiSWT)** [Low intensity shock wave therapy] to stimulate angiogenesis
- **PRP** to enhance microvascular repair
- **Stem cell therapy** (where available) for severe microvascular disease

Phase 4 — Maintenance

- Periodic shockwave booster sessions
- Continued cardiovascular optimisation

If pelvic floor dysfunction is the primary issue

Phase 1 — Pelvic floor assessment

- Identify weakness vs. overactivity
- Evaluate coordination and endurance

Phase 2 — Targeted therapy

- **Weak pelvic floor:**
  - Neuromuscular electrical stimulation
  - EM-based pelvic floor strengthening
  - Biofeedback training
- **Overactive pelvic floor:**
- Relaxation training
- Myofascial release
- Breathing and down-training protocols

Phase 3 — Integration

- Combine pelvic floor training with PDE5 inhibitors or shockwave for synergistic effect

If hormonal imbalance is the primary issue

(Low testosterone, high SHBG, metabolic syndrome)

Phase 1 — Identify the pattern

- Low T with high LH → primary hypogonadism
- Low T with low LH → secondary hypogonadism
- High SHBG → reduced free testosterone

Phase 2 — Correct the imbalance

- Testosterone replacement therapy (if clinically indicated)
- Address sleep, stress, and metabolic factors
- Manage comorbidities (thyroid, prolactin, insulin resistance)

Phase 3 — Combine with vascular therapy

- TRT + PDE5 inhibitors often restores full function

If nerve injury or neuropathy is the primary issue

(Diabetes, pelvic surgery, cycling trauma)

Phase 1 — Neuro-regeneration support

- PRP injections
- Stem cell therapy (where available)
- Shockwave therapy (improves nerve signalling)

Phase 2 — Neuromuscular rehabilitation

- Pelvic floor neuromuscular stimulation
- Biofeedback
- Coordination training

Phase 3 — Adjunctive pharmacology

- PDE5 inhibitors
- Alpha-lipoic acid (general antioxidant support — not medical advice)

If psychological or relational factors dominate

(Performance anxiety, stress, relationship strain)

Phase 1 — Psychological support

- Cognitive behavioural therapy
- Sex therapy
- Stress-reduction strategies

Phase 2 — Combined approach

- PDE5 inhibitors to break the anxiety cycle
- Gradual exposure and confidence rebuilding

Advanced or Refractory ED Pathway

If first-line and regenerative therapies fail:

Option 1 — Vacuum erection device (VED)

- Non-invasive
- Useful for men who cannot take medications

Option 2 — Intracavernosal injections

- Alprostadil
- Trimix (where available)

Option 3 — Penile implant

- Inflatable or malleable
- High satisfaction rates
- Reserved for severe, long-standing ED

Option 4. Integrated, Multi-Modal Pathway (Most Effective)

Modern ED clinics increasingly use **combined protocols**:

Example integrated plan

- Daily low-dose tadalafil
- Shockwave therapy (6–12 sessions)
- PRP (1–3 sessions)

- Pelvic floor neuromuscular training
- Lifestyle optimisation
- Hormonal correction if needed

This approach treats **vascular, muscular, neurological, and hormonal** components simultaneously.

Step 1: Understanding What's Causing the Problem

ED can happen for different reasons. Before choosing treatment, a clinician usually checks:

- Blood flow to the penis
- Hormone levels (especially testosterone)
- Pelvic floor muscle strength
- Nerve function
- Stress, anxiety, or relationship factors
- Lifestyle habits (sleep, smoking, alcohol, exercise)

This helps match the treatment to the cause.

Step 2: Your Personalised Treatment Plan

Below are the main pathways depending on what's going on in the body.

If the issue is blood flow (the most common cause)

What helps:

- Improving fitness and weight
- Reducing smoking and alcohol
- Medications like Viagra or Cialis
- Shockwave therapy to improve blood supply
- PRP or stem cell treatments to help repair tissue (available in some clinics)

Why it works:

Better blood flow makes it easier to get and keep an erection.

If the pelvic floor muscles are weak or too tight

What helps:

- Pelvic floor exercises
- Electrical or electromagnetic stimulation
- Relaxation techniques if the muscles are overactive

Why it works:

Strong, well-coordinated pelvic muscles help trap blood in the penis and maintain firmness.

If hormones are low (especially testosterone)

What helps:

- Testosterone replacement (only if levels are genuinely low)
- Improving sleep, stress, and weight

Why it works:

Healthy testosterone levels support libido, energy, and erectile function.

If nerves are affected (diabetes, surgery, injury)

What helps:

- Shockwave therapy
- PRP or stem cell treatments
- Pelvic floor rehabilitation
- Medications to support erections

Why it works:

These treatments help nerves heal and improve communication between the brain and the penis.

If stress, anxiety, or relationship issues are involved

What helps:

- Talking therapy or sex therapy

- Relaxation techniques
- Short-term use of ED medication to rebuild confidence

Why it works:

Reducing anxiety breaks the cycle of "worry → poor erection → more worry".

Step 3: If first-line treatments don't work

There are still effective options:

Vacuum pump

Draws blood into the penis and helps maintain an erection.

Penile injections

Very effective for men who don't respond to tablets.

Penile implant

A long-term solution for severe ED that hasn't improved with other treatments.

Step 4: The Most Effective Approach

Many men benefit from a **combined plan**, such as:

- A daily low-dose ED tablet
- Shockwave therapy
- Pelvic floor strengthening
- Lifestyle improvements

- **Simple Erectile Dysfunction Treatment Flow Chart**

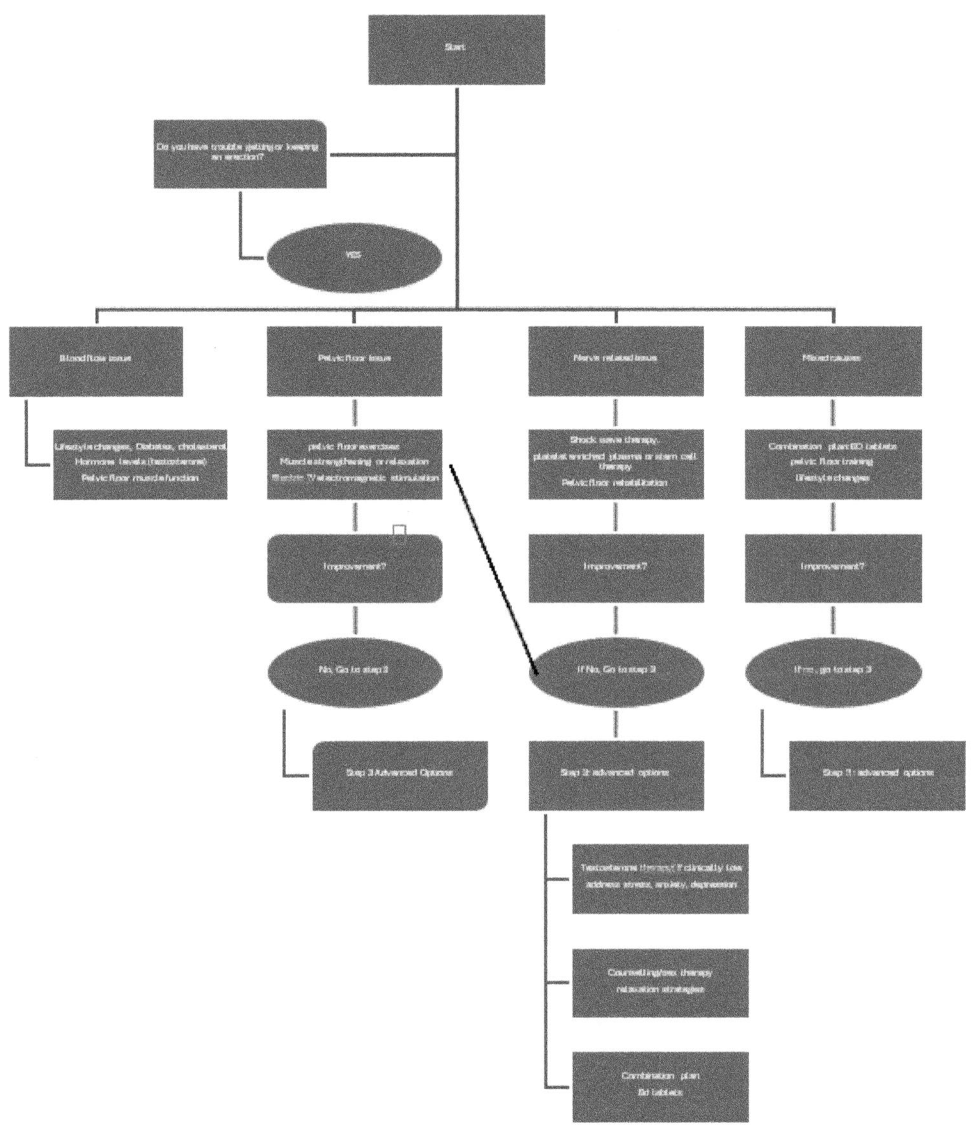

Pause for thought

- Modern erectile dysfunction treatment incorporates much more than tablets. It involves a range of options from lifestyle optimisation, oral medications and regenerative therapy such as shock wave therapy, platelet enriched plasma, stem cells, and neuromuscular stimulation.
- The modern approach to erectile dysfunction treatment aims to identify underlying causes such as vascular, neurological, hormonal, and muscular causes, it then aims to target the relevant cause, thus it goes beyond just symptomatic treatment.
- Lifestyle and foundational interventions are first line options because they directly improve vascular and metabolic health, the most common cause of erectile dysfunction. These lifestyle interventions include regular aerobic exercise, weight reduction, smoking cessation, reduction in alcoholic intake, better sleep and stress management.
- These approaches aim to improve endothelial function and nitric oxide availability, reduced inflammation and insulin resistance and enhanced testosterone levels without the use of pharmacological materials.
- Oral medications, such as the PDE5 inhibitors are still the most used treatment. These include sildenafil (Viagra), tadalafil (Cialis), and vardenafil (Levitra). They work by blocking the enzyme PDE5, thus allowing nitric oxide to work more effectively. The result is blood flow to the penis is increased during sexual stimulation.

- Low intensity shock wave therapy is among the most modern of advances which reputedly works by stimulating angiogenesis and activates stem cells and growth factors. It is also claimed that this repairs microvascular damage.
- The benefits of low intensity shock wave therapy is that it is non-invasive, provides long lasting improvements up to two years and it is particularly effective for vascular erectile dysfunction. It is believed that this therapy improves blood flow and promotes tissue regeneration.
- Platelet rich plasma (PRP) therapy is a regenerative, injection-based treatment. This procedure involves the harvesting of a sample of the patient's blood which is processed to concentrate platelets, growth factors are then injected into penile tissue which is believed to stimulate tissue repair and nerve regeneration. It improves erectile function nerve for 12 – 18 months and is useful for men with nerve or tissue damage. It is believed to improve erectile function and repair damaged tissue.
- Stem cell therapy is still emerging but highly promising. It uses mesenchymal stem cells derived from fat or bone marrow. It is believed to work by generating smooth muscle, nerves and blood vessels. While simultaneously reducing fibrosis in penile tissues. Its effect is long lasting (usually over 1-2 years) and addresses root causes rather than symptoms. They work at the cellular level.
- Botox injections is now gaining traction, it is believed to work by relaxing smooth muscle in penile arteries, thus improving blood flow; it may also

be helpful in the treatment of premature ejaculation and last for about 6-9 months.

Take Home Nuggets

- Electromagnetic/Neuromuscular stimulation is often used in multimodal erectile dysfunction clinics. It uses focussed electromagnetic pulses, the objective being to strengthen pelvic floor muscles. It improves nerve signalling and venous occlusion. It is non-invasive and useful for men with pelvic floor weakness.
- Testosterone replacement therapy is useful for men with clinically low testosterone. This improves libido, energy and erectile function. It can be delivered as gels, injections or patches.
- The vacuum erectile devices provide a mechanical, non-invasive option. This works through the creation of negative pressure to draw blood into the penis, the use of constriction rings maintains the erection. It is considered safe for men who cannot take medication. These are effective non-invasive tools for erectile dysfunction management.
- The surgical option of a penile implant is reserved for severe or treatment resistant erectile dysfunction. They can be inflatable implants or malleable rods. These work by producing a mechanically induced erection on demand.

- Clinicians employ pathways which tries to identify which system is failing. The vascular health is assessed along the lines of the patients' blood pressure, lipid profile, diabetes risk. A hormonal profile should be explored assessing testosterone levels, sex hormone binding globulin (SHBG), Luteinising hormone follicle stimulating hormone ratio, prolactin levels. The strength of the pelvic also needs to be assessed, so too is its coordination and hypertonicity, neurological integrity assessing the pudendal nerve, post-surgical changes as well as lifestyle factors: sleep, stress, alcohol usage and smoking as well as medications in use such as selective serotonin reuptake inhibitors (SSRI) and antihypertensive medications to inform management.
- If vascular insufficiency is the primary cause; several approaches can be explored, among them aerobic exercise programmes, weight optimisation, smoking/alcohol reduction and the inclusion of a Mediterranean style diet.
- Pharmacological support may also be considered with PDE 5 inhibitors sildenafil (Viagra), tadalafil (Cialis); a daily low dose of tadalafil offers support to the vascular endothelium.
- Further supplementation can be had through regenerative vascular therapies such as low intensity shock wave therapy and platelet enriched plasma and the now emerging stem cell therapy.

- Once success has been achieved, there is need for maintenance in the form of periodic shock wave booster sessions and continued cardiovascular optimisation.
- If erectile dysfunction has a psychological or relational cause such as performance anxiety, stress, or relationship strain, psychological support becomes necessary and may take the form of cognitive behavioural therapy, sex therapy, and stress reduction strategies.

Chapter 10
Introduction to Testicular Diseases

Overview of Testicular Health

Testicular health is a crucial aspect of male well-being, encompassing a variety of conditions that can significantly affect reproductive health and overall quality of life. Understanding the anatomy and function of the testis is essential for recognising potential health issues. The testis is responsible for the production of sperm and the secretion of hormones such as testosterone, both of which are vital for male fertility and sexual health. Awareness of the common diseases that can affect the testis is important for timely diagnosis and treatment.

Testicular cancer is one of the most significant concerns regarding testicular health, with various types, such as seminomas and non-seminomas, each requiring specific treatment protocols. Early detection through regular self-examinations and professional assessments can lead to better outcomes. Healthcare professionals should educate men on the importance of being vigilant for any unusual changes in the testicular area, as this can facilitate early intervention and improve prognosis.

Conditions such as orchitis and epididymitis, often stemming from infections, can cause considerable discomfort and complications if left untreated. Orchitis, an inflammation of the testis, may be caused by viral or bacterial infections, while epididymitis affects the epididymis and can result from sexually transmitted infections. Both conditions necessitate prompt medical attention to manage symptoms and prevent long-term health issues.

Testicular torsion, a medical emergency characterised by the twisting of the spermatic cord, can lead to severe consequences if not addressed swiftly. Diagnosis often involves clinical evaluation and imaging techniques, and immediate surgical intervention is typically required to restore blood flow. Understanding the signs and symptoms of testicular torsion is vital for both men and healthcare providers to ensure timely treatment and preserve testicular function.

Additionally, congenital anomalies of the testis and hormonal disorders can lead to infertility and other reproductive issues. Diagnostic imaging techniques play a key role in identifying testicular conditions, allowing for accurate diagnosis and tailored treatment options. By promoting awareness and understanding of these various aspects of testicular health, men can better navigate their health needs, while healthcare professionals can provide more effective care.

Importance of Awareness and Early Detection

Awareness and early detection of testicular diseases are crucial for effective management and treatment. Men should regularly perform self-examinations to identify any unusual changes in their testicles. Such changes can include lumps, swelling, or pain, which may indicate potential issues such as testicular cancer or infections. By recognising these signs early, individuals can seek timely medical advice, significantly improving their chances of favourable outcomes.

Healthcare professionals, particularly urologists, play a vital role in promoting awareness about testicular health. Educational initiatives targeting men of all ages can help dispel myths and encourage proactive health behaviours. Regular check-ups and discussions about testicular health should be part of routine healthcare, as many men are often reluctant to address these sensitive topics. Ensuring that men feel comfortable discussing their concerns can lead to earlier diagnoses and interventions.

Testicular cancer, for instance, is one of the most treatable forms of cancer when detected early. The prognosis is significantly improved for patients whose cancer is diagnosed at an early stage. Understanding the various types of testicular cancer and their symptoms can empower men to seek help without delay. Awareness campaigns can highlight risk factors, such as family history and undescended testicles, which can predispose individuals to this disease.

In addition to cancer, other testicular conditions such as orchitis, epididymitis, and testicular torsion require prompt attention to avoid complications. Early detection of these conditions can prevent severe outcomes, including infertility or long-term damage to the testicles. Men should be educated on the importance of recognising symptoms like swelling, redness, or acute pain, which may indicate these urgent issues that warrant immediate medical evaluation.

The integration of diagnostic imaging techniques in the evaluation of testicular diseases has further enhanced early detection. Imaging modalities, such as ultrasound, can help identify abnormalities that may not be palpable during a physical examination. As technology advances, these tools become more accessible, allowing for quicker and more accurate diagnoses. Ultimately, fostering a culture of awareness and early detection is essential for improving men's health outcomes related to testicular diseases.

Risk Factors and Epidemiology

Testicular diseases encompass a range of conditions that vary significantly in their aetiology and impact on male reproductive health. Understanding the risk factors associated with these diseases is crucial for early detection and effective management. Factors such as age, family history, and certain genetic predispositions can increase the likelihood of developing conditions like testicular cancer. Furthermore, lifestyle choices, including smoking and exposure to environmental toxins, have been implicated in the aetiology of these diseases, necessitating a comprehensive approach to risk assessment.

Epidemiologically, testicular cancer is one of the most common malignancies among young men, particularly those aged 15 to 35. The incidence of this cancer has been rising in many parts of the world, although the reasons for this increase remain unclear. In contrast, conditions such as orchitis and epididymitis, which are often linked to infections, are more prevalent in specific demographics, such as sexually active young men. Understanding these epidemiological trends helps healthcare professionals tailor screening and preventive strategies effectively.

Another significant aspect of testicular diseases is the relationship between hormonal disorders and testicular function. Conditions such as hypogonadism can lead to infertility and have been associated with an increased risk of developing testicular cancer. This interplay between hormonal health and testicular conditions highlights the need for a multidisciplinary approach in diagnosing and treating these diseases. Urologists and healthcare professionals must remain vigilant in recognising symptoms that may indicate underlying hormonal imbalances.

Moreover, the implications of testicular trauma cannot be overlooked. Injuries to the testis can result from various activities, including sports or accidents, and can lead to acute conditions requiring immediate intervention. The management of testicular trauma often necessitates a thorough understanding of both the physical and psychological impacts on the patient, as these events can profoundly affect male reproductive health and self-esteem. Prompt diagnosis and appropriate treatment are essential to preserve testicular function and prevent long-term complications.

Lastly, congenital anomalies of the testis, although less common, represent an important area of concern in the field of urology. Conditions such as undescended testes can predispose individuals to various complications, including infertility and cancer. Early identification and surgical intervention are critical in managing these anomalies to reduce associated risks. Continuous research into the epidemiology and risk factors of testicular diseases is vital for improving outcomes and enhancing the quality of care for affected individuals.

Testicular Cancer Types and Treatments

Types of Testicular Cancer

Testicular cancer is a significant concern for men, particularly those aged between 15 and 35. It is essential to understand the various types of testicular cancer to facilitate early detection and treatment. The two primary categories of testicular cancer are seminomas and non-seminomas, each exhibiting distinct characteristics and treatment responses. Recognising these differences can aid healthcare professionals in tailoring effective management strategies for their patients.

Seminomas are a type of testicular cancer that typically grows slowly and is more responsive to radiation therapy. These tumours arise from germ cells and are often diagnosed at an early stage. There are two subtypes of seminomas: classic seminomas and spermatocytic seminomas. Classic seminomas are the most common, while spermatocytic seminomas are rare and usually affect older men. Early-stage seminomas have a high cure rate, making them a critical focus in testicular cancer treatment.

On the other hand, non-seminomas encompass a group of testicular cancers that include embryonal carcinoma, yolk sac tumour, and teratoma, among others. Non-seminomas tend to grow more quickly and may spread to other parts of the body at an earlier stage compared to seminomas. These types can be more challenging to treat, particularly if not detected early. The treatment typically involves a combination of surgery, chemotherapy, and in some cases, radiation therapy, depending on the specific type and stage of the cancer.

In addition to the classification based on histology, the staging of testicular cancer is crucial in determining the prognosis and treatment options. The staging system evaluates the extent of cancer spread, which significantly influences the treatment strategy. Understanding the staging and the type of testicular cancer helps both men and healthcare professionals in making informed decisions about management and potential outcomes.

In conclusion, familiarity with the different types of testicular cancer, such as seminomas and non-seminomas, is vital for effective treatment and management. Men and healthcare professionals should work closely to ensure early detection and appropriate intervention. As research continues to evolve, it is imperative to stay informed about the latest treatment options and guidelines to improve survival rates and quality of life for those affected by this disease.

Staging and Grading of Testicular Cancer

The staging and grading of testicular cancer are crucial processes that determine the extent of the disease and the appropriate treatment options. Testicular cancer is primarily classified into two main types: seminomas and non-seminomas. Each type has different characteristics and behaviours, which significantly influence the staging process. By understanding these classifications, healthcare professionals can more effectively plan treatment strategies tailored to individual patient needs.

Staging involves assessing the size of the tumour, whether it has spread to lymph nodes, and if there are metastases to other organs. The most used staging system for testicular cancer is the American Joint Committee on Cancer (AJCC) system, which categorises the disease into stages I through IV. Each stage reflects the severity of the cancer, providing critical information that guides treatment decisions and prognosis. For instance, stage I indicates a confined tumour, while stage IV signifies advanced disease with distant spread.

Grading, on the other hand, refers to the histological characteristics of the tumour cells, indicating how aggressive the cancer may be. Testicular tumours are graded based on their appearance under a microscope, with higher grades suggesting a more aggressive disease. This information helps urologists and oncologists predict the likely course of the disease and decide on the intensity of the treatment required. Understanding grading is essential for men diagnosed with testicular cancer, as it can affect their overall outlook and treatment options.

In addition to staging and grading, diagnostic imaging techniques play a vital role in assessing testicular cancer. Imaging modalities such as ultrasound, CT scans, and MRI are utilised to evaluate the presence of tumours and their potential spread. These techniques not only assist in staging but also help in monitoring the response to treatment, enabling healthcare professionals to make informed decisions throughout the patient's care journey. Accurate imaging is essential for ensuring optimal outcomes for men facing this diagnosis.

Finally, it is important for both men and healthcare professionals to engage in discussions about the implications of staging and grading on fertility and hormonal function. Testicular cancer and its treatments can have significant effects on a man's reproductive health. Understanding these factors is vital for managing patients holistically, ensuring that their concerns about fertility, sexual function, and overall health are addressed as part of their treatment plan.

Treatment Modalities

Treatment modalities for testicular diseases encompass a wide array of approaches tailored to specific conditions. For instance, testicular cancer management often involves a combination of surgery, chemotherapy, and radiation therapy, depending on the type and stage of cancer. Surgical options may include orchiectomy, where the affected testis is removed, which can significantly impact fertility and hormonal balance. Healthcare professionals must discuss these implications with patients to ensure informed decision-making.

In cases of orchitis, treatment focuses on addressing the underlying cause, which may be viral or bacterial. Antibiotics are prescribed for bacterial infections, while supportive care such as rest, ice, and pain relief is recommended for viral cases. Men experiencing orchitis should be monitored closely to prevent complications such as abscess formation or infertility. Effective communication between healthcare providers and patients is crucial for successful management.

Testicular torsion is a surgical emergency that requires immediate intervention to salvage the affected testis. The diagnosis is typically made based on clinical history and physical examination, with imaging techniques such as Doppler ultrasound aiding in the assessment of blood flow. Prompt surgical detorsion and fixation are essential to prevent irreversible damage. Understanding the urgency of this condition can help men recognise its symptoms and seek timely medical assistance.

Epididymitis, often resulting from infections or sexually transmitted diseases, is treated with antibiotics and analgesics. Patients are advised to abstain from sexual activity during treatment and to follow up with their healthcare provider to ensure resolution of symptoms. Chronic cases may require further investigation to identify underlying causes, including congenital anomalies or hormonal disorders. Education on preventive measures is crucial in reducing recurrence rates.

Finally, the management of testicular trauma varies significantly based on the severity of the injury. In minor cases, conservative treatment may suffice, while severe injuries may necessitate surgical intervention to repair damage and preserve testicular function. Proper assessment through diagnostic imaging techniques is vital to guide treatment strategies. Healthcare professionals should remain vigilant about the long-term implications of testicular trauma on fertility and overall health.

Follow-Up and Survivorship

Follow-up care and survivorship are critical components in the management of testicular diseases, particularly after a diagnosis of testicular cancer. Regular monitoring allows healthcare providers to detect any recurrence of cancer early, which can significantly improve outcomes. Men who have undergone treatment for testicular cancer should have a structured follow-up plan that includes physical examinations and imaging tests, tailored to their specific treatment history and risk factors.

In addition to cancer, other testicular conditions require diligent follow-up. Orchitis, epididymitis, and testicular torsion can lead to complications if not managed properly. For instance, chronic pain or infertility can arise from untreated infections or torsion. Therefore, men experiencing symptoms such as persistent pain, swelling, or changes in testicular size should seek medical attention promptly. Healthcare professionals should educate patients about the importance of follow-up visits, ensuring they understand the potential long-term effects of their conditions.

Hormonal disorders related to testicular function also necessitate ongoing evaluation. Conditions such as hypogonadism can impact a man's overall health, leading to issues such as decreased libido, fatigue, and mood disturbances. Regular assessments of testosterone levels, along with other relevant hormones, should be part of the follow-up plan for men with a history of testicular diseases. This proactive approach can help address any hormonal imbalances that may contribute to further health complications.

Infertility linked to testicular diseases is another area where follow-up is crucial. Men diagnosed with conditions such as varicocele or previous testicular trauma may face challenges in fathering children. Fertility assessments should be integrated into follow-up care, with referrals to specialists as needed. Additionally, men should be educated on potential assisted reproductive technologies that can help them achieve their family planning goals despite underlying testicular issues.

Finally, survivorship care should extend beyond physical health to encompass mental and emotional wellbeing. The psychological impact of a testicular disease diagnosis, particularly cancer, can be profound. Survivorship programmes should include support for mental health, addressing anxiety and depression that may arise during and after treatment. By providing comprehensive care that includes both physical and psychological support, healthcare professionals can greatly enhance the quality of life for men navigating life after testicular disease.

Orchitis: Causes and Management

Definition and Types of Orchitis

Orchitis is defined as the inflammation of one or both testicles, which can result from various infectious or non-infectious causes. This condition often presents with symptoms such as testicular pain, swelling, and redness. Understanding the underlying causes of orchitis is essential for effective management and treatment, making it crucial for both men and healthcare professionals to recognise its implications on reproductive health.

There are primarily two types of orchitis: viral and bacterial. Viral orchitis, often associated with infections like mumps, tends to be self-limiting and requires supportive care. In contrast, bacterial orchitis can stem from sexually transmitted infections or urinary tract infections, necessitating prompt antibiotic treatment to prevent complications such as abscess formation or infertility.

In addition to these infectious types, non-infectious orchitis can occur due to trauma, autoimmune conditions, or even following certain medical procedures. This type may present similarly to infectious orchitis but often requires a different approach in terms of diagnosis and management. Identifying the type of orchitis is pivotal in tailoring the treatment plan appropriately.

The diagnosis of orchitis typically involves a thorough clinical examination, patient history, and diagnostic imaging techniques such as ultrasound. These methods help differentiate orchitis from other testicular conditions, including testicular torsion and epididymitis, which may present with similar symptoms.

Accurate diagnosis is vital to implement the correct treatment strategy and to avoid unnecessary complications.

In conclusion, understanding the definition and types of orchitis is crucial for effective management of testicular diseases. Both men and healthcare professionals should be educated about the signs, causes, and treatment options available for this condition. Timely intervention can significantly improve outcomes and preserve fertility, making awareness a key element in testicular health.

Causes of Orchitis

Orchitis, an inflammation of one or both testicles, can arise from a variety of causes. The most common culprits are viral infections, particularly mumps, which can lead to significant testicular swelling and pain. Mumps orchitis tends to occur in post-pubertal males and can result in complications such as infertility. Other viral agents, such as the Coxsackie virus, can also induce similar symptoms, emphasising the need for awareness of viral aetiologies in orchitis cases.

Bacterial infections constitute another significant cause of orchitis, often resulting from sexually transmitted infections (STIs) such as gonorrhoea and chlamydia. These infections can ascend from the urethra or epididymis, leading to inflammation of the testicular tissue. Timely recognition and treatment of these bacterial infections are crucial, as they can not only cause acute discomfort but also pose long-term risks, including infertility and chronic pain if left untreated.

In addition to infectious causes, orchitis may also be linked to non-infectious factors, such as trauma or injury to the testicles. Physical trauma can result from sports injuries, accidents, or even vigorous sexual activity, leading to inflammation and subsequent pain. Understanding the role of trauma in orchitis is important for both patients and healthcare professionals as it emphasises the need for protective measures in high-risk activities.

Autoimmune conditions are another potential cause of orchitis, where the body's immune system mistakenly attacks its own testicular tissue. This can occur in various autoimmune disorders, leading to chronic inflammation and fertility issues. Identifying autoimmune causes requires a comprehensive evaluation by healthcare professionals, ensuring that patients receive appropriate management strategies to mitigate symptoms and preserve testicular function.

Lastly, certain congenital anomalies or anatomical variations can predispose individuals to orchitis. Conditions such as testicular torsion or hernias can compromise blood supply to the testicles, resulting in inflammation. Awareness of these congenital factors is essential for urologists and healthcare professionals, as early intervention can prevent significant complications and enhance patient outcomes.

Clinical Presentation

The clinical presentation of testicular diseases encompasses a wide range of symptoms and signs that can indicate underlying pathologies. Men may experience pain, swelling, or changes in the size of the testis, which can be indicative of conditions such as testicular torsion or orchitis. Additionally, the presence of lumps or masses in the scrotal area should raise suspicion for testicular cancer and warrants further investigation. Accurate assessment of these symptoms is crucial for timely diagnosis and management, especially in cases where immediate intervention may be necessary.

Testicular cancer often presents with a painless lump in the testicle, which may be accompanied by a feeling of heaviness in the scrotum. Men may also report other symptoms such as discomfort or an ache in the lower abdomen or groin area. Clinical examination and ultrasound imaging are vital in distinguishing between benign and malignant lesions. Understanding the specific types of testicular cancer, including seminomas and non-seminomas, is essential for determining the appropriate treatment course and ensuring better patient outcomes.

Orchitis, an inflammation of the testis, may present with sudden onset of testicular pain, swelling, and warmth. This can be caused by viral infections, such as mumps, or bacterial infections, often linked to sexually transmitted diseases. Management of orchitis typically involves supportive care, including analgesics and antibiotics if a bacterial cause is identified. Prompt diagnosis and treatment are necessary to prevent complications, such as infertility or chronic pain.

Testicular torsion is a surgical emergency characterised by the twisting of the spermatic cord, leading to ischaemia of the testicle. It often manifests with acute onset of severe scrotal pain, nausea, and vomiting. Diagnosis is primarily clinical, supported by imaging studies if needed. Immediate surgical intervention is critical to salvage the affected testis and prevent long-term complications, including loss of testicular function.

Epididymitis, an inflammation of the epididymis, typically presents with scrotal pain and swelling, often associated with urinary symptoms. The condition can be caused by bacterial infections, including sexually transmitted infections, and may require antibiotic therapy based on the underlying cause. Diagnostic imaging may also be employed to exclude other conditions, such as testicular torsion or abscess formation. Understanding these clinical presentations enables healthcare professionals to provide effective and timely care to men experiencing testicular issues.

Management Strategies

Management strategies for testicular diseases are essential for both healthcare professionals and patients. Understanding the various conditions that can affect the testes, such as testicular cancer, orchitis, and testicular torsion, allows for the formulation of effective treatment plans. Early diagnosis and intervention are crucial, as they significantly improve outcomes and quality of life for the affected individuals. Here we will explore the key management strategies associated with these conditions, focusing on prevention, diagnosis, treatment, and follow-up care.

For testicular cancer, the management strategy typically involves a multidisciplinary approach. This includes urologists, oncologists, and radiologists working together to establish the best course of action. Treatment options may include surgery, chemotherapy, and radiation therapy, depending on the type and stage of cancer. Regular monitoring through imaging techniques and serum tumour markers is vital to assess treatment effectiveness and detect any recurrence early.

Orchitis and epididymitis management strategies often focus on identifying and treating the underlying causes, which may include infections or trauma. Antibiotics are commonly prescribed for bacterial infections, while pain management and anti-inflammatory medications are used to alleviate symptoms. In some cases, surgical intervention may be necessary to address complications or persistent issues. Patient education on preventive measures, such as safe sexual practices and proper hygiene, is also a vital component of effective management.

Testicular torsion represents a surgical emergency that requires prompt diagnosis and intervention to save the affected testis. The management strategy involves immediate surgical detorsion and fixation of the testis to prevent future occurrences. Healthcare professionals must be vigilant in recognising the symptoms of torsion to initiate timely treatment, as delayed intervention can lead to significant complications, including loss of the testis.

In managing infertility linked to testicular diseases, a thorough assessment of hormonal function, testicular health, and potential infections is necessary. Treatment options may include hormonal therapy, surgical correction of anatomical anomalies, or assisted reproductive technologies such as in vitro fertilisation. Comprehensive follow-up care is crucial for monitoring progress and addressing any emerging concerns, ensuring that patients receive the support they need throughout their treatment journey.

Testicular Torsion: Diagnosis and Intervention

Understanding Testicular Torsion

Testicular torsion is a medical emergency that occurs when the spermatic cord becomes twisted, cutting off the blood supply to the testis. This condition can lead to severe pain and, if not promptly treated, may result in the loss of the affected testis. Understanding the anatomy of the testis and the mechanism behind torsion is crucial for both men and healthcare professionals, as early recognition and intervention are essential for preserving testicular function.

The symptoms of testicular torsion typically include sudden onset of severe testicular pain, swelling, and sometimes nausea or vomiting. Men may also notice a change in the position of the testis, which can appear higher in the scrotum. It is important for healthcare professionals to differentiate between torsion and other causes of acute scrotal pain, such as epididymitis or trauma, as the management strategies differ significantly.

Diagnosis is often made through a combination of clinical examination and imaging studies, such as Doppler ultrasound, which can assess blood flow to the testis. In some cases, a surgical exploration may be necessary to confirm the diagnosis. The urgency of the situation cannot be overstated; studies indicate that the testis can become necrotic within hours of torsion onset, highlighting the importance of immediate medical attention.

Treatment for testicular torsion usually involves surgical intervention to untwist the spermatic cord and restore blood flow. Surgical fixation of the testis is often performed to prevent recurrence of torsion. Post-operative care and counselling regarding the risk of infertility or hormonal issues related to testicular health should be discussed with the patient, as these factors can significantly impact quality of life.

In conclusion, understanding testicular torsion is vital for both men and healthcare professionals. Awareness of the symptoms, timely diagnosis, and prompt surgical management can greatly influence outcomes and preserve testicular health. Continuous education and training in recognising this condition are necessary to improve awareness and response rates among both patients and healthcare providers.

Symptoms and Signs

Recognising the symptoms and signs associated with testicular diseases is crucial for early diagnosis and effective management. Men may experience various symptoms that could indicate underlying conditions, such as swelling or lumps in the testicular region. Additionally, changes in size or shape of the testicles, accompanied by pain or discomfort, should prompt immediate medical consultation to rule out serious issues like testicular cancer or torsion.

Testicular cancer can present with non-specific symptoms such as a feeling of heaviness in the scrotum or persistent back pain. It is essential for healthcare professionals to educate patients about self-examination techniques, enabling them to identify any abnormalities early. Regular check-ups and awareness of family history can also aid in early detection, significantly improving treatment outcomes.

Orchitis, an inflammation of the testis, often develops following a viral infection, leading to symptoms like acute pain, swelling, and fever. In some cases, men may experience nausea and vomiting due to the severity of the discomfort. Management of orchitis involves addressing the underlying infection and providing symptomatic relief, highlighting the importance of recognising these signs promptly.

Epididymitis, characterised by inflammation of the epididymis, can also present with similar symptoms, including pain in the lower abdomen and fever. It is frequently caused by sexually transmitted infections, making awareness and education about sexual health vital in preventing such conditions. Treatment typically involves antibiotics and pain management, underscoring the need for timely intervention to prevent complications.

In addition to these conditions, hormonal disorders linked to testicular function may exhibit symptoms such as changes in libido or fertility issues. Men experiencing these signs should seek evaluation from a urologist, who can perform diagnostic imaging techniques to assess testicular health. Understanding these symptoms and signs is a key aspect of managing testicular diseases effectively, ensuring better health outcomes for men.

Diagnostic Approaches

Diagnostic approaches for testicular diseases are crucial in ensuring timely and effective treatment. A thorough understanding of the various diagnostic techniques available can aid healthcare professionals in differentiating between diverse conditions such as testicular cancer, orchitis, and testicular torsion.

Traditional methods such as physical examinations and patient history taking are often complemented by advanced imaging techniques to provide a comprehensive assessment of testicular health.

Ultrasound imaging has emerged as a key diagnostic tool in evaluating testicular conditions. This non-invasive procedure allows for real-time visualization of the testes and surrounding structures, enabling the detection of abnormalities such as masses, cysts, or signs of torsion. In cases of suspected testicular cancer, ultrasound findings can guide further investigations, including fine-needle aspiration or biopsy, which are essential for confirming malignancy and determining the appropriate treatment plan.

In addition to imaging, laboratory tests play a significant role in the diagnostic process. Serum tumour markers, including alpha-fetoprotein (AFP) and human chorionic gonadotropin (hCG), are particularly useful in diagnosing testicular cancer and monitoring treatment response. Moreover, hormone level assessments can provide insights into underlying hormonal disorders related to testicular function, which may contribute to infertility issues in men.

When diagnosing conditions such as epididymitis or orchitis, a thorough clinical evaluation is essential. This may involve urine tests to identify potential infections, including sexually transmitted diseases. In cases of testicular trauma, imaging studies combined with a detailed clinical history are critical to assessing the extent of injury and guiding management decisions to prevent complications.

Lastly, understanding congenital anomalies of the testis requires a multidisciplinary approach, where genetic counselling and imaging may be necessary for accurate diagnosis. Ultimately, an integrated approach that combines clinical evaluation, imaging, and laboratory tests is vital for effective diagnosis and management of testicular diseases. This comprehensive strategy not only aids in the identification of specific conditions but also enhances patient outcomes through timely interventions.

Surgical Intervention

Surgical intervention plays a crucial role in the management of various testicular diseases, particularly when conservative treatments fail or when immediate action is required. In cases of testicular torsion, for example, prompt surgical intervention is essential to salvage the affected testis and prevent irreversible damage. The surgical procedure typically involves untwisting the spermatic cord and securing the testis to prevent recurrence, highlighting the importance of timely diagnosis and intervention in preserving testicular health.

Testicular cancer is another area where surgical intervention is critical. Different types of testicular cancer may require distinct surgical approaches, such as radical inguinal orchiectomy, which involves the removal of the affected testis and surrounding tissue. This procedure not only provides a definitive diagnosis through histopathological examination but also serves as a primary treatment modality for localized tumours. Post-operative management may include further treatments like chemotherapy or radiotherapy, depending on the cancer stage and type.

In cases of orchitis and epididymitis, surgical intervention may be less common but is sometimes necessary. Severe cases that do not respond to medical management or present with abscess formation may require drainage or, in rare instances, surgical removal of affected tissues. Understanding when to escalate to surgical options is vital for healthcare professionals to ensure optimal patient outcomes and reduce complications associated with untreated infections.

Testicular trauma, whether from blunt force or penetrating injuries, often necessitates surgical intervention to repair damaged tissues or to address complications such as testicular rupture. The approach to managing testicular trauma can vary based on the severity and type of injury, with the goal of preserving testicular function and fertility whenever possible. This underscores the importance of rapid assessment and intervention to mitigate long-term consequences for affected individuals.

Lastly, congenital anomalies of the testis may also require surgical correction. Conditions such as undescended testis (cryptorchidism) can lead to infertility and increase the risk of testicular cancer if left untreated. Surgical intervention is typically performed during childhood to position the testis in the scrotum, ensuring normal development and function. This proactive approach reflects the essential role of surgery in addressing testicular diseases and preserving men's health throughout their lives.

Epididymitis: Symptoms and Treatment Options

Overview of Epididymitis

Epididymitis is an inflammation of the epididymis, a coiled tube located at the back of the testis responsible for the storage, maturation, and transport of sperm.

This condition can affect men of all ages, but it is most commonly seen in sexually active males between the ages of 14 and 35. The inflammation can be caused by various factors, including infections, trauma, or even certain medical conditions. Understanding the underlying causes and implications of epididymitis is crucial for effective diagnosis and treatment.

The most common infectious agents responsible for epididymitis include sexually transmitted infections (STIs) such as Chlamydia trachomatis and Neisseria gonorrhoeae, as well as non-sexually transmitted bacteria. In older men, urinary tract infections can also lead to epididymitis. Symptoms typically manifest as unilateral scrotal pain, swelling, and tenderness, often accompanied by fever and dysuria. Early recognition of these symptoms is vital to prevent complications such as abscess formation or chronic pain.

Diagnosis of epididymitis generally involves a combination of clinical evaluation, patient history, and laboratory tests, including urinalysis and STI screening. Ultrasound may be employed to assess the extent of inflammation and rule out other potential conditions such as testicular torsion. Accurate diagnosis is essential, as it informs the appropriate management strategies and helps differentiate epididymitis from other testicular disorders.

Treatment of epididymitis typically involves the use of antibiotics, tailored to the specific causative organism identified through laboratory tests. Non-steroidal anti-inflammatory drugs (NSAIDs) may be prescribed to alleviate pain and inflammation. In cases where an abscess forms, surgical intervention may be necessary. Patient education regarding safe sexual practices and regular follow-ups are also critical components of management to prevent recurrence and address any potential complications.

Overall, understanding epididymitis is crucial for both men and healthcare professionals as it highlights the importance of timely diagnosis and treatment. Awareness of the condition can lead to improved health outcomes and a better quality of life for affected individuals. By recognising the symptoms and seeking appropriate care, men can mitigate the risks associated with this condition and contribute to their overall reproductive health.

Causes and Risk Factors

Understanding the causes and risk factors associated with testicular diseases is crucial for both men and healthcare professionals. Various factors can contribute to the development of these conditions, ranging from genetic predispositions to environmental influences. For instance, a family history of testicular cancer can significantly increase an individual's risk, highlighting the importance of awareness and regular check-ups for those with affected relatives.

In addition to genetic factors, hormonal disorders play a significant role in testicular health. Conditions such as hypogonadism, which leads to low testosterone levels, can affect the function of the testis and may predispose individuals to various diseases, including infertility and cancer. Men experiencing symptoms related to hormonal imbalances should seek medical advice to manage these issues effectively.

Environmental factors are also noteworthy when discussing testicular diseases. Exposure to certain chemicals, such as pesticides or heavy metals, has been linked to an increased risk of testicular cancer. Additionally, lifestyle factors such as smoking and excessive alcohol consumption can exacerbate these risks, underlining the need for healthy lifestyle choices to mitigate potential harm.

Infections and sexually transmitted diseases (STDs) represent another significant cause of testicular complications. Conditions like epididymitis and orchitis can arise from infections, leading to inflammation and discomfort. Understanding these infections and their transmission routes can help in early diagnosis and treatment, reducing the risk of long-term consequences such as infertility.

Lastly, congenital anomalies of the testis can lead to various complications later in life, including an increased risk of malignancy. Conditions such as undescended testis (cryptorchidism) require careful monitoring and potential surgical intervention to prevent future health issues. Awareness of these congenital factors is essential for healthcare professionals in guiding patients towards appropriate management strategies.

Clinical Manifestations

Clinical manifestations of testicular diseases can vary significantly, often presenting with a range of symptoms that may indicate underlying conditions. One of the most common issues is testicular pain, which can arise from various causes such as torsion, trauma, or infections. Men experiencing acute or severe pain should seek immediate medical attention, as timely intervention is crucial for preserving testicular function. Additionally, swelling or enlargement of the testis may signal conditions like epididymitis or orchitis, necessitating a thorough evaluation by a healthcare professional.

Testicular cancer is another critical concern with distinct clinical manifestations. Patients may notice a painless lump or swelling in the testis, which is often the first sign prompting medical consultation. Other symptoms may include changes in the shape or texture of the testicle, discomfort in the scrotum, or a feeling of heaviness. Early detection is vital for effective treatment, making awareness of these signs essential for men, particularly those in higher risk categories such as younger males.

Infections of the testis, such as epididymitis and orchitis, frequently present with characteristic symptoms including pain, swelling, and redness. These infections can be caused by sexually transmitted diseases or bacterial infections, and they often require prompt medical treatment to prevent complications. Men experiencing fever, chills, or discharge should seek medical help, as these symptoms can indicate a more serious underlying issue.

Testicular torsion, a surgical emergency, typically manifests through sudden acute pain and swelling. It often occurs in adolescents and young adults and can lead to irreversible damage if not addressed quickly. Diagnosis is typically made through clinical evaluation and ultrasound imaging, which helps confirm the presence of blood flow issues. Immediate surgical intervention is essential to salvage the affected testis and prevent long-term complications.

Lastly, congenital anomalies of the testis can present with various clinical manifestations from birth or during adolescence. Conditions such as cryptorchidism, where one or both testicles fail to descend, may lead to fertility issues or increased cancer risk later in life. Regular check-ups and awareness of these conditions can help in early diagnosis and management, ensuring better health outcomes for affected individuals.

Treatment and Management

The management of testicular diseases requires a multi-faceted approach that encompasses accurate diagnosis, tailored treatment plans, and ongoing support. For testicular cancer, early detection is crucial, and treatment options may include surgery, chemotherapy, and radiation therapy, depending on the type and stage of cancer. Healthcare professionals must remain vigilant in monitoring patients for recurrence and managing the long-term side effects of treatment, which can significantly impact quality of life.

In cases of orchitis, the underlying causes must be identified to determine the appropriate management strategies. Viral infections often resolve on their own, while bacterial orchitis may necessitate antibiotic therapy. Pain management and supportive care are essential components of treatment, and healthcare professionals should educate patients about the importance of rest and hydration during recovery.

Testicular torsion is a surgical emergency that demands immediate intervention to salvage the affected testis. Prompt diagnosis through clinical examination and imaging techniques can facilitate timely surgical correction. Post-operative care involves monitoring for complications and addressing any concerns regarding fertility, particularly in younger patients.

Epididymitis presents with a range of symptoms, including swelling and pain, and its treatment hinges on the underlying cause. Antibiotics are often prescribed for bacterial infections, while non-steroidal anti-inflammatory drugs can alleviate discomfort. Patients should be counselled on preventive measures to reduce the risk of recurrence, such as safe sexual practices and regular medical check-ups.

Testicular trauma can have significant implications, from acute injury to chronic complications such as infertility. Proper assessment and management are essential, including imaging studies to evaluate for internal damage. Healthcare professionals must provide comprehensive care that addresses both the physical and emotional aspects of recovery, ensuring that patients receive the support they need during this challenging time.

Testicular Trauma and Its Implications

Types of Testicular Trauma

Testicular trauma can manifest in various forms, each with distinct causes and implications. The most common type is blunt trauma, which often results from sports injuries, accidents, or physical altercations. Such incidents may lead to bruising, swelling, or even rupture of the testicles. Recognising the signs of blunt trauma is crucial for timely intervention and treatment to prevent further complications.

Another significant type of testicular trauma is penetrating injury, typically seen in cases involving sharp objects or gunshot wounds. These injuries can lead to severe damage, not only to the testis but also to surrounding structures, potentially resulting in significant blood loss and infection. Prompt surgical evaluation is essential to address the extent of the injury and to preserve testicular function, which can be crucial for fertility.

Testicular torsion, while primarily a condition involving the twisting of the spermatic cord, can also be classified under traumatic events. This condition is often triggered by an injury or even vigorous physical activity. It requires immediate medical attention to restore blood flow to the affected testis, as prolonged torsion can lead to necrosis. Understanding the symptoms, such as severe pain and swelling, is vital for men and healthcare professionals to facilitate swift diagnosis and intervention.

In the context of trauma, the implications for fertility and overall testicular health are significant. Injuries that lead to testicular loss or dysfunction can have long-term effects, including infertility. Men experiencing any form of testicular trauma should be aware of the potential risks and seek medical advice to explore options for preservation of fertility and overall reproductive health.

Finally, diagnostic imaging plays a critical role in assessing testicular trauma. Techniques such as ultrasound are essential for evaluating the extent of injury and guiding treatment decisions. Healthcare professionals must be adept at interpreting these images to ensure appropriate management of testicular trauma, thereby optimising outcomes for affected individuals. This comprehensive understanding of types of testicular trauma is paramount for both men and healthcare providers in promoting reproductive health and addressing any related complications.

Assessment and Diagnosis

Assessment and diagnosis of testicular diseases is crucial for effective management and treatment. The first step in this process typically involves a thorough medical history and physical examination. Healthcare professionals must be vigilant in asking about symptoms such as pain, swelling, and changes in size or texture of the testicles, as these can indicate underlying conditions. A detailed history of any previous infections, trauma, or family history of testicular cancer is also essential for a comprehensive assessment.

Laboratory tests play a significant role in the evaluation of testicular diseases. In cases of suspected testicular cancer, serum tumour markers such as alpha-fetoprotein (AFP), human chorionic gonadotropin (hCG), and lactate dehydrogenase (LDH) can provide valuable diagnostic information. Additionally, routine blood tests may help identify infections or hormonal imbalances that could be contributing to testicular dysfunction. These tests, coupled with physical findings, guide the clinician towards a more accurate diagnosis.

Diagnostic imaging techniques are indispensable tools in the assessment of testicular conditions. Ultrasound is often the first-line imaging modality used to evaluate scrotal abnormalities, providing real-time images that can help distinguish between different types of lesions, such as cysts, tumours, or signs of torsion. In certain cases, more advanced imaging like MRI or CT scans may be employed to gain further insight into complex situations, especially in the context of suspected malignancy or trauma.

In addition to imaging and laboratory studies, specialist referrals may be necessary for comprehensive management. Urologists, who have advanced training in male reproductive health, are essential in diagnosing and treating conditions like orchitis, epididymitis, and testicular torsion. Their expertise is vital not only in surgical interventions but also in managing the long-term implications of these diseases, including fertility concerns and hormonal disorders linked to testicular function.

Ultimately, timely assessment and accurate diagnosis of testicular diseases are paramount for successful treatment outcomes. Men experiencing symptoms related to testicular health should be encouraged to seek medical advice promptly. By fostering an environment where open discussions about testicular health are normalised, healthcare professionals can significantly improve early detection and treatment of potentially serious conditions, ensuring better health and quality of life for their patients.

Management and Surgical Considerations

Management of testicular diseases requires a comprehensive understanding of the various conditions that can affect testicular health. This includes not only testicular cancer but also infections such as epididymitis and orchitis, as well as traumatic injuries and congenital anomalies. Each condition presents unique challenges for diagnosis and treatment, necessitating a tailored approach to patient care. Healthcare professionals must be adept at recognising symptoms that may indicate serious underlying issues, ensuring timely intervention to mitigate complications.

In the case of testicular cancer, management strategies can vary significantly based on the type and stage of the disease. Urologists play a crucial role in determining the most effective treatment options, which may include surgery, chemotherapy, or radiation therapy. Early detection is key, and healthcare providers must employ appropriate diagnostic imaging techniques to identify malignancies at the earliest possible stage. Additionally, discussions surrounding fertility preservation should be a routine part of the management plan, as many treatments can impact reproductive function.

Orchitis and epididymitis, often caused by infections, require prompt diagnosis and management to prevent long-term complications such as infertility. Antibiotic therapy is typically the first line of treatment, and in cases of severe pain or abscess formation, surgical intervention may be necessary. It is essential for healthcare professionals to educate patients about the importance of recognising symptoms early, as well as the potential for sexually transmitted infections to exacerbate these conditions.

Testicular torsion is another urgent condition that demands immediate surgical intervention. The diagnosis is often made based on clinical examination and imaging studies, and time is of the essence to salvage the affected testis. Urologists must be prepared to perform emergency surgery to untwist the spermatic cord and restore blood flow, highlighting the importance of prompt recognition of the symptoms by both patients and healthcare providers.

Finally, congenital anomalies and hormonal disorders related to testicular function require a multidisciplinary approach for effective management. Infertility linked to testicular diseases can often be addressed through assisted reproductive technologies, but it is vital for healthcare professionals to understand the underlying causes. This involves thorough diagnostic evaluation and long-term follow-up to optimise the management of these complex conditions, ultimately improving outcomes for affected individuals.

Congenital Anomalies of the Testis

Overview of Congenital Anomalies

Congenital anomalies of the testis refer to a range of developmental disorders that affect the normal structure and function of the testes. These anomalies can manifest in various forms, including undescended testes, testicular hypoplasia, or the presence of additional testicular tissue. Understanding these conditions is crucial, as they can significantly impact male reproductive health and increase the risk of associated complications, such as infertility and testicular cancer.

One of the most common congenital anomalies is cryptorchidism, where one or both testes fail to descend into the scrotum during foetal development. This condition is not only a cosmetic concern but also poses a risk for testicular cancer later in life. Early diagnosis and intervention are essential for managing cryptorchidism, often involving surgical procedures to relocate the testes to their proper position, thereby minimising potential long-term consequences.

Another significant anomaly is testicular agenesis, where one or both testes are absent. This condition can lead to hormonal imbalances and infertility. It often requires a multidisciplinary approach for management, including hormone replacement therapy and assisted reproductive technologies for those seeking to conceive. Urologists and healthcare professionals must be well-versed in these conditions to provide appropriate care and counselling to affected individuals.

The implications of congenital anomalies extend beyond physical appearance and fertility. Many of these conditions are associated with psychological effects, as men may experience feelings of inadequacy or distress related to their reproductive health. Therefore, healthcare professionals must adopt a holistic approach, addressing both the medical and psychological aspects of these anomalies to support men effectively.

In conclusion, congenital anomalies of the testis are critical conditions that warrant attention from both healthcare professionals and patients. Early detection and management can lead to improved outcomes, reducing the risks of infertility and malignancy. As our understanding of these conditions evolves, it is imperative for urologists and other health professionals to stay informed about the latest diagnostic and treatment options available to enhance patient care.

Types of Anomalies

Anomalies of the testis can broadly be classified into several categories, each with unique characteristics and implications. Congenital anomalies, for example, are present at birth and may include conditions such as cryptorchidism, where one or both testes fail to descend into the scrotum. These conditions often require careful management to prevent complications such as infertility or increased risk of testicular cancer later in life. Understanding these anomalies is crucial for both patients and healthcare professionals in order to provide timely intervention and appropriate treatment options.

Another significant category is testicular trauma, which can result from various causes including sports injuries, accidents, or surgical interventions. The implications of testicular trauma can be severe, leading to conditions such as testicular torsion or even loss of the testis. Prompt diagnosis and intervention are vital to preserving testicular function and preventing long-term consequences. Healthcare providers must be equipped to recognise the signs of trauma and implement immediate care strategies to mitigate risks.

Infections represent another critical type of anomaly affecting the testis, commonly seen in conditions such as epididymitis and orchitis. These infections can lead to significant discomfort and potential fertility issues if not treated effectively. The management of testicular infections often involves a combination of antibiotic therapy and supportive care. Recognising the symptoms early and understanding the underlying causes are essential for effective treatment and patient education.

Testicular cancer is a serious concern that encompasses various types of neoplasms, each with distinct treatment protocols. The most common types include seminomas and non-seminomas, which require different approaches to management and follow-up care. Awareness of the risk factors and early symptoms of testicular cancer is essential for early detection, which can significantly improve treatment outcomes. Health care professionals play a vital role in educating patients about self-examination and the importance of seeking medical advice for any abnormalities.

Lastly, hormonal disorders related to testicular function can lead to a range of health issues, including infertility. Conditions such as hypogonadism can disrupt normal hormonal balance and affect overall health. Understanding these disorders and their impact on testicular health is crucial for both diagnosis and management. Men facing such challenges should be encouraged to discuss their symptoms openly with healthcare providers to explore potential treatment options and support systems.

Clinical Implications and Management

Understanding the clinical implications of testicular diseases is crucial for both men and healthcare professionals. These conditions can significantly affect quality of life, fertility, and overall health. Early diagnosis and appropriate management are essential to mitigate long-term consequences. This subchapter will explore various testicular diseases, including testicular cancer, orchitis, testicular torsion, epididymitis, and congenital anomalies, highlighting their implications and management strategies.

Testicular cancer remains a significant concern, particularly among younger men. Awareness of the types of testicular cancer and their respective treatments is vital for effective management. Regular self-examinations and prompt medical consultation for any abnormalities can lead to early detection. Healthcare professionals should provide guidance on risk factors and the importance of vigilance in monitoring changes in testicular health.

Orchitis, often caused by infections or autoimmune conditions, can lead to pain and swelling. Management typically involves addressing the underlying cause, whether it be antibiotics for bacterial infections or supportive care for viral origins. Understanding the triggers and symptoms of orchitis enables healthcare providers to offer tailored treatment plans, minimising the impact on fertility and overall testicular function.

Testicular torsion is a surgical emergency that requires swift intervention to prevent necrosis of the affected testis. Recognising the clinical signs, such as sudden severe pain and swelling, is critical for timely diagnosis and treatment. Urologists play a pivotal role in the surgical management of this condition, and public awareness campaigns can help educate men about the signs and urgency of this serious condition.

Lastly, testicular infections and sexually transmitted diseases pose additional challenges in testicular health. Treatment options vary depending on the specific infection and its severity. Diagnostic imaging techniques are essential in evaluating testicular conditions, providing clarity in cases of trauma or suspected malignancy. Healthcare professionals must stay informed about the latest diagnostic and treatment advancements to offer the best care for their patients.

Hormonal Disorders Related to Testicular Function

Overview of Hormonal Regulation

Hormonal regulation plays a crucial role in the functioning of the testis and overall male reproductive health. The hypothalamic-pituitary-gonadal (HPG) axis is central to this process, beginning with the release of gonadotropin-releasing hormone (GnRH) from the hypothalamus. This hormone stimulates the pituitary gland to release luteinising hormone (LH) and follicle-stimulating hormone (FSH), which are essential for testicular function. LH primarily stimulates the Leydig cells to produce testosterone, while FSH is vital for spermatogenesis in the Sertoli cells. This delicate interplay of hormones ensures the maintenance of male reproductive capabilities and contributes to secondary sexual characteristics.

Testosterone, the principal male sex hormone, has far-reaching effects on the body beyond reproduction. It influences muscle mass, bone density, and even mood. Disorders of hormonal regulation can lead to conditions such as hypogonadism, where the body does not produce enough testosterone, potentially resulting in infertility and diminished quality of life. Understanding the hormonal balance is essential for diagnosing and managing various testicular diseases, including those linked to hormonal disorders.

In addition to testosterone, other hormones such as inhibin B and anti-Müllerian hormone (AMH) play significant roles in testicular function. Inhibin B, produced by Sertoli cells, provides negative feedback to the pituitary gland to regulate FSH secretion. AMH, produced during foetal development, is crucial for male sexual differentiation. An imbalance in these hormones can lead to a range of testicular issues, including congenital anomalies and infertility, highlighting the importance of a comprehensive hormonal assessment in men facing reproductive challenges.

Moreover, testicular diseases such as infections, torsion, and trauma can also impact hormonal regulation. Conditions like orchitis and epididymitis can lead to inflammation and subsequent hormonal dysregulation, affecting testosterone production and sperm quality. Prompt diagnosis and intervention are essential to mitigate the long-term effects these conditions may have on hormonal health and fertility. Urologists and healthcare professionals must remain vigilant in assessing hormonal levels when managing testicular diseases to provide optimal patient care.

In summary, a thorough understanding of hormonal regulation is vital for recognising and treating testicular diseases effectively. The interplay between various hormones and their impact on testicular function is essential knowledge for healthcare professionals. Addressing hormonal disorders not only aids in the management of testicular diseases but also enhances the overall reproductive health of men. Future research in this area may lead to improved diagnostic and therapeutic strategies, ultimately benefiting patients with testicular conditions.

Common Hormonal Disorders

Hormonal disorders related to testicular function can significantly impact men's health, influencing various physiological processes. These conditions often arise from imbalances in testosterone and other hormones produced by the testes.

Understanding the common hormonal disorders is essential for both men and healthcare professionals, as these issues can lead to infertility, reduced libido, and other health complications if left untreated.

One prevalent hormonal disorder is hypogonadism, characterised by insufficient testosterone production. This condition can be primary, resulting from testicular dysfunction, or secondary, caused by issues in the hypothalamus or pituitary gland. Symptoms often include fatigue, decreased muscle mass, and mood changes. Diagnosis typically involves blood tests to measure hormone levels, followed by appropriate treatment options, which may include hormone replacement therapy.

Another common disorder is hyperprolactinaemia, where elevated levels of prolactin can interfere with testosterone production. This condition can lead to sexual dysfunction and infertility in men. Causes can range from pituitary tumours to certain medications. Treatment usually focuses on addressing the underlying cause, which may involve medication or surgical intervention, thereby restoring hormonal balance and normal testicular function.

Androgen insensitivity syndrome (AIS) is another notable hormonal disorder that affects testicular function. In this condition, individuals with male XY chromosomes have a reduced response to androgens, leading to incomplete masculinisation. Diagnosis is often made in adolescence or adulthood when individuals present with atypical genitalia or infertility. Management may involve hormone therapy and psychological support to aid in coping with the condition's implications.

Lastly, hormonal disorders can also manifest in the form of testicular tumours, which can produce hormones such as human chorionic gonadotropin (hCG) or oestrogen, leading to hormonal imbalances. These tumours may cause symptoms such as gynecomastia or signs of precocious puberty in younger males. Early detection through diagnostic imaging and blood tests is vital for effective management and treatment, ensuring optimal outcomes for affected individuals.

Diagnosis and Treatment

The diagnosis of testicular diseases involves a comprehensive assessment that includes patient history, physical examination, and diagnostic imaging. Men presenting with symptoms such as lumps, pain, or changes in size require thorough evaluation. A detailed medical history can reveal potential risk factors, while a physical examination helps to identify any abnormalities. Ultrasound is commonly employed as the first-line imaging technique due to its non-invasive nature and ability to differentiate between solid and cystic lesions.

Testicular cancer is one of the most critical conditions to diagnose early, as it is highly treatable when detected promptly. Various types of testicular cancer, such as seminomas and non-seminomas, have distinct characteristics and treatment protocols. After imaging studies suggest malignancy, a biopsy may be performed to confirm the diagnosis. Following diagnosis, staging is essential to determine the extent of the disease and tailor the treatment plan effectively.

Orchitis, characterized by inflammation of the testis, can result from infections or autoimmune conditions. Management typically involves addressing the underlying cause, which may include antibiotics for bacterial infections or anti-inflammatory medications for viral infections. Proper diagnosis is crucial to prevent complications such as infertility or chronic pain. In cases of testicular torsion, immediate diagnosis and intervention are vital to salvage the testis and prevent irreversible damage.

Epididymitis, often linked to sexually transmitted infections, presents with specific symptoms such as swelling and pain in the scrotum. Treatment usually involves antibiotics and anti-inflammatory drugs to alleviate symptoms and eradicate the infection. In certain cases, scrotal support and rest may also be recommended. Understanding the spectrum of testicular infections is essential for healthcare professionals to provide appropriate care and counselling for affected men.

In addition to infections and malignancies, congenital anomalies of the testis, hormonal disorders, and trauma can significantly impact testicular function and male fertility. Diagnostic imaging techniques play a crucial role in identifying these conditions, allowing for timely and effective management. For instance, conditions such as varicocele or testicular trauma require different approaches based on their presentation, highlighting the importance of a tailored treatment strategy to optimise patient outcomes.

Infertility Linked to Testicular Diseases

Understanding Male Infertility

Male infertility is a complex issue that affects a significant proportion of men worldwide. It is primarily defined as the inability to conceive after one year of unprotected intercourse. Understanding the underlying causes of male infertility is crucial not only for affected individuals but also for healthcare professionals who aim to provide effective treatment options. Various factors can contribute to male infertility, including hormonal imbalances, anatomical abnormalities, and environmental influences.

One of the most common causes of male infertility is hormonal disorders that affect testicular function. Conditions such as hypogonadism, where the body does not produce enough testosterone, can lead to reduced sperm production and quality. Additionally, disorders of the hypothalamus or pituitary gland, which regulate hormone secretion, can also impact fertility. Identifying these hormonal issues through appropriate diagnostic tests is essential for developing a tailored treatment plan.

Testicular diseases, including infections, torsion, and trauma, can significantly impact a man's fertility. Orchitis, an inflammation of the testes, and epididymitis, an inflammation of the epididymis, can both lead to scarring and impaired sperm transport. Moreover, testicular torsion, a condition where the spermatic cord becomes twisted, requires immediate medical intervention to prevent permanent damage. Understanding these conditions allows healthcare providers to manage symptoms effectively and improve fertility outcomes.

Congenital anomalies of the testis, such as undescended testes, can also contribute to infertility issues. These conditions may lead to abnormal testicular development, impacting sperm production. Furthermore, testicular cancer and its treatments can have long-term effects on fertility. It is essential for men diagnosed with testicular cancer to discuss fertility preservation options prior to undergoing treatment, as certain therapies may adversely affect their reproductive capabilities.

Lastly, lifestyle factors and environmental exposures play a critical role in male fertility. Factors such as obesity, smoking, and exposure to toxins can negatively affect sperm quality and quantity. Healthcare professionals should encourage men to adopt healthier lifestyles to enhance their fertility potential. By understanding the multifaceted nature of male infertility, both men and healthcare providers can work collaboratively to address and manage this significant health concern.

Testicular Factors Affecting Fertility

The male reproductive system is intricately linked to the health of the testes, which play a crucial role in fertility. Various testicular factors can significantly impact a man's ability to conceive, including hormonal imbalances, infections, and anatomical anomalies. Understanding these factors is essential for healthcare professionals and men alike, as they can lead to infertility or complicate existing reproductive issues. This chapter delves into the various testicular conditions that can affect fertility, providing insights into diagnosis, management, and treatment options.

Hormonal disorders related to testicular function are a common concern among men facing infertility. The testes produce testosterone and other hormones vital for sperm production and overall reproductive health. Conditions such as hypogonadism can result in low testosterone levels, leading to decreased sperm production and, consequently, fertility challenges. Effective management often involves hormone replacement therapy, which can help restore normal hormonal levels and improve fertility outcomes.

Infections and inflammation of the testes, such as orchitis and epididymitis, are also significant factors affecting fertility. These conditions can arise from bacterial or viral infections, leading to swelling, pain, and potential damage to the sperm-producing structures. Prompt diagnosis and treatment are crucial to mitigate long-term impacts on fertility. Antibiotics or anti-inflammatory medications may be prescribed depending on the underlying cause, and in some cases, surgery may be necessary to address complications.

Anatomical issues, including testicular torsion and trauma, can acutely compromise testicular function and fertility. Testicular torsion is a surgical emergency that requires immediate intervention to restore blood flow to the affected testis. Delayed treatment can result in irreversible damage, making awareness and rapid response essential. Similarly, testicular trauma from accidents or injuries can lead to complications that affect fertility, necessitating a thorough evaluation and appropriate management strategies by healthcare professionals.

Lastly, congenital anomalies of the testis may also play a role in male infertility. Conditions such as undescended testes can hinder normal testicular function and sperm production. Early diagnosis and surgical intervention are vital to correct these anomalies and improve fertility potential. Through comprehensive understanding and timely management of these testicular factors, men can enhance their reproductive health and address infertility issues more effectively.

Evaluation and Treatment Options

Evaluation of testicular diseases begins with a thorough medical history and physical examination. Healthcare professionals assess symptoms such as pain, swelling, or changes in size of the testicles, which can indicate various underlying conditions. Diagnostic imaging techniques, including ultrasound, are often employed to evaluate the structure and blood flow in the testis, helping to differentiate between potential diseases like testicular cancer, torsion, and infections. Blood tests measuring tumour markers can further aid in the diagnosis of testicular cancer, ensuring timely and appropriate treatment decisions.

Treatment options for testicular cancer vary depending on the type and stage of the disease. Common approaches include surgical removal of the affected testicle, known as orchiectomy, which is typically followed by chemotherapy or radiation therapy in more advanced cases. For less aggressive forms of cancer, active surveillance may be recommended, allowing for monitoring of the disease without immediate intervention. This tailored approach ensures that individuals receive the most effective treatment while minimising unnecessary procedures and side effects.

In the case of orchitis and epididymitis, the management focuses on addressing the underlying cause, whether it be viral, bacterial, or sexually transmitted infections. Antibiotics are frequently prescribed for bacterial infections, while supportive care, including pain relief and anti-inflammatory medications, plays a crucial role in managing symptoms. Education on safe sexual practices is also vital to prevent the recurrence of sexually transmitted infections, which can lead to these conditions.

Testicular torsion requires immediate intervention to prevent loss of the testicle. Diagnosis is often made through clinical evaluation and imaging studies. The standard treatment involves surgical detorsion and fixation of the affected testicle, ensuring that blood supply is restored promptly. Delayed treatment can result in irreversible damage, highlighting the importance of recognising the signs and symptoms early to optimise outcomes.

Congenital anomalies of the testis, such as undescended testis or testicular agenesis, may necessitate surgical correction to prevent complications like infertility or malignancy in later life. Hormonal disorders affecting testicular function can also impact fertility and overall health. Consequently, a multidisciplinary approach involving urologists, endocrinologists, and fertility specialists is essential in managing these complex conditions. Regular follow-up and patient education are key components of effective management strategies, ensuring that men are informed and empowered regarding their reproductive health.

Testicular Infections and Sexually Transmitted Diseases

Overview of Testicular Infections

Testicular infections represent a significant concern in men's health, affecting various aspects of reproductive and overall well-being. They can arise due to a range of pathogens, including bacteria, viruses, and fungi, leading to conditions such as epididymitis and orchitis. Understanding these infections is crucial for both men and healthcare professionals, as timely diagnosis and treatment can prevent complications such as infertility and chronic pain.

Epididymitis, an inflammation of the epididymis, is often linked to sexually transmitted infections (STIs) such as chlamydia and gonorrhoea. Symptoms may include swelling, pain in the scrotum, and fever, which require prompt medical attention. Orchitis, on the other hand, is characterised by inflammation of the testis itself and can be caused by viral infections, notably mumps. Both conditions can lead to significant discomfort and long-term issues if not managed correctly.

The diagnosis of testicular infections typically involves a thorough clinical evaluation, which may include physical examinations, urine tests, and imaging studies. Ultrasound is a useful diagnostic tool, helping to differentiate between infections and other testicular conditions, such as torsion or tumours. Accurate diagnosis is vital, as the treatment varies greatly depending on the underlying cause.

Treatment options for testicular infections often include antibiotics for bacterial infections and supportive care for viral cases. Pain management and rest are also crucial in the recovery process. In some cases, surgical intervention may be necessary, particularly if an abscess develops or if there is suspicion of testicular torsion, which requires immediate attention to prevent permanent damage.

In conclusion, awareness and understanding of testicular infections can empower men and healthcare professionals to recognise symptoms early and seek appropriate care. Given the potential implications on fertility and overall health, addressing these infections promptly is essential for maintaining reproductive health and preventing long-term complications.

Common Infections and STDs

Common infections and sexually transmitted diseases (STDs) can significantly impact male reproductive health, particularly concerning the testis and surrounding structures. Orchitis, epididymitis, and other infections can arise from bacterial or viral agents, often presenting with acute pain and swelling. Awareness of these conditions is crucial for both men and healthcare professionals, as early diagnosis and treatment can prevent complications such as infertility or chronic pain.

Orchitis, primarily caused by viral infections such as mumps, can lead to inflammation of the testis and may result in testicular atrophy if left untreated. Symptoms typically include unilateral swelling and tenderness, accompanied by fever and malaise. Management often involves symptomatic relief, including analgesics and anti-inflammatory medications, although severe cases may require hospitalisation for further intervention.

Epididymitis, another common infection, is predominantly caused by sexually transmitted infections like chlamydia and gonorrhoea. Men may experience acute onset of scrotal pain, often with associated urinary symptoms such as dysuria or increased frequency of urination. Treatment generally involves the use of antibiotics targeting the specific pathogen, and in some cases, supportive care to alleviate discomfort.

Testicular torsion, while not an infection, is a critical condition that can arise in conjunction with infections. It requires immediate surgical intervention to prevent irreversible damage to the testis. Additionally, testicular trauma, whether from sports or accidents, can also lead to secondary infections that complicate the clinical picture, necessitating comprehensive evaluation and management.

Understanding the link between testicular infections and STDs is essential for promoting reproductive health. Regular screenings and education regarding safe sexual practices can help reduce the incidence of these infections. For healthcare professionals, recognising the signs and symptoms early is key to ensuring effective treatment and minimising long-term complications, thus maintaining the overall health of male patients.

Diagnosis and Treatment Strategies

Diagnosing testicular diseases requires a comprehensive approach that integrates patient history, physical examinations, and advanced diagnostic imaging techniques. Healthcare professionals must be vigilant in noting symptoms such as swelling, pain, or changes in size, which may indicate underlying issues like testicular cancer, orchitis, or epididymitis. A thorough examination often includes a scrotal ultrasound, which can provide vital information about the structure and condition of the testis, allowing for accurate identification of abnormalities.

Once a diagnosis is established, treatment strategies vary significantly depending on the specific condition. For instance, testicular cancer treatment may involve a combination of surgery, chemotherapy, and radiation, tailored to the type and stage of cancer. In cases of orchitis or epididymitis, where inflammation is the primary concern, conservative management with antibiotics and anti-inflammatory medications is often effective. Urologists play a crucial role in determining the most appropriate intervention based on individual patient needs.

Testicular torsion represents a surgical emergency that requires prompt diagnosis and intervention to prevent long-term complications, including infertility. The classic presentation of acute onset scrotal pain should prompt immediate evaluation. Surgical detorsion and fixation are typically performed within a few hours of symptom onset to preserve testicular viability. Awareness of this condition is vital among both patients and healthcare professionals to ensure timely treatment.

In addition to acute conditions, chronic issues such as hormonal disorders and congenital anomalies may also necessitate management strategies. Hormonal imbalances can significantly affect testicular function and overall male health, requiring endocrinological assessment and potential hormonal therapy. Congenital anomalies may need surgical correction or careful monitoring, depending on their nature and severity, underscoring the importance of a multidisciplinary approach to treatment.

Infertility linked to testicular diseases presents another challenging aspect of management, necessitating thorough evaluation of both partners. Advanced techniques, such as assisted reproductive technologies, may be considered for couples facing infertility due to testicular dysfunction. Additionally, ongoing research and developments in the field of testicular health promise to enhance treatment options and improve outcomes for men affected by these conditions, highlighting the necessity for continuous education among healthcare providers.

Diagnostic Imaging Techniques for Testicular Conditions

Importance of Imaging in Testicular Health

Imaging plays a crucial role in assessing testicular health, enabling healthcare professionals to diagnose a variety of conditions accurately. Whether it's detecting testicular cancer, evaluating the severity of testicular torsion, or understanding the underlying causes of orchitis, imaging techniques provide essential insights. The advancement of technology in imaging has paved the way for more precise examinations, leading to timely interventions and better patient outcomes. This is particularly significant given the rising incidence of testicular diseases, which necessitates thorough and effective diagnostic methods.

Ultrasound is often the first-line imaging modality employed in the evaluation of testicular conditions. Its non-invasive nature and ability to provide real-time results make it an invaluable tool for urologists. Ultrasound can effectively identify abnormal masses, fluid collections, and changes in the testicular structure, allowing for the differentiation between benign and malignant lesions. Moreover, the use of Doppler ultrasound enhances the assessment of blood flow, which is critical in diagnosing conditions such as testicular torsion and epididymitis.

In cases where ultrasound findings are inconclusive, advanced imaging techniques such as MRI and CT scans may be employed. These modalities offer a more comprehensive view of the testicular region and can help in staging testicular cancer or evaluating the extent of traumatic injuries. MRI, in particular, is beneficial in assessing soft tissue structures and can provide detailed information on the presence of lymphadenopathy, which is essential for determining the appropriate treatment plan.

The implications of diagnostic imaging extend beyond mere detection; they play a significant role in managing testicular health. Accurate imaging informs treatment decisions, whether it involves surgical intervention for torsion or targeted therapy for malignancies. Furthermore, imaging can assist in monitoring the effectiveness of treatment and identifying any recurrence of disease. Thus, the integration of imaging into routine clinical practice is fundamental for optimising outcomes for men facing testicular health issues.

In conclusion, the importance of imaging in testicular health cannot be overstated. It serves as a cornerstone in the diagnosis and management of various testicular conditions, facilitating early detection and intervention. As technology continues to evolve, the reliance on imaging will likely increase, providing healthcare professionals with the necessary tools to combat testicular diseases effectively. An informed approach to imaging not only enhances patient care but also contributes to better long-term health outcomes for men.

Ultrasound in Testicular Diagnosis

Ultrasound has become an indispensable tool in the diagnosis of testicular diseases, offering a non-invasive means of visualising the internal structures of the testes. It is particularly effective in differentiating between various conditions such as testicular cancer, orchitis, and torsion. By utilising high-frequency sound waves, ultrasound provides real-time images that aid in the assessment of testicular masses, fluid collections, and other abnormalities. This diagnostic technique is essential for urologists and healthcare professionals in making informed decisions regarding patient management.

In cases of testicular cancer, ultrasound plays a pivotal role in identifying the presence of tumours and determining their characteristics. By assessing the size, shape, and echogenicity of testicular masses, healthcare providers can distinguish between benign and malignant lesions. This differentiation is crucial for establishing an appropriate treatment plan. Furthermore, ultrasound can guide biopsy procedures, ensuring accurate sampling of tissues for histological analysis, thereby enhancing diagnosis accuracy.

Ultrasound is also vital in the evaluation of acute conditions such as testicular torsion and epididymitis. In torsion, time is of the essence, and ultrasound can quickly confirm the diagnosis by revealing reduced blood flow to the affected testicle. Similarly, in cases of epididymitis, ultrasound can demonstrate the presence of swelling and increased vascularity, facilitating timely intervention. The speed and precision of ultrasound imaging significantly improve patient outcomes by enabling rapid diagnosis and treatment initiation.

Beyond acute conditions, ultrasound is instrumental in managing chronic testicular issues such as orchitis and testicular trauma. For orchitis, ultrasound can identify changes in testicular echogenicity and the presence of associated fluid collections. In cases of testicular trauma, imaging can help assess the extent of injury and guide surgical intervention if necessary. Regular ultrasound examinations may also be warranted in patients with congenital anomalies or hormonal disorders affecting testicular function, allowing for ongoing monitoring and timely intervention.

Overall, the integration of ultrasound into the diagnostic pathway for testicular diseases has transformed the landscape of urological practice. Its ability to provide detailed imaging without the need for invasive procedures underscores its value in both acute and chronic conditions. As technology advances, the role of ultrasound is likely to expand further, offering even greater diagnostic capabilities and enhancing patient care in the field of urology.

Other Imaging Modalities

In the realm of testicular diseases, various imaging modalities play a crucial role in diagnosis and management. Beyond the commonly used ultrasound, techniques such as magnetic resonance imaging (MRI) and computed tomography (CT) scans are valuable in assessing testicular conditions. MRI is particularly beneficial for soft tissue evaluation, providing detailed images that can help differentiate between benign and malignant lesions. Meanwhile, CT scans can be instrumental in staging testicular cancer and identifying metastases, enabling healthcare professionals to devise appropriate treatment plans.

Ultrasound remains the first-line imaging technique for evaluating testicular abnormalities due to its accessibility, cost-effectiveness, and lack of ionising radiation. It is particularly useful in diagnosing conditions such as testicular torsion, epididymitis, and orchitis. The real-time imaging capability of ultrasound allows for rapid assessment, which is vital in emergency situations where timely intervention can save the affected testis.

In addition to standard imaging techniques, advanced modalities like Doppler ultrasound can provide additional insights into blood flow dynamics within the testis. This is especially relevant in cases of testicular torsion, where the absence of blood flow can indicate an emergency requiring immediate surgical intervention. Doppler studies can also assist in evaluating the vascularity of testicular masses, aiding in the differential diagnosis between benign and malignant conditions.

Nuclear medicine techniques, such as positron emission tomography (PET) scans, are increasingly being explored for their role in the management of testicular cancer. PET scans can detect metabolic activity associated with cancer cells, providing information about tumour aggressiveness and potential recurrence. This information is invaluable for urologists and oncologists in tailoring personalised treatment strategies and monitoring patient outcomes post-therapy.

As our understanding of testicular diseases evolves, so too does the technology available for their diagnosis. The integration of these imaging modalities enhances the ability of healthcare professionals to accurately diagnose and effectively manage testicular conditions. By employing a multimodal imaging approach, clinicians can ensure that men receive comprehensive care tailored to their specific needs, ultimately improving outcomes in testicular health.

Interpreting Imaging Results

Interpreting imaging results is a critical aspect of diagnosing various testicular diseases. Imaging techniques such as ultrasound, MRI, and CT scans provide valuable insights into the structural and functional status of the testis. Each modality has its strengths and weaknesses, and understanding these can aid healthcare professionals in making more accurate diagnoses. For instance, ultrasound is the first-line imaging technique for evaluating testicular abnormalities due to its safety and ability to provide real-time images.

In the context of testicular cancer, imaging plays a pivotal role in staging the disease and determining the appropriate treatment plan. Radiologists assess the size and extent of tumours, lymph node involvement, and potential metastasis. Accurate interpretation of imaging results can significantly influence patient management and outcomes. For example, the distinction between seminomatous and non-seminomatous germ cell tumours can be made using imaging features, which is crucial for tailoring treatment strategies.

Orchitis, an inflammation of the testis, can be evaluated using imaging to rule out other conditions such as testicular torsion or abscess formation. The imaging results can reveal characteristic signs of inflammation and help guide the management approach. Careful interpretation is essential, as misdiagnosis can lead to unnecessary surgical interventions or delayed treatment.

In cases of testicular torsion, timely imaging is vital for diagnosis. An ultrasound with Doppler studies can assess blood flow to the affected testis, providing crucial information regarding the viability of the tissue. Rapid interpretation of these results can facilitate urgent surgical intervention, which is paramount to preserving testicular function and preventing complications such as infertility.

Lastly, imaging is also instrumental in identifying congenital anomalies and other testicular conditions. For men presenting with infertility linked to testicular diseases, imaging can reveal structural anomalies that may contribute to their condition. By understanding the implications of imaging results, healthcare professionals can better educate patients about their conditions and the available management options, ultimately leading to improved health outcomes.

Conclusion and Future Perspectives

Summary of Key Points

Here, we summarise the key points regarding testicular diseases that are crucial for both men and healthcare professionals. Understanding the various types of testicular cancer, including seminomas and non-seminomas, helps in early diagnosis and treatment planning. The importance of recognising symptoms and the role of timely interventions cannot be overstated, as they significantly impact patient outcomes.

Orchitis, an inflammation of the testis, arises from various causes such as viral infections or sexually transmitted diseases. Management strategies range from symptomatic relief to specific treatments targeting the underlying cause. Awareness of the signs and symptoms is essential for both patients and healthcare providers to ensure prompt care and prevent complications.

Testicular torsion is a critical emergency that requires immediate attention. The swift diagnosis and intervention can save the affected testis and preserve fertility. Understanding the clinical presentation and the urgency of surgical intervention is vital for practitioners to improve patient prognosis in such cases.

Epididymitis, often linked to infections, presents with specific symptoms that require appropriate treatment options. Differentiating between acute and chronic forms of the condition is crucial for effective management. Men should be educated about the risk factors and the importance of seeking medical help at the onset of symptoms.

Finally, the implications of testicular trauma, congenital anomalies, and hormonal disorders must not be overlooked. These conditions can lead to infertility and other significant health issues. Diagnostic imaging techniques play a pivotal role in the assessment of testicular conditions, enhancing the accuracy of diagnoses and the effectiveness of treatment plans.

Advances in Research and Treatment

Advancements in research and treatment for testicular diseases have significantly improved outcomes for men facing these conditions. With a deeper understanding of testicular cancer types and their treatments, healthcare professionals can offer tailored therapies that enhance survival rates and quality of life. Recent studies have elucidated the molecular pathways involved in testicular cancer, leading to the development of targeted therapies that are more effective and have fewer side effects compared to traditional chemotherapy.

Furthermore, research into orchitis, an inflammation of the testes, has revealed various causes, including viral and bacterial infections. This has allowed for better management strategies that not only address the immediate symptoms but also target the underlying infections. Current treatment protocols now include a combination of antibiotics and anti-inflammatory medications, which have proven to reduce recovery times and complications associated with orchitis.

Testicular torsion remains a surgical emergency, and advancements in diagnostic imaging techniques have revolutionised the speed and accuracy of diagnosis. Ultrasound with Doppler flow studies is now a standard practice, enabling clinicians to assess blood flow to the testes quickly. Timely intervention has been emphasised through research that shows the necessity of prompt surgical correction to preserve testicular viability, reducing the risk of infertility.

In addition to acute conditions, chronic issues such as epididymitis have also seen improvements in treatment options. Understanding the aetiology of epididymitis, which can stem from infections or trauma, has led to more effective treatment regimens that include both pharmacological and non-pharmacological interventions. Men are now more informed about the signs and symptoms, facilitating earlier diagnosis and treatment, which is crucial in preventing chronic pain and complications.

Lastly, hormonal disorders related to testicular function have gained attention in recent research. These disorders can significantly impact fertility and overall health. Advances in hormonal therapies and lifestyle interventions are being explored, providing hope for men experiencing infertility linked to testicular diseases. With ongoing research, there is a strong emphasis on holistic approaches that encompass both medical treatments and lifestyle modifications to enhance reproductive health.

Importance of Ongoing Education for Healthcare Professionals

Ongoing education is crucial for healthcare professionals, particularly in fields like urology where advancements occur rapidly. With the emergence of new research and treatment protocols, healthcare providers must stay informed to offer the best care for patients suffering from testicular diseases. This commitment to lifelong learning not only enhances clinical skills but also improves patient outcomes by ensuring that professionals are well-versed in the latest diagnostic techniques and therapies available.

For urologists and other healthcare professionals dealing with testicular conditions, understanding the nuances of diseases such as testicular cancer, orchitis, and epididymitis is paramount. Continuous education programmes provide updated insights into the evolving landscape of these diseases, including the latest treatment modalities and management strategies. This knowledge is essential for making informed decisions when diagnosing and treating patients, particularly in cases of complex conditions such as testicular torsion or trauma.

Furthermore, ongoing education fosters a deeper understanding of the hormonal disorders related to testicular function and their implications for male fertility. As new studies emerge, healthcare providers must be equipped to address the latest findings regarding infertility linked to testicular diseases. By engaging in continuous professional development, practitioners can better support their patients through evidence-based interventions and counselling.

The importance of diagnostic imaging techniques in the evaluation of testicular conditions cannot be overstated. Healthcare professionals must stay abreast of advancements in imaging technology to accurately diagnose conditions like testicular infections and congenital anomalies. This ongoing education not only enhances diagnostic accuracy but also ensures that practitioners can effectively collaborate with radiologists and other specialists to optimise patient care.

In conclusion, the commitment to ongoing education is fundamental for healthcare professionals in the field of urology. As they navigate the complexities of testicular diseases, their ability to stay informed about current research, treatment options, and diagnostic techniques is vital. By prioritising lifelong learning, healthcare providers can improve their practice and deliver high-quality care to men facing various testicular health issues.

Pause for thought

- Testicular health is a crucial aspect of male wellbeing, encompassing a variety of conditions that can significantly affect reproductive health and overall quality of life. The testes is responsible for the production of sperm and the secretion of hormones such as testosterone.
- Testicular cancer is a most significant cancer in testicular health of which there are two general types, seminomas and non-seminomas, each requiring specific treatment protocols. Early detection through regular self-examinations and professional assessments will lead to better outcomes.
- Conditions such as orchitis and epididymitis often are the result of infections and can cause considerable discomfort and complications if left untreated. Orchitis is an inflammatory process of the testes which may be caused by viral or bacterial infections, while epididymitis affects the epididymis and can result from sexually transmitted infections. Both conditions require prompt medical attention to manage symptoms and prevent long term health issues.
- Testicular torsion is a medical emergency which is characterised by the twisting of the spermatic cord which can lead to severe consequences if not addressed swiftly. Diagnosis often involves clinical evaluation and imaging techniques, followed by immediate intervention to restore blood flow.

- Congenital anomalies of the testes and hormonal disorders can lead to infertility and other reproductive issues. Diagnostic imaging techniques play a key role in identifying testicular conditions, allowing for accurate diagnosis and tailored treatment options.
- Men should regularly perform self-examination to identify any unusual changes in their testicles. Changes can include lumps, swelling, or pain which can indicate testicular cancer or infections.
- Risk factors for testicular disease include age, family history, genetic predisposition, this is further influenced by lifestyle choices such as smoking and exposure to environmental toxins.
- Testicular cancer is one of the most common malignancies among young men, particularly those aged 15 to 35. The incidence of this can has been rising in many parts of the world though the reasons remain unclear. Conditions like orchitis and epididymitis which are often linked to infection are more prevalent among sexually active young men.
- Testicular trauma cannot be ignored. Injuries to the testes can result from various activities, including sports or accidents and can lead to acute conditions requiring immediate intervention. The management of testicular trauma often necessitates a thorough understanding of both the physical and psychological impacts on the patient as these events can profoundly affect male reproductive health and self-esteem. Prompt diagnosis and appropriate treatment are essential to preserve testicular function and prevent long term complications.

- There are two primary categories of testicular cancers, the seminomas and the non-seminoma's, each of which exhibit distinct characteristic and treatment responses. Seminomas are typically slow growing and arise from germ cells, these are usually diagnosed early. And are usually responsive to radiotherapy. There are two subtypes of seminomas-classical seminomas, the most common type, and spermatocytic seminomas which are rare and usually affect older men. The non-seminomas include embryonal cancers, yolk sac tumours and teratomas among others. These tend to grow more quickly and may spread to other parts of the body at an earlier stage.

Take Home Nuggets

- The staging and grading of testicular cancers are crucial processes that determine the extent of the disease and the appropriate treatment options. Each stage reflects the severity of the cancer, stage 1 for example describes a tumour that is confined to the organ from which it arose whereas stage iv cancer describes advanced disease with distant spread. Grading on the other hand talks about the histological characteristics of the tumour cells indicating the aggressiveness of the cancer.
- Imaging modalities such as ultrasound scans, cat scans, and magnetic resonance imaging are utilized in evaluating the presence of tumours and their potential spread. Treatment modalities may involve a combination of

surgery, chemotherapy, and radiation treatment depending on the type and stage of cancer.

- In cases of orchitis treatment focuses on addressing the underlying cause which may be viral or bacterial. Antibiotics are prescribed for bacterial infections. Whilst supportive care – rest, ice, and pain relief is recommended for viral cases. Close monitoring is necessary in these cases to prevent abscess formation or infertility. Testicular torsion is a surgical emergency that requires immediate intervention to salvage the affected testes. The diagnosis is based on clinical history and physical examination while imaging techniques such as doppler ultrasound will help in assessing blood flow. Prompt surgical detorsion and fixation are essential to avert irreversible damage.
- Epididymitis resulting from infections or sexually transmitted diseases is treated with antibiotics and analgesics. Patients are advised to abstain from sexual activity during treatment and to follow up with their health care provider to ensure resolution. Chronic cases may require further investigations to identify underlying causes including congenital abnormalities or hormonal disorders.
- Management of testicular trauma is guided by the severity of the injury. In minor cases, conservative treatment may suffice, while in severe injuries surgical intervention may be required to repair damage and to preserve testicular function.

- Chronic pain or infertility can arise from untreated infections or torsion; therefore men experiencing symptoms such as persistent pain, swelling or changes in testicular size should seek prompt medical attention.
- Hypogonadism can impact men's overall health leading to issues of decreased libido, fatigue, and mood disturbances. This necessitates regular hormonal assessments. Since infertility is linked to testicular disease, men diagnosed with conditions such as varicocele or previous testicular trauma may face challenges in fathering children.
- Congenital abnormalities of the testes refer to a range of developmental disorders that affect the normal structure and function of the testes. These can manifest in various forms such as undescended testis, testicular hypoplasia, or the presence of additional testicular tissue. These can adversely affect male reproductive health and increase the risk of associated complications such as infertility and testicular cancer.
- Types of congenital anomalies include cryptorchidism in which one or both testes fail to descend to the scrotum. This is both a cosmetic issue as well as it poses a risk of infertility and cancer in later life. This condition can be corrected surgically. Testicular agenesis is another congenital abnormality. Here one or both testes are absent from the scrotum. The implications of this are hormonal imbalance and, infertility and cancer.

Chapter 11
Understanding Prostate Health

The Anatomy of the Prostate

The prostate is a small gland located just below the bladder, surrounding the urethra. Its primary function is to produce seminal fluid, which nourishes and transports sperm. Understanding the anatomy of the prostate is crucial for men, especially as they age, because changes in this gland can significantly impact urinary and sexual health. The prostate's position and size make it susceptible to various medical conditions, including benign prostatic hyperplasia and prostate cancer, which can affect quality of life for aging men.

As men reach their advanced years, the prostate undergoes natural changes. It often enlarges, a condition known as benign prostatic hyperplasia (BPH), which can lead to urinary difficulties such as frequent urination or incomplete bladder emptying. Hormonal changes, particularly the decrease in testosterone levels, also play a significant role in the health of the prostate. These alterations can lead to various symptoms that may require lifestyle modifications, dietary adjustments, and, in some cases, medical interventions.

Dietary supplements have garnered attention for their potential benefits in maintaining prostate health. Nutrients such as zinc, selenium, and omega-3 fatty acids are believed to support prostate function and may reduce the risk of prostate-related issues. Additionally, natural remedies and herbs, like saw palmetto and pygeum, are often explored for their therapeutic effects on prostate wellness. Incorporating these supplements into a balanced diet can be a proactive approach for men seeking to enhance their prostate health as they age.

Exercise and lifestyle modifications are also vital for promoting prostate wellness. Regular physical activity can help maintain a healthy weight, reduce inflammation, and improve overall well-being, which are essential factors in managing prostate health. Furthermore, engaging in stress-reducing practices such as yoga or meditation can have positive psychological effects, contributing to better prostate function and sexual health.

Early detection through prostate health screenings is critical in preventing severe complications, including prostate cancer. Men should discuss with their healthcare provider when to begin screenings based on personal risk factors. Awareness of prostate health, including potential symptoms and the importance of regular check-ups, can empower aging men to take charge of their health, ensuring they live their lives with confidence and vitality.

Common Prostate Issues in Aging Men

As men age, the prostate gland undergoes a series of changes that can lead to various health issues. Common problems include benign prostatic hyperplasia (BPH), which is characterized by an enlarged prostate that can cause urinary difficulties. Men may experience symptoms such as a frequent need to urinate, especially at night, and a weak urine stream. Understanding these symptoms is crucial for early intervention and maintaining quality of life.

Prostate cancer is another significant concern for aging men. It often progresses slowly, making regular screenings essential for early detection. Men should discuss their risk factors with healthcare providers to determine the appropriate age to begin screenings. Awareness of family history and lifestyle factors can help in making informed decisions regarding prostate health.

Dietary supplements and natural remedies play a vital role in supporting prostate health. Nutrients like saw palmetto and zinc are often recommended to help manage symptoms associated with BPH. Additionally, a diet rich in fruits, vegetables, and healthy fats can contribute to overall prostate wellness. Men should consider integrating these dietary changes into their daily routines for optimal health benefits.

Exercise and lifestyle modifications are equally important for maintaining prostate health. Regular physical activity not only helps manage weight but also supports hormonal balance, which is crucial as testosterone levels decline with age. Engaging in activities such as walking, swimming, or yoga can enhance overall well-being and reduce the risk of prostate-related issues.

Finally, the psychological aspects of prostate health cannot be overlooked. Men may experience anxiety or depression related to prostate issues, affecting their sexual health and overall quality of life. It is essential to address these emotional factors through support groups or counselling, ensuring that aging men feel empowered and informed about their prostate health journey.

Importance of Prostate Health

Prostate health is a critical aspect of overall wellness for mature men, particularly as they age. The prostate gland, although small, plays a significant role in male reproductive health and can be affected by a variety of factors including hormonal changes, lifestyle choices, and genetics. Understanding the importance of maintaining prostate health can empower men to take proactive steps in their health journey, ultimately enhancing their quality of life. Regular screenings and awareness about potential issues can lead to early detection and better treatment outcomes.

Dietary supplements and lifestyle modifications can greatly influence prostate health. Nutrients such as zinc, selenium, and omega-3 fatty acids have been shown to support prostate function and may reduce the risk of prostate-related issues. Furthermore, engaging in regular exercise can help manage weight and improve hormonal balance, both of which are beneficial for prostate health. Men who adopt a balanced diet rich in fruits, vegetables, and whole grains often report fewer prostate-related problems as they age.

Natural remedies and herbs have also gained popularity as complementary approaches to supporting prostate health. Ingredients such as saw palmetto, Pygeum, and green tea extract have been researched for their potential benefits in promoting prostate function and reducing symptoms associated with benign prostatic hyperplasia (BPH). However, it is essential for men to consult healthcare professionals before starting any supplement regimen to ensure safety and efficacy.

Prostate health screenings and awareness of prostate cancer are vital components of male healthcare. Routine check-ups can help detect abnormalities early, which is crucial for effective treatment. Men are encouraged to discuss their risk factors and family history with their healthcare providers to determine the appropriate screening schedule. Awareness campaigns focusing on prostate cancer prevention can significantly impact early detection rates and improve survival outcomes.

Finally, the psychological aspects of prostate health should not be overlooked. Issues related to prostate function can affect a man's self-esteem and intimate relationships. Open communication about these concerns and seeking support can play a vital role in mental wellness. By prioritizing prostate health, mature men can navigate the challenges of aging with confidence and maintain a fulfilling lifestyle.

Dietary Supplements for Prostate Health

Key Nutrients for Prostate Wellness

Prostate wellness is crucial for aging men, and understanding the key nutrients that support prostate health is a vital step towards maintaining overall well-being. A diet rich in specific vitamins, minerals, and antioxidants can play a significant role in reducing the risk of prostate issues, including benign prostatic hyperplasia and prostate cancer. Nutrients such as zinc, selenium, and omega-3 fatty acids are particularly important, as they have been shown to promote healthy prostate function and may even aid in reducing inflammation.

Zinc is essential for testosterone metabolism and is found in high concentrations in the prostate. Studies suggest that adequate zinc levels may protect against prostate enlargement and cancer. Men should consider incorporating zinc-rich foods like oysters, beef, and pumpkin seeds into their diets, or explore dietary supplements if they struggle to meet their nutritional needs through food alone. This mineral not only supports prostate health but also enhances immune function, making it a dual-benefit nutrient.

Another key nutrient is selenium, an antioxidant that helps combat oxidative stress in the body. Research has indicated that adequate selenium intake may be linked to a lower risk of prostate cancer. Foods such as Brazil nuts, fish, and whole grains are excellent sources of selenium. For men concerned about their prostate health, ensuring sufficient selenium intake can be a proactive measure in their dietary regimen.

Omega-3 fatty acids, primarily found in fatty fish, walnuts, and flaxseeds, have anti-inflammatory properties that can be beneficial for prostate health. These healthy fats may help lower the risk of prostate cancer and improve overall prostate function. Incorporating omega-3-rich foods into the diet or considering fish oil supplements could be advantageous for mature men looking to enhance their prostate wellness.

In addition to focusing on these essential nutrients, men should also consider lifestyle modifications such as regular exercise and maintaining a healthy weight. Physical activity not only supports overall health but also aids in hormone regulation, which is crucial for prostate health as men age. By understanding and integrating key nutrients alongside healthy lifestyle choices, aging men can take significant steps towards promoting their prostate wellness and reducing the risk of related health issues.

Popular Supplements and Their Benefits

In the realm of prostate health, several dietary supplements have gained popularity due to their potential benefits for mature men. These supplements often contain natural ingredients that are believed to support prostate function and overall wellness. Among the most discussed are saw palmetto, which has been linked to improved urinary function, and beta-sitosterol, known for its ability to alleviate urinary symptoms associated with benign prostatic hyperplasia (BPH). Incorporating these supplements into a daily routine may offer men a proactive approach to managing their prostate health as they age.

Another key supplement is Pygeum africanum, derived from the bark of an African plum tree. Research suggests that this natural remedy can help reduce nighttime urination and improve overall urinary tract health. Additionally, zinc is an essential mineral that plays a crucial role in maintaining prostate health, with studies indicating that adequate levels of zinc may help mitigate the risk of prostate issues. Men may benefit from considering these supplements as part of a comprehensive strategy for prostate wellness.

In recent years, the importance of lifestyle modifications has become increasingly evident in the context of prostate health. Regular exercise, combined with a balanced diet rich in fruits, vegetables, and healthy fats, can significantly influence prostate function. Supplements such as omega-3 fatty acids, commonly found in fish oil, are recognized for their anti-inflammatory properties, which may further enhance prostate health. By integrating these lifestyle changes with the use of dietary supplements, men can work towards achieving optimal prostate wellness.

Moreover, the psychological aspects of maintaining prostate health cannot be overlooked. Men may experience stress and anxiety regarding prostate health issues, which can affect their overall well-being. Herbal supplements like ashwagandha and rhodiola rosea have been studied for their adaptogenic properties, helping to manage stress and improve mental clarity. Addressing both the physical and psychological components of prostate health is essential for mature men aiming to age gracefully and healthfully.

In conclusion, while dietary supplements offer potential benefits for prostate health, it is vital for men to consult with healthcare professionals before beginning any new regimen. This ensures that they choose the most suitable supplements for their individual health needs and conditions. As research continues to advance in this field, staying informed about the latest findings can empower men to make proactive decisions about their prostate health and overall wellness.

Guidelines for Supplement Use

As men age, the importance of maintaining prostate health becomes increasingly vital. Dietary supplements can play a significant role in supporting prostate function and overall well-being. However, it is crucial to approach supplement use with caution and awareness. Understanding what supplements are effective and how they fit into a broader health strategy is essential for mature men seeking to age gracefully.

When considering supplements for prostate health, it is advisable to consult with a healthcare professional. This step ensures that the chosen supplements do not interfere with any medications or existing health conditions. Professionals can provide personalized recommendations based on individual health profiles and help identify supplements that may be beneficial, such as saw palmetto or beta-sitosterol, which have shown promise in supporting prostate health.

In addition to dietary supplements, lifestyle modifications can significantly enhance prostate wellness. Regular exercise, a balanced diet rich in fruits and vegetables, and hydration are fundamental components of a healthy lifestyle. Incorporating physical activity not only aids in maintaining a healthy weight but also improves hormonal balance, which can positively impact prostate function. Men should strive for at least 150 minutes of moderate exercise each week to support their prostate health effectively.

Natural remedies and herbal supplements can also provide additional support for prostate health. Herbs like Pygeum, stinging nettle, and pumpkin seed extract have been traditionally used to promote urinary health and reduce symptoms associated with prostate enlargement. However, it is essential to use these herbs responsibly and under the guidance of a healthcare professional to avoid potential side effects and interactions with other treatments.

Lastly, understanding the psychological aspects of prostate health is crucial. Men may experience anxiety or stress related to prostate health issues, which can affect their overall quality of life. Engaging in support groups or counselling can be beneficial for emotional well-being. By addressing both the physical and psychological aspects of prostate health, men can take a holistic approach to their well-being, ensuring they age gracefully while maintaining their prostate health.

Exercise and Lifestyle Modifications for Prostate Wellness

The Role of Physical Activity

Physical activity plays a crucial role in maintaining prostate health, especially for aging men. Regular exercise can help manage weight, reduce inflammation, and improve circulation, all of which are vital for prostate function. Engaging in activities such as walking, swimming, or resistance training can enhance overall well-being, making it easier to cope with the changes that come with age. For men concerned about prostate health, incorporating physical activity into daily routines is an essential strategy.

In addition to its physical benefits, exercise has been shown to have positive effects on mental health. Many men experience anxiety or depression when facing prostate health challenges. Regular physical activity releases endorphins, which can help alleviate stress and improve mood. This psychological aspect of exercise can encourage men to stay proactive about their health and well-being, fostering a more positive outlook on life as they age.

Exercise also plays a significant role in the prevention of prostate cancer. Research suggests that men who engage in regular physical activity may have a lower risk of developing prostate cancer. Specifically, activities that promote cardiovascular health and increase muscle strength can contribute to hormonal balance, which is crucial for prostate health. By staying active, men can take an important step towards reducing their cancer risk.

Furthermore, lifestyle modifications that include physical activity can enhance the effectiveness of dietary supplements and natural remedies for prostate support. For instance, while supplements may provide essential nutrients, their absorption and efficacy can be improved through a healthy lifestyle that includes regular exercise. This holistic approach not only supports prostate health but also promotes overall wellness, making it easier for men to manage their health proactively.

In conclusion, the role of physical activity in promoting prostate health cannot be overstated. As men age, incorporating regular exercise into their routines can lead to numerous health benefits, from improved physical function to better mental health. By recognizing the importance of staying active, men can embrace a healthier lifestyle that supports their prostate health and well-being as they navigate the aging process.

Recommended Exercises for Prostate Health

Maintaining prostate health is crucial for aging men, and incorporating regular exercise into daily routines can significantly contribute to overall wellness. Aerobic exercises, such as walking, swimming, and cycling, are particularly beneficial. These activities help improve circulation, reduce body fat, and enhance hormonal balance, all of which are vital for prostate function. Engaging in at least 150 minutes of moderate-intensity aerobic exercise each week is recommended to support prostate health and overall physical conditioning.

Strength training is another essential component of a comprehensive exercise regimen for prostate health. Incorporating resistance exercises, such as weightlifting or bodyweight workouts, helps build muscle mass and improve metabolic function. This is particularly important as men age and experience hormonal changes that can affect prostate health. Aim for strength training sessions at least two times a week, ensuring to target all major muscle groups for balanced development.

Flexibility and balance exercises, such as yoga and tai chi, also play a significant role in promoting prostate health, especially for older men. These practices not only enhance physical flexibility but also reduce stress and improve mental well-being. Stress management is crucial, as elevated stress levels can negatively impact prostate health. Incorporating these exercises into weekly routines can promote relaxation and improve quality of life.

In addition to structured exercise, incorporating more movement into daily life is important. Simple changes, such as taking the stairs instead of the elevator, standing while working, or walking during breaks, can contribute to overall activity levels. These lifestyle modifications can have a cumulative effect, improve cardiovascular health and supporting prostate wellness. Staying active contributes to maintaining a healthy weight, which is associated with a lower risk of prostate issues.

Lastly, it is essential to combine physical activity with a balanced diet and regular health screenings. Nutritional support, including dietary supplements rich in vitamins and minerals, can bolster exercise efforts. Regular check-ups and prostate screenings can help detect any issues early, ensuring timely intervention if needed. By weaving together exercise, nutrition, and proactive health management, aging men can take significant steps towards maintaining their prostate health and overall well-being.

Lifestyle Changes to Support Prostate Function

Maintaining prostate health is crucial for adult males, especially as they age. Lifestyle changes play a significant role in supporting prostate function and overall well-being. By adopting a balanced diet rich in antioxidants, healthy fats, and fibre, men can promote better prostate health. Foods such as tomatoes, broccoli, and fish provide essential nutrients that may help reduce the risk of prostate issues and support hormonal balance.

Incorporating regular physical activity into daily routines can greatly benefit prostate function. Exercise helps improve circulation, reduces inflammation, and supports hormonal regulation, all of which are vital for prostate health. Men should aim for at least 150 minutes of moderate aerobic activity each week, along with strength training exercises. Activities like walking, swimming, and yoga not only enhance physical fitness but also contribute to mental wellness, reducing stress and anxiety levels associated with prostate concerns.

Dietary supplements can also play a supportive role in maintaining prostate health. Natural remedies such as saw palmetto, Pygeum, and pumpkin seed oil have been studied for their potential benefits on prostate function. These supplements may help alleviate urinary symptoms and support hormone balance in aging men. However, it is essential to consult a healthcare professional before starting any new supplements to ensure they are appropriate and safe for individual health needs.

Screenings and early detection are vital components of proactive prostate health management. Men should discuss with their healthcare providers about appropriate screening tests, such as PSA levels and digital rectal exams, especially as they reach their 50s or earlier if they have a family history of prostate issues. Regular check-ups can lead to early intervention, which is crucial in managing any potential health concerns effectively.

Lastly, understanding the psychological aspects of prostate health is essential for holistic wellness. The impact of hormonal changes and the fear of prostate-related diseases can lead to emotional distress. Men are encouraged to seek support from healthcare professionals, support groups, or mental health resources to address any psychological challenges. Emphasizing a proactive approach to both physical and mental health can help men age gracefully while maintaining prostate wellness.

Natural Remedies and Herbs for Prostate Support

Overview of Natural Remedies

Natural remedies have gained popularity among men seeking to maintain their prostate health as they age. These remedies often draw from traditional practices and natural sources, providing holistic alternatives to conventional treatments. Many mature men are particularly interested in options that can complement their existing health strategies, especially as they navigate hormonal changes that can affect prostate function. Understanding what natural remedies are available and their potential benefits is crucial for informed decision-making regarding prostate health.

Dietary supplements play a significant role in the realm of natural remedies for prostate health. Ingredients such as saw palmetto, beta-sitosterol, and Pygeum africanum have shown promise in supporting prostate function and alleviating symptoms associated with benign prostatic hyperplasia (BPH). These supplements can help improve urinary flow and reduce discomfort, making them appealing for aging men experiencing prostate-related issues. However, it is essential to consult with healthcare professionals before starting any new supplement regimen to ensure safety and efficacy.

In addition to dietary supplements, exercise and lifestyle modifications are vital components of a holistic approach to prostate health. Regular physical activity can improve overall health, enhance mood, and reduce the risk of prostate diseases. Engaging in activities such as walking, strength training, and yoga can also help manage weight, which is linked to prostate health. Men should consider incorporating exercise into their daily routines as a proactive measure for maintaining prostate wellness.

Natural herbs also play a significant role in supporting prostate health. Herbs like nettle root, turmeric, and green tea extract have been researched for their anti-inflammatory and antioxidant properties. These natural compounds may help protect prostate cells from damage and support the body's overall defence mechanisms. By integrating these herbs into their diet, men can explore additional avenues for promoting prostate health and enhancing their well-being as they age.

Finally, awareness of prostate health screenings and early detection methods cannot be overstated. Regular check-ups and discussions with healthcare providers about prostate-specific antigen (PSA) tests are essential for monitoring prostate health. Detecting changes early can lead to more effective management of prostate conditions, including prostate cancer. By combining natural remedies with regular screenings, men can take a proactive stance on their prostate health, leading to improved quality of life and longevity.

Effective Herbs for Prostate Health

Prostate health is an essential aspect of aging gracefully, and certain herbs have shown promising benefits for maintaining prostate function. Saw palmetto is one of the most widely recognized herbs for prostate health, known for its ability to support urinary function and reduce symptoms associated with benign prostatic hyperplasia (BPH). This herb works by inhibiting the conversion of testosterone to dihydrotestosterone (DHT), a hormone that can contribute to prostate enlargement. Incorporating saw palmetto into your daily routine may help alleviate discomfort and improve overall prostate health.

Another effective herb is Pygeum africanum, derived from the bark of the African plum tree. Research indicates that Pygeum may help reduce inflammation and improve urinary flow in men suffering from prostate issues. Its ability to influence hormonal balance and reduce symptoms of BPH makes it a valuable addition to any prostate health regimen. Regular use of Pygeum can enhance quality of life by addressing urinary difficulties and supporting prostate wellness.

Pumpkin seed oil is another natural remedy that offers significant support for prostate health. Rich in zinc and fatty acids, pumpkin seeds can help maintain hormonal balance and reduce the risk of prostate-related issues. The oil extracted from these seeds has been linked to improved urinary function and may play a role in preventing prostate cancer. Including pumpkin seeds in your diet can provide essential nutrients that promote prostate health.

In addition to these herbs, lifestyle modifications can further enhance prostate wellness. Regular exercise, a balanced diet rich in fruits and vegetables, and stress management techniques are crucial for maintaining a healthy prostate. Engaging in activities that promote physical health can complement the benefits of herbal remedies, leading to improved overall well-being. Combining these approaches creates a holistic strategy for managing prostate health as men age.

Lastly, it's important to stay informed about prostate health screenings and early detection. Regular check-ups and consultations with healthcare providers can help identify potential issues before they escalate. Awareness of the psychological aspects of prostate health is also vital, as emotional well-being can significantly influence physical health. By prioritizing both natural remedies and proactive health measures, men can take charge of their prostate health and age gracefully with confidence.

Integrating Natural Remedies into Daily Life

Integrating natural remedies into daily life can significantly enhance prostate health for mature men. Many herbs and dietary supplements have been shown to support prostate function and overall wellness. These natural options, when combined with healthy lifestyle choices, can lead to improved quality of life and may help mitigate some of the side effects of aging and hormonal changes that affect the prostate. For instance, incorporating saw palmetto and Pygeum can help manage urinary symptoms associated with an enlarged prostate, a common concern for older men.

Dietary changes also play a crucial role in prostate health. Consuming a diet rich in fruits, vegetables, and omega-3 fatty acids can provide essential nutrients that promote prostate wellness. Foods such as tomatoes, which are high in lycopene, and cruciferous vegetables like broccoli can support hormonal balance and may even reduce the risk of developing prostate cancer. Making small, consistent changes in diet can lead to significant benefits over time.

Exercise is another vital component in the integration of natural remedies. Regular physical activity not only helps maintain a healthy weight but also improves hormone regulation and circulation, which are essential for prostate health. Engaging in activities like walking, swimming, or strength training can enhance overall well-being and reduce the risk of prostate-related issues. Establishing a routine that includes both aerobic and resistance training can provide the best results.

Incorporating mindfulness practices such as yoga and meditation can also benefit psychological aspects of prostate health. Stress management is crucial, as high stress levels can negatively impact hormonal balance and prostate health. These practices promote relaxation and mental clarity, which can improve overall health outcomes. By integrating these natural remedies and lifestyle modifications, men can take proactive steps to support their prostate health.

Lastly, regular prostate health screenings are essential, especially as men age. While natural remedies can provide support, they should not replace professional medical advice or routine check-ups. Staying informed about prostate health and engaging in open discussions with healthcare providers can lead to early detection of any issues. By combining natural approaches with regular medical care, mature men can effectively manage their prostate health and enhance their quality of life.

Prostate Health Screenings and Early Detection

Importance of Regular Screenings

Regular screenings are crucial for maintaining prostate health, especially as men age. These screenings help detect potential issues early, allowing for timely intervention and management. Prostate health screenings often include tests such as the prostate-specific antigen (PSA) test and digital rectal exams (DRE), which can provide valuable insights into a man's prostate condition. By prioritizing these screenings, men can take proactive steps towards their health and well-being.

The impact of hormonal changes on prostate health cannot be overstated. As men age, fluctuations in hormone levels can lead to various prostate-related issues, including benign prostatic hyperplasia (BPH) and, in some cases, prostate cancer. Regular screenings play a significant role in monitoring these hormonal changes and their effects on prostate health. Understanding how these changes affect prostate function is essential for making informed lifestyle and dietary choices that can support overall wellness.

In addition to screenings, lifestyle modifications, including diet and exercise, significantly contribute to prostate health. Incorporating dietary supplements rich in antioxidants and anti-inflammatory properties can provide added support. Regular physical activity not only helps maintain a healthy weight but also promotes hormonal balance, reducing the risk of prostate issues. By combining regular screenings with a proactive approach to diet and exercise, men can enhance their prostate health and overall quality of life.

Awareness and education about prostate cancer are vital components of preventive health strategies. Regular screenings not only help in early detection but also empower men with knowledge about their health. Understanding risk factors, symptoms, and the importance of early intervention can lead to better outcomes. Prostate cancer awareness campaigns often emphasize the significance of screenings, encouraging men to discuss their prostate health with healthcare providers and take charge of their well-being.

Lastly, the psychological aspects of prostate health should not be overlooked. The stress and anxiety associated with prostate health concerns can impact overall mental well-being. Regular screenings can alleviate some of this anxiety by providing reassurance or early detection of potential issues. Creating a supportive environment for discussions about prostate health can foster a positive approach to aging gracefully and maintaining sexual health, ultimately contributing to a fulfilling life for mature men.

Types of Prostate Health Screenings

Prostate health screenings are essential for early detection and prevention of prostate-related issues, especially for aging men. As men grow older, the risk of prostate conditions, including benign prostatic hyperplasia (BPH) and prostate cancer, increases significantly. Regular screenings can help identify these issues before they progress, allowing for timely intervention and better outcomes. Understanding the different types of screenings available is crucial for making informed health decisions.

One common method of screening is the prostate-specific antigen (PSA) test, which measures the level of PSA in the blood. Elevated PSA levels can indicate potential problems with the prostate, prompting further investigation. While the PSA test is a valuable tool, it is important to interpret the results in conjunction with other factors, such as age and family history, to avoid unnecessary anxiety and invasive procedures.

Digital rectal exams (DRE) are another vital component of prostate health screenings. During this exam, a healthcare provider manually checks the prostate for any abnormalities. Although it may seem uncomfortable, the DRE is a quick procedure that can provide important information about the prostate's size and texture. Together with the PSA test, DREs enhance the accuracy of prostate health assessments.

Additionally, imaging tests, such as ultrasound and MRI, may be used to obtain more detailed information about the prostate's condition. These advanced imaging techniques can help identify tumours or other abnormalities that may not be detectable through blood tests or physical examinations. Men should discuss with their healthcare providers the appropriateness of these tests based on personal risk factors and symptoms.

Ultimately, proactive screening and regular check-ups are key to maintaining prostate health as men age. Engaging in preventive measures, exploring dietary supplements, and adopting lifestyle modifications can further enhance prostate wellness. By staying informed and participating in regular screenings, men can take significant steps toward ensuring their prostate health and overall well-being for years to come.

Understanding Screening Results

Understanding screening results is crucial for older men aiming to maintain prostate health. Prostate screenings, including PSA tests and digital rectal exams, provide valuable insights into the condition of the prostate. These tests can reveal abnormalities that may indicate potential issues, such as benign prostatic hyperplasia or prostate cancer. Therefore, grasping the meaning of these results empowers men to make informed decisions about their health and treatment options.

When men receive their screening results, it is important to interpret them within the context of their overall health and lifestyle. Elevated PSA levels may not necessarily indicate cancer; factors such as age, race, and family history play a significant role. Understanding these nuances helps men avoid unnecessary anxiety and encourages them to engage in discussions with healthcare providers about the implications of their results.

In addition to understanding individual results, men should consider the importance of regular screening as part of their health maintenance routine. Early detection of prostate issues can lead to more effective treatment and better outcomes. Incorporating dietary supplements, exercise, and lifestyle modifications can also enhance prostate health and mitigate risks associated with aging.

Moreover, the psychological aspects of receiving screening results cannot be overlooked. Many men experience a range of emotions, from fear to relief, upon learning their prostate health status. Addressing these feelings through support groups or counselling can be beneficial, fostering a proactive approach to health and wellness.

Finally, staying informed about advancements in prostate health treatments and research is essential. As new information emerges, men can better navigate their health journeys and advocate for themselves. By understanding screening results and their implications, older men can take significant steps toward maintaining their prostate health and overall well-being.

Impact of Hormonal Changes on Prostate Health

Hormonal Changes with Aging

As men age, hormonal changes significantly impact their overall health, particularly concerning prostate health. The most notable change is the gradual decline in testosterone levels, which can lead to various physical and psychological effects. These hormonal shifts can influence not only sexual function but also the risk of developing prostate conditions, including benign prostatic hyperplasia (BPH) and prostate cancer. Understanding these changes is crucial for mature men to manage their health proactively.

The decline in testosterone often leads to symptoms such as reduced libido, fatigue, and mood swings. These changes can affect a man's quality of life and may lead to increased stress and anxiety. It is essential for men to recognize these signs and consider lifestyle modifications, including exercise and dietary adjustments, that can help mitigate the effects of hormonal changes. Engaging in regular physical activity and maintaining a balanced diet can support hormonal balance and promote overall well-being.

In addition to lifestyle modifications, dietary supplements may play a pivotal role in supporting prostate health as men age. Nutrients such as zinc, vitamin D, and omega-3 fatty acids have been shown to benefit prostate function. Some natural remedies and herbs, like saw palmetto and Pygeum, are also popular among those seeking alternative support for prostate health. However, it's crucial to consult with healthcare professionals before starting any new supplement regimen to ensure safety and efficacy.

Regular screenings and early detection of prostate health issues are vital, especially as hormonal changes can increase the risk of prostate cancer. Men should discuss with their healthcare providers the appropriate age to begin screenings and the frequency of these tests based on individual risk factors. Awareness and preventive measures can substantially impact outcomes, making it essential for men to stay informed and proactive regarding their prostate health.

Lastly, the psychological aspects of dealing with hormonal changes and prostate health cannot be overlooked. Many men may experience feelings of vulnerability or fear regarding their health, which can affect their mental well-being. Support groups, counselling, and open discussions with healthcare providers can help address these concerns. By fostering a holistic approach to health, including physical, emotional, and psychological support, men can navigate the complexities of aging with greater confidence and assurance.

Effects on Prostate Function

The prostate gland plays a crucial role in male reproductive health, particularly as men age. Changes in prostate function can significantly impact urinary health and sexual function, leading to conditions such as benign prostatic hyperplasia (BPH) and prostate cancer. Understanding these effects is vital for mature men to maintain their quality of life and overall wellness.

Dietary supplements have emerged as a popular option for supporting prostate health. Nutrients such as zinc, selenium, and omega-3 fatty acids are known to promote prostate function. Additionally, herbal remedies like saw palmetto and Pygeum africanum have shown promise in alleviating symptoms associated with prostate enlargement, providing a natural approach to management.

Regular exercise and lifestyle modifications are also key components of maintaining prostate health. Engaging in physical activity can reduce the risk of prostate-related issues by improving circulation and hormonal balance. Furthermore, adopting a balanced diet rich in fruits, vegetables, and whole grains can help mitigate the adverse effects of aging on prostate function.

Hormonal changes, particularly the decline in testosterone levels, can have a profound impact on prostate health. This reduction can lead to various symptoms, including decreased libido and erectile dysfunction. Men should be aware of these changes and consider discussing them with their healthcare providers to explore potential treatments and lifestyle adjustments.

Lastly, regular screenings and awareness of prostate cancer are essential for early detection and prevention. Understanding the risks and symptoms of prostate cancer can empower men to take proactive steps in their health management. Combining knowledge of dietary, lifestyle, and medical strategies can significantly enhance prostate health, ensuring that aging men can maintain their sexual health and overall well-being.

Managing Hormonal Imbalances

Managing hormonal imbalances is crucial for maintaining prostate health, especially as men age. Hormones like testosterone and oestrogen play significant roles in various bodily functions, including sexual health and prostate function. An imbalance in these hormones can lead to problems such as enlarged prostate, reduced libido, and even increased risk of prostate cancer. Thus, understanding how to identify and manage these imbalances can significantly enhance overall well-being for mature men.

One effective approach to managing hormonal imbalances is through dietary modifications. Consuming a balanced diet rich in antioxidants, healthy fats, and essential vitamins can support hormone production and balance. Foods such as fatty fish, nuts, seeds, and leafy greens are particularly beneficial. Additionally, specific dietary supplements like saw palmetto and zinc have been shown to promote prostate health and may help in stabilizing hormonal fluctuations.

Regular exercise is another pivotal strategy for managing hormonal levels. Engaging in physical activity not only helps in maintaining a healthy weight but also improves hormone regulation. Activities such as strength training, aerobic exercises, and yoga can enhance testosterone levels while reducing stress hormones. Incorporating a consistent workout routine tailored to individual fitness levels can contribute significantly to hormonal balance and overall prostate wellness.

Natural remedies and herbs also provide alternative options for addressing hormonal imbalances. Herbal supplements like Pygeum and stinging nettle have been traditionally used to support prostate health and may help in regulating hormonal levels. These remedies, combined with lifestyle changes, can create a holistic approach to health that is particularly beneficial for aging men.

Lastly, regular screenings and awareness of hormonal changes are essential for early detection of potential prostate issues. Routine check-ups can help monitor hormone levels and prostate health, allowing for timely intervention if necessary. By staying informed and proactive about hormonal management, mature men can significantly improve their quality of life and reduce the risk of prostate-related health concerns.

Prostate Cancer Awareness and Prevention

Understanding Prostate Cancer

Prostate cancer is one of the most common types of cancer affecting men, particularly those over the age of 50. Understanding the disease is crucial for early detection and effective treatment. Prostate cancer develops in the prostate gland, which is responsible for producing seminal fluid. Factors such as age, family history, and certain genetic mutations can significantly increase the risk of developing this condition. Awareness and education about prostate health are essential for mature men to navigate their health journeys effectively.

Dietary choices and lifestyle modifications play a vital role in supporting prostate health. Incorporating a balanced diet rich in fruits, vegetables, and healthy fats can contribute to overall wellness and potentially reduce the risk of prostate cancer. Additionally, specific dietary supplements, such as zinc and saw palmetto, are often explored for their benefits in maintaining prostate health. Regular exercise is also recommended as it helps manage weight and improves hormonal balance, further supporting prostate function.

Natural remedies and herbs have garnered interest as complementary approaches to prostate health. Some studies suggest that certain herbs, like

Pygeum and stinging nettle, may help alleviate symptoms of benign prostatic hyperplasia and enhance overall prostate wellness. While these remedies can be beneficial, it is crucial for men to consult healthcare professionals before starting any new regimen. Understanding the balance between natural and conventional treatments can empower men to make informed decisions about their health.

Regular screenings and early detection are key components in the fight against prostate cancer. Men are encouraged to discuss prostate health screenings with their healthcare providers, especially as they age. Tests such as the PSA (Prostate-Specific Antigen) blood test and digital rectal exams are common methods for monitoring prostate health. Early detection can lead to more effective treatment options and significantly improve outcomes for those diagnosed with prostate cancer.

Lastly, it's essential to consider the psychological aspects of prostate health and cancer. The diagnosis of prostate cancer can impact a man's mental and emotional well-being significantly. Support groups and counselling can provide valuable resources for coping with the psychological challenges associated with prostate cancer. Maintaining open communication with healthcare providers, family, and friends can help men navigate these challenges while promoting overall prostate health and wellness.

Importance of Early Detection

The importance of early detection in prostate health cannot be overstated, especially for adult males and older men. As men age, the risk of developing prostate-related issues, including benign prostatic hyperplasia and prostate cancer, increases significantly. Regular screenings and awareness of potential symptoms can lead to timely interventions, greatly enhancing the chances of successful treatment and improved quality of life. Understanding the significance of early detection empowers men to take proactive steps in managing their health.

Prostate health screenings, such as prostate-specific antigen (PSA) tests and digital rectal exams (DRE), play a crucial role in identifying potential problems at an early stage. These screenings allow healthcare providers to monitor changes in prostate health over time and initiate necessary interventions before conditions worsen. Regular check-ups not only aid in early diagnosis but also serve as an opportunity for men to discuss their health concerns with their doctors, fostering a collaborative approach to wellness.

In addition to screenings, lifestyle modifications can also enhance early detection efforts. A balanced diet rich in antioxidants, regular physical activity, and maintaining a healthy weight contribute to overall prostate health. Certain dietary supplements can support prostate function and provide additional protection against age-related changes. By integrating these practices into their daily routines, men can create an environment conducive to early detection and prevention of prostate issues.

Moreover, understanding the impact of hormonal changes on prostate health is essential for older men. Testosterone levels naturally decline with age, which can influence prostate size and function. Awareness of these changes enables men to recognize symptoms early and seek medical advice promptly. This proactive attitude towards hormonal health can lead to better management of prostate conditions, reducing the risk of complications.

Finally, fostering awareness around prostate cancer and its prevention is crucial today. Education about risk factors, symptoms, and the importance of early detection can save lives. Psychological aspects also play a role; men should feel encouraged to speak openly about their prostate health concerns. A supportive environment can help reduce stigma and promote proactive health management, ultimately leading to improved outcomes for aging men.

Sexual Health and Prostate Function

Relationship Between Prostate Health and Sexual Function

The relationship between prostate health and sexual function is a significant concern for aging men. As men age, the prostate undergoes various changes that can impact not only urinary function but also sexual health. Conditions such as benign prostatic hyperplasia (BPH) and prostate cancer can lead to complications that interfere with sexual performance and satisfaction. Understanding this relationship is vital for men who wish to maintain a healthy sexual life as they grow older.

Dietary supplements play a crucial role in supporting prostate health and, by extension, sexual function. Nutrients like zinc, selenium, and omega-3 fatty acids have been shown to promote prostate health, potentially reducing the risk of disorders that affect sexual performance. Additionally, herbal remedies such as saw palmetto and Pygeum may aid in alleviating symptoms associated with prostate enlargement, allowing for improved sexual function. Men should consider consulting with healthcare providers to identify suitable supplements that support both prostate and sexual health.

Regular exercise and lifestyle modifications are equally important in maintaining prostate health and enhancing sexual function. Engaging in physical activities can improve blood circulation, reduce stress, and promote hormonal balance, all of which contribute to better sexual performance. Furthermore, adopting a balanced diet rich in fruits, vegetables, and whole grains can positively impact prostate health, thereby supporting sexual wellness. Men are encouraged to embrace an active lifestyle as a preventive measure against age-related prostate issues.

Prostate health screenings and early detection are vital components in safeguarding sexual function. Regular check-ups can help identify potential health problems early, allowing for timely interventions that may prevent more severe complications. Men should not shy away from discussing prostate health with their healthcare providers, as proactive measures can lead to better outcomes and an enhanced quality of life, including sexual health.

Lastly, the psychological aspects of prostate health cannot be overlooked, as emotional well-being significantly impacts sexual performance. Anxiety about prostate health, especially concerning potential diagnoses like cancer, can lead to decreased libido and performance anxiety. It is essential for men to address these psychological factors, either through counselling or support groups, to foster a healthier mindset towards aging and sexual function. By focusing on both physical and mental aspects of prostate health, men can improve their overall quality of life as they age.

Common Sexual Health Issues

As men age, they often face various sexual health issues that can significantly impact their quality of life. Common problems include erectile dysfunction, decreased libido, and changes in sexual function, all of which can be related to the aging process and underlying prostate health. These issues are not only physical but can also have psychological effects, leading to anxiety and stress in intimate relationships. Understanding these challenges is crucial for mature men to seek appropriate support and maintain their sexual health as they age.

Erectile dysfunction (ED) is one of the most prevalent sexual health concerns for older men, often linked to prostate health. Conditions such as benign prostatic hyperplasia (BPH) and prostate cancer treatments can contribute to ED. Lifestyle factors, including diet and exercise, play a significant role in managing this condition. Incorporating dietary supplements and engaging in regular physical activity can improve circulation and hormonal balance, potentially alleviate the symptoms of ED and enhancing overall prostate health.

Another common issue is the decrease in libido, which can be influenced by hormonal changes that occur with aging. Testosterone levels typically decline in older men, affecting sexual desire and function. It's essential for aging men to monitor these changes and consult healthcare professionals for guidance on maintaining hormonal balance through lifestyle modifications and, if necessary, hormone replacement therapies. Addressing these hormonal shifts can help improve sexual health and well-being.

Additionally, awareness of prostate cancer risks is vital for mature men. Regular screenings and early detection strategies can significantly improve outcomes for those diagnosed with prostate cancer. Engaging in discussions about prostate health with healthcare providers can empower men to make informed decisions about their health. Understanding the importance of screening and being proactive about prostate health can reduce anxiety surrounding potential diagnoses and contribute to better overall wellness.

Lastly, exploring natural remedies and herbs for prostate support can benefit sexual health. Many men find that incorporating specific dietary supplements, like saw palmetto or Pygeum, may provide relief from symptoms related to prostate enlargement and improve urinary function. However, it is essential to approach these remedies with caution and consult with a healthcare provider before starting any new supplement regimen. By combining knowledge of common sexual health issues with proactive health strategies, mature men can enhance their quality of life as they age gracefully.

Strategies for Maintaining Sexual Health

Maintaining sexual health is a crucial aspect of overall well-being for aging men, particularly concerning prostate health. As men age, they may experience various changes that can impact their sexual function and prostate health. Understanding these changes and implementing effective strategies can help mitigate potential issues. This includes adopting a balanced diet rich in nutrients that support prostate health, such as antioxidants and healthy fats, while considering dietary supplements that may provide additional support.

Incorporating regular exercise into daily routines is another vital strategy for enhancing sexual health. Exercise promotes healthy blood circulation, which is essential for sexual function, and helps maintain a healthy weight, reducing the risk of prostate-related issues. Activities such as walking, swimming, and strength training not only contribute to physical fitness but also support mental health by reducing stress and anxiety, which can further impact sexual health.

Natural remedies and herbs have gained popularity for their potential benefits in supporting prostate health. For instance, saw palmetto and Pygeum are often recommended for their possible effects on urinary function and prostate size. However, it is essential to consult a healthcare professional before starting any herbal regimen to ensure safety and effectiveness, especially when combining with other treatments.

Regular screenings and early detection are paramount in managing prostate health, particularly for those at increased risk of prostate cancer. Men should engage in discussions with their healthcare providers about the appropriate age to begin screenings and the frequency of tests. Early detection can significantly improve treatment outcomes and enhance the quality of life, emphasizing the importance of proactive health management.

Lastly, addressing the psychological aspects of prostate health is essential for holistic wellness. Many men may experience anxiety or depression related to changes in sexual function or the fear of prostate disease. Seeking support from mental health professionals or participating in support groups can provide valuable resources and coping strategies, fostering a healthier outlook on aging and prostate health. Engaging in open conversations about these issues can also help lessen stigma and encourage more men to prioritize their sexual health.

Prostate Health for Aging Men

Unique Challenges Faced by Aging Men

As men age, they encounter a variety of unique challenges that can significantly impact their overall health, particularly concerning prostate health. One of the most pressing issues is the increased risk of prostate enlargement and benign prostatic hyperplasia (BPH), which can lead to uncomfortable urinary symptoms. These conditions often require careful management through lifestyle adjustments, dietary changes, and possibly medical interventions. Understanding these challenges is crucial for aging men to maintain their quality of life and health.

Dietary supplements have become a focal point for many aging men looking to support their prostate health. Nutrients such as zinc, selenium, and certain herbal extracts are believed to play vital roles in promoting prostate wellness. However, it is essential to consult healthcare professionals to ensure that any supplements taken do not interfere with existing medications or conditions. Proper guidance can help men make informed choices that align with their health goals.

Another significant challenge is the impact of hormonal changes that occur with aging. Testosterone levels naturally decline, which can affect sexual health and prostate function. These hormonal shifts may lead to changes in mood, energy levels, and overall vitality. Understanding these changes allows men to seek appropriate interventions, whether through lifestyle modifications, exercise, or medical treatments, to maintain their physical and emotional well-being.

Prostate health screenings and early detection are critical components of managing prostate health as men age. Regular check-ups can lead to the early identification of potential issues, including prostate cancer, which remains a significant concern for older men. Awareness and education about the importance of screenings can empower men to take charge of their health, leading to better outcomes and increased survival rates.

Lastly, the psychological aspects of prostate health cannot be overlooked. Aging men may experience anxiety or depression related to their health status, especially when faced with prostate-related issues. Support groups and counseling can offer valuable resources to navigate these emotional challenges, fostering a sense of community and understanding. By addressing both the physical and psychological aspects of prostate health, aging men can age gracefully while maintaining their well-being and vitality.

Tailoring Health Strategies for Older Adults

As men age, tailoring health strategies specifically for older adults becomes increasingly vital, particularly concerning prostate health. The aging process brings about various hormonal changes that can significantly impact prostate function and overall wellness. It is essential to recognize that everyone may experience these changes differently; hence, personalized approaches to health strategies are crucial in promoting prostate health and enhancing quality of life.

Dietary supplements can play a pivotal role in supporting prostate health for mature men. Research has shown that certain vitamins and minerals, such as zinc, selenium, and vitamin D, can contribute to healthier prostate function. Additionally, natural remedies and herbs, like saw palmetto and Pygeum, have been traditionally used to alleviate symptoms associated with an enlarged prostate. Incorporating these supplements into a balanced diet, alongside regular meals rich in fruits, vegetables, and healthy fats, can provide a comprehensive approach to prostate wellness.

Exercise and lifestyle modifications are equally important in fostering prostate health among older adults. Engaging in regular physical activity can help manage weight, improve hormonal balance, and enhance overall vitality. Activities such as walking, swimming, or gentle yoga can be particularly beneficial. Furthermore, reducing stress through mindfulness practices and maintaining social connections can contribute to a positive mental outlook, which is essential for psychological well-being and prostate health.

Regular prostate health screenings and early detection are crucial components of any health strategy for aging men. Routine check-ups allow for the monitoring of prostate-specific antigen (PSA) levels and can help in identifying potential issues before they become severe. Awareness of prostate cancer risks and the importance of early intervention can empower men to take charge of their health. Understanding the psychological aspects of prostate health, including the emotional impact of diagnoses, is also essential to provide holistic support.

As research continues to advance in the field of prostate health treatments, staying informed about new findings and therapeutic options is vital for older adults. Engaging with healthcare professionals who specialize in prostate health can provide guidance tailored to individual needs. By embracing a proactive approach that includes dietary management, physical activity, regular screenings, and emotional support, older men can significantly enhance their prostate health and overall well-being, allowing them to age gracefully.

Support Systems for Prostate Health

Prostate health is an essential aspect of aging gracefully, and establishing robust support systems can significantly enhance well-being for mature men. These systems encompass lifestyle modifications, dietary supplements, and regular screenings that contribute to maintaining prostate function. Understanding the importance of these elements is crucial for preventing complications related to prostate health, including the potential for prostate cancer. A proactive approach towards prostate wellness not only helps in early detection but also empowers men to take charge of their health as they age.

Dietary supplements play a vital role in supporting prostate health. Nutrients such as zinc, selenium, and omega-3 fatty acids have been shown to promote prostate function and reduce inflammation. Additionally, herbal remedies like saw palmetto and Pygeum africanum are popular choices among men seeking natural support for their prostate. Incorporating these supplements into a balanced diet can help mitigate risks associated with prostate issues and contribute to overall wellness.

Exercise and lifestyle changes are equally important in maintaining prostate health. Regular physical activity can improve circulation, reduce stress, and promote hormonal balance, all of which are beneficial for prostate function. Activities such as walking, swimming, or weight training not only enhance physical fitness but also support emotional well-being. Adopting a healthy lifestyle, including a balanced diet and regular exercise regimen, is essential for aging men looking to sustain their prostate health over the long term.

Prostate health screenings and early detection are paramount in identifying potential issues before they escalate. Regular check-ups, including PSA tests and digital rectal exams, are essential for monitoring prostate health and catching abnormalities early. Awareness of personal risk factors and family history can guide men in discussing screening options with their healthcare providers. Emphasizing the importance of early detection can lead to better outcomes and increased survival rates in cases of prostate cancer.

Finally, understanding the psychological aspects of prostate health is crucial for overall wellness. The impact of hormonal changes and the stress associated with prostate issues can affect mental health, leading to anxiety or depression. Support systems, including counselling and support groups, can provide men with the tools to navigate these challenges. By fostering a supportive environment and promoting open discussions about prostate health, men can improve their quality of life and maintain a positive outlook as they age.

Research Advancements in Prostate Health Treatments

Overview of Current Research

As research on prostate health continues to evolve, there is an increasing focus on understanding how various factors contribute to the overall well-being of mature men. Studies are focusing on the role of dietary supplements, lifestyle modifications, and natural remedies in supporting prostate health. This has led to a significant interest in identifying which strategies are most effective for preventing prostate issues, including benign prostatic hyperplasia and prostate cancer. The integration of these elements into daily routines can empower men to take charge of their health as they age.

Recent advancements in research have highlighted the importance of regular screenings and early detection of prostate-related conditions. Prostate health screenings, including PSA tests and digital rectal exams, are crucial for identifying issues before they progress. Awareness campaigns emphasizing the need for early detection are becoming more prevalent, encouraging men to prioritize their health. The psychological aspects of undergoing these screenings also play a role in how men perceive their prostate health and overall wellness.

Moreover, hormonal changes that occur with aging significantly impact prostate health. Research indicates that testosterone levels decline as men age, which can influence prostate function and overall health. Understanding the relationship between hormones and prostate health is essential for developing effective treatment and prevention strategies. This area of study is crucial for informing mature men about the implications of hormonal changes and how they can manage their health proactively.

Exercise and lifestyle modifications are also key components of current research into prostate wellness. Regular physical activity has been shown to have positive effects on prostate health, potentially reducing the risk of prostate cancer and other issues. Researchers are investigating specific types of exercise that may offer the most benefit, as well as the impact of diet and nutrition on prostate health. These findings are vital for developing comprehensive health strategies that men can adopt into their daily lives.

In conclusion, the landscape of prostate health research is rapidly changing, with a strong emphasis on holistic approaches that encompass diet, exercise, and psychological well-being. As more studies emerge, they will continue to inform men about how to navigate the complexities of prostate health throughout their aging process. Staying informed about these developments will empower men to make better choices for their health and enhance their quality of life as they grow older.

Promising Treatments on the Horizon

As research into prostate health continues to advance, promising treatments are emerging that offer hope for aging men concerned about prostate issues. Innovations in dietary supplements designed specifically for prostate support have gained traction. These supplements often include natural ingredients known for their anti-inflammatory properties, which can help reduce the risk of prostate enlargement and improve overall health. The focus on incorporating such supplements into daily routines reflects a growing recognition of the importance of nutrition in maintaining prostate health.

Exercise and lifestyle modifications are also proving essential in the prevention and management of prostate-related conditions. Recent studies have highlighted the benefits of regular physical activity in reducing prostate cancer risk and improving recovery outcomes for those diagnosed. Simple lifestyle adjustments, such as increasing daily activity and adopting a balanced diet rich in fruits and vegetables, can significantly impact prostate wellness. These changes not only enhance physical health but also contribute to psychological well-being, thereby creating a holistic approach to health.

Natural remedies and herbs have long been used in traditional medicine, and recent scientific studies are beginning to validate some of these practices. Ingredients like saw palmetto and Pygeum have shown efficacy in alleviating symptoms associated with benign prostatic hyperplasia (BPH). Furthermore, these natural treatments often come with fewer side effects compared to conventional medications, making them an attractive option for many men. The rise in interest surrounding these remedies encourages further research into their benefits and potential applications in prostate health.

Prostate health screenings and early detection remain critical components in the fight against prostate cancer. Awareness campaigns are increasingly focusing on educating men about the importance of regular screenings, which can lead to earlier intervention and better outcomes. As more men embrace these screenings, healthcare providers are improving methods to make them more accessible and less daunting. This proactive approach to health can alleviate fears and promote a culture of openness regarding prostate health issues.

In conclusion, the landscape of prostate health treatments is evolving, with promising advancements on the horizon. From dietary innovations to lifestyle changes and natural remedies, men now have a variety of options to support their prostate health. As research continues to uncover the complexities of prostate conditions and hormonal changes, the future looks bright for aging men eager to maintain their wellness and quality of life. Staying informed and proactive is essential in this journey, ensuring that men can age gracefully while managing their prostate health effectively.

Future Directions in Prostate Health

As advancements in medical research continue to unfold, the future of prostate health looks promising. New dietary supplements, specifically formulated to support prostate wellness, are being developed based on the latest scientific findings. These supplements are designed to target the unique needs of aging men, offering a proactive approach to maintaining prostate health. The importance of a balanced diet rich in antioxidants and essential nutrients cannot be overstated, as it plays a crucial role in combating age-related prostate issues.

In addition to dietary changes, exercise and lifestyle modifications are gaining traction as key components of prostate health strategies. Regular physical activity not only improves overall wellness but also has specific benefits for the prostate gland. Engaging in activities such as walking, swimming, or yoga can enhance blood circulation and hormonal balance, which are vital for prostate function.

Encouraging men to adopt healthier lifestyles will be instrumental in reducing the risk of prostate-related diseases.

Natural remedies and herbal supplements are also emerging as popular choices for men seeking alternative support for their prostate health. Herbal treatments, such as saw palmetto and Pygeum, have shown promise in alleviating symptoms associated with benign prostatic hyperplasia (BPH). The integration of these natural solutions into daily routines can provide a holistic approach to prostate care, especially for those who prefer to avoid conventional medications.

Screenings and early detection remain crucial in the fight against prostate cancer. Future directions in prostate health will emphasize the importance of regular check-ups and awareness campaigns to educate men about the signs and symptoms of prostate issues. Increased access to screening tests, such as prostate-specific antigen (PSA) tests, will facilitate early diagnosis, leading to better treatment outcomes and improved survival rates.

Finally, addressing the psychological aspects of prostate health is essential for a comprehensive approach. Men often experience emotional challenges related to prostate disorders, including anxiety and diminished self-esteem. Future initiatives should focus on providing support systems and resources that promote mental well-being alongside physical health. By fostering an environment that encourages open discussions about prostate health and its implications, we can help men navigate the complexities of aging with confidence and resilience.

Psychological Aspects of Prostate Health and Wellness

Mental Health and Prostate Issues

Mental health plays a critical role in the overall well-being of aging men, especially when facing prostate issues. Many men experience anxiety, depression, and stress as they navigate the complexities of prostate health. The connection between mental health and prostate conditions is profound; emotional distress can exacerbate physical symptoms, leading to a cycle of discomfort that affects quality of life. Understanding this relationship is vital for promoting comprehensive care strategies that address both mental and physical health needs.

Dietary supplements and lifestyle modifications are essential components in managing prostate health, yet they can also impact mental health. Nutrients such as omega-3 fatty acids and antioxidants have been linked to improved mood and cognitive function. Moreover, regular physical activity not only supports prostate wellness but also helps alleviate symptoms of anxiety and depression. As men adopt healthier lifestyles, they may find a boost in their mental resilience, enhancing their ability to cope with prostate-related challenges.

Natural remedies and herbs for prostate support can contribute to both physical health and emotional stability. Ingredients like saw palmetto and pygeum have shown promise in supporting prostate function, while herbal supplements like ashwagandha may help in reducing stress and improving mood. Integrating these remedies into a holistic approach can empower aging men to take charge of their health, fostering a sense of control and well-being that is crucial for mental health.

Prostate health screenings and early detection are not only about physical health; they can also alleviate mental burdens associated with uncertainty and fear of the unknown. Regular check-ups and discussions with healthcare providers about prostate health can reduce anxiety and empower men to make informed decisions about their health. Awareness of prostate cancer risks and preventive measures can further alleviate concerns, promoting a more relaxed and proactive approach to health management.

Finally, hormonal changes significantly affect both prostate health and mental well-being in aging men. Fluctuations in testosterone levels can lead to mood swings, fatigue, and decreased libido, all of which can impact mental health. By addressing these hormonal changes through appropriate medical interventions and lifestyle adaptations, men can improve their mental health, leading to better prostate health outcomes. This interconnectedness underscores the importance of a comprehensive approach to health that considers both the physical and psychological aspects of aging, prostate issues, and overall wellness.

Coping Strategies for Emotional Well-Being

As men age, coping with the emotional challenges associated with prostate health becomes increasingly important for overall well-being. The emotional toll of health concerns, such as potential prostate issues or cancer, can lead to feelings of anxiety and depression. Developing effective coping strategies can help individuals maintain a positive outlook and improve their quality of life. By addressing the psychological aspects of prostate health, men can empower themselves to manage their emotions more effectively.

One effective strategy is to engage in regular physical activity. Exercise not only supports prostate health but also releases endorphins, which are natural mood lifters. Activities such as walking, swimming, or yoga can provide both physical benefits and an emotional boost. Incorporating exercise into daily routines can serve as a vital coping mechanism, helping to alleviate stress and improve mental clarity.

Additionally, maintaining a balanced diet rich in nutrients can play a significant role in emotional well-being. Dietary supplements that support prostate health, such as omega-3 fatty acids, zinc, and antioxidants, may also contribute to improved mood. A diet that emphasizes whole foods, including fruits, vegetables, and lean proteins, can enhance overall health and resilience against emotional stressors.

Mindfulness and relaxation techniques are other valuable coping tools. Practices such as meditation, deep breathing exercises, and progressive muscle relaxation can help men manage anxiety and promote a sense of calm. These techniques encourage a focus on the present moment, reducing worries about health concerns and fostering a more balanced emotional state.

Finally, seeking support from healthcare professionals or support groups can provide a crucial outlet for sharing experiences and feelings. Open discussions about prostate health and associated emotions can lessen the burden of isolation. Building a network of support not only enhances emotional well-being but also helps men navigate the complexities of prostate health with greater confidence and understanding.

Importance of Support Networks

Support networks play a crucial role in the lives of mature men, particularly when it comes to prostate health. As men age, they often face various health challenges, including prostate issues, which can be daunting. Having a solid support network, including family, friends, and healthcare professionals, can provide the emotional and informational resources necessary to navigate these challenges. These connections foster a sense of community and belonging, which is vital for mental and emotional well-being during the aging process.

In addition to emotional support, these networks can offer practical advice on lifestyle modifications that promote prostate health. Engaging with peers who share similar experiences can be beneficial for discussing dietary supplements, exercise routines, and natural remedies that may aid in prostate wellness. Sharing tips and strategies among friends or support groups can lead to better choices and increased motivation to maintain a healthy lifestyle. This communal approach to health can help alleviate feelings of isolation and encourage a proactive attitude towards prostate health.

Furthermore, support networks play an essential role in raising awareness about prostate health screenings and early detection. Mature men often delay seeking medical advice due to stigma or fear. However, a strong support system can encourage individuals to pursue regular check-ups and screenings, which are vital for early detection of potential issues, including prostate cancer. By discussing these topics openly within a network, men can become more informed and empowered to take charge of their health.

The psychological aspects of prostate health cannot be overlooked either. Emotional support from a network can help men cope with the anxiety and stress that often accompany prostate health concerns. Talking openly about fears, expectations, and experiences with others who understand can provide relief and clarity. This shared understanding fosters resilience and promotes a healthier mindset when facing the challenges of aging and prostate health.

In summary, the importance of support networks for mature men regarding prostate health is multifaceted. These networks provide emotional, practical, and psychological support that is essential for navigating health challenges. Encouraging open conversations about prostate health within these circles can lead to better health outcomes, improved mental well-being, and a stronger sense of community. Men are encouraged to cultivate and rely upon these supportive relationships as they age, ensuring they maintain their health and wellness effectively.

Pause for thought

- The prostate is a small gland located just below the bladder sounding the urethra. Its primary function is to produce seminal fluids, which nourishes and transports sperm. As men age, there are age related changes in the gland that can significantly impact urinary and sexual health, among which are benign prostatic hypertrophy (BPH) and prostate cancer.

- As a natural effect of aging the prostate may enlarge, the result is BPH which can lead to urinary difficulties such as frequent urination or incomplete bladder emptying.
- Hormonal changes particularly the decrease in testosterone which inevitably accompany the aging process play a significant role in the health of the prostate. There are however, dietary supplements which have potential benefits in maintaining prostate health. Among those nutrients are zinc, selenium, and omega-3 fatty acids. Natural remedies like saw palmetto and Pygeum are also deserving of mention.
- Exercise and lifestyle modifications are vital for promoting prostate wellness. Regular physical activity not only help in weight maintenance, but reduces inflammation and improves overall wellbeing, essential factors in managing prostate health. Additionally, engaging in stress reducing practices such as yoga, or meditation can have positive psychological effects which contribute to better prostate function and sexual health.
- Early detection through prostate health screening is critical in preventing severe complications, including prostate cancer. Awareness of prostate health, including potential symptoms and the importance of regular check ups can empower aging men to take charge of their health.
- Diets rich in vitamins, selenium and omega-3 fatty acids are particularly important in promoting a healthy prostate function and may aid in reducing inflammation. Zinc is essential for testosterone metabolism. It is

believed that adequate levels of zinc can protect against prostate enlargement and prostate cancer. Additives to diet such as oysters, beef and pumpkin seeds offer a source of zinc.

- Selenium is an antioxidant which helps to combat oxidative stress, research suggest that adequate selenium intake may be linked to a lower risk of prostate cancer. Foods such as Brazil nuts, fish and whole grains are excellent sources of selenium. Omega-3 fatty acids found primarily in fish, walnuts, and flaxseeds, can be beneficial to prostate health because of their anti-inflammatory properties.
- Natural remedies and herbal supplements can provide support for prostate health. Herbs like turmeric, Pygeum, stinging nettle, and pumpkin seed extract have been used to promote urinary health and reduce symptoms associated with prostate enlargement. These however should only be used under the supervision of your health care provider.
- By adopting a balanced diet rich in antioxidants, healthy fats, and fibre, men can promote better prostatic health. Foods such as tomatoes, broccoli and fish provide essential nutrients that may help reduce the risk of prostatic issues and support hormonal balance.
- Saw palmetto, is among the most widely recognised herbs for prostate health, it is associated with supporting urinary function and reducing symptoms associated with BPH. It reputedly works by inhibiting the conversion of testosterone to dihydrotestosterone (DHT), a hormone which contributes to prostate enlargement. By the addition of this to

men's daily routine, discomfort may be relieved and there may be overall improvement in prostate health.

Take Home Nuggets

- Regular screening is crucial for maintaining prostate health as men age. Prostate health screening often includes blood test such as prostate specific antigen (PSA) test and digital rectal examinations (DRE) which can provide insights into a man's prostate condition.
- Additional screening tools involves imaging test such as ultrasound and Magnetic resonance imaging (MRI) which can give more detailed information about the condition of the prostate. These imaging techniques can help identify tumours or other abnormalities that may not be detectable through blood test or physical examinations. Proactive screening and regular check ups are key to maintaining prostate health as men age. One can further enhance prostate wellness by engaging in preventative measures, using dietary supplements and adopting lifestyle modifications.
- Elevated PSA values may not necessarily indicate the presence of prostatic cancer, factors such as age, race, and family history must also be considered.
- Hormonal imbalances can adversely affect prostate health. Hormones like testosterone and oestrogen play significant roles in various bodily functions including sexual health and prostate function. An imbalance in

these hormones can lead to problems such as an enlarged prostate, reduced libido, and increased risk of prostate cancer.

- Prostate cancer is among the most common types of cancers affecting men over the age of 50. This is influenced by age, family history, and genetic mutations. Early-stage prostate conditions often present with minimal signs. It is therefore, vitally important that men should be screened regularly as early detection and appropriate treatment yields the best results.
- Maintaining sexual health is a crucial aspect of overall wellbeing for aging men Particularly, concerning prostate health. As men age, they may experience various changes that can impact sexual function and prostate health.
- Current research on prostate health has an increasing focus on understanding how various factors contribute to overall wellbeing of mature men. Studies are focusing on the role of dietary supplements, lifestyle modifications, and natural remedies in supporting prostate health.
- Recent advancements in research have highlighted the importance of regular screening, including PSA testing and DRE as crucial in the identifying issues with the prostate before they progress. Awareness campaigns emphasising the need for early detection are becoming more prevalent, encouraging men to prioritize their health.

- The landscape of prostate health research is rapidly changing, with a strong emphasis on holistic approaches that encompass diet, exercise, and psychological wellbeing. As the results of studies become available, they will inform men about how to navigate the complexities of prostate health throughout the aging process.
- Recent studies have highlighted the benefits of regular physical activity in reducing prostate cancer risk and improving recovery outcomes for those diagnosed. Simple lifestyle adjustments such as increasing daily activity and adopting a balanced diet rich in fruit and vegetables can significantly impact prostate wellness.

Chapter 12
Genetics and prostate health

Importance of Prostate Health in Aging Men

Prostate health is a critical concern for aging men, as the prostate gland undergoes significant changes over time. Two of the most common conditions affecting this demographic are benign prostatic hypertrophy (BPH) and prostate cancer. BPH, which involves the enlargement of the prostate, can lead to uncomfortable urinary symptoms and significantly impact quality of life. On the other hand, prostate cancer remains one of the most prevalent forms of cancer among men, making understanding its risks and management essential for older males.

Early detection and screening methods play a vital role in managing prostate health. Regular check-ups can help identify potential issues before they develop into more serious conditions. Screening practices such as prostate-specific antigen (PSA) testing and digital rectal exams are crucial for early diagnosis. These methods can facilitate timely interventions that may improve outcomes and reduce the risk of complications associated with prostate diseases.

Lifestyle modifications can greatly assist men in managing benign prostatic hypertrophy. Engaging in regular physical activity, maintaining a healthy weight, and avoiding irritants such as caffeine and alcohol can help alleviate symptoms associated with BPH. Additionally, incorporating specific exercises targeting pelvic floor muscles can enhance urinary control and improve overall prostate health, leading to a better quality of life.

Nutritional interventions also play a significant role in promoting prostate health. A diet rich in fruits, vegetables, and healthy fats, particularly omega-3 fatty acids, has been linked to a lower risk of prostate issues. Foods high in antioxidants, such as tomatoes and broccoli, may also provide protective benefits against prostate cancer. By focusing on nutrition, aging men can take proactive steps toward better prostate health and overall well-being.

The psychological impact of a prostate cancer diagnosis can be profound, affecting not just the patient but also their families. Support groups and resources are essential in providing emotional support and guidance through treatment and recovery. Furthermore, advancements in prostate cancer treatments, including targeted therapies and immunotherapy, offer hope for improved outcomes. Regular medical check-ups, coupled with lifestyle changes and support systems, empower aging men to maintain their prostate health and navigate the complexities of prostate conditions effectively.

Two Common Diseases of the Aging Male

Benign Prostatic Hypertrophy

Benign Prostatic Hypertrophy (BPH) is a common condition that affects many aging males, characterized by the enlargement of the prostate gland. As men age, the risk of developing BPH increases due to hormonal changes that occur in the body. This condition can lead to uncomfortable urinary symptoms, including frequent urination, urgency, and difficulty starting or maintaining urination. Understanding BPH is essential for older men, as it can significantly impact quality of life and may require medical intervention.

The relationship between BPH and prostate cancer is an important consideration for aging men. While BPH is not cancerous, its symptoms can mimic those of prostate cancer, leading to confusion and anxiety. Regular screenings and early detection methods, such as PSA tests and digital rectal exams, are crucial for distinguishing between these two conditions. Men are encouraged to discuss their risk factors with healthcare providers to ensure timely diagnosis and appropriate management.

Lifestyle modifications play a vital role in managing the symptoms of BPH. Adopting a healthy diet, maintaining a regular exercise routine, and reducing alcohol and caffeine intake can help alleviate urinary issues associated with BPH. Additionally, techniques such as bladder training and pelvic floor exercises may also provide benefits. By making these changes, men can improve their overall health and reduce the impact of BPH on their daily lives.

Nutritional interventions are another key aspect of prostate health. Diets rich in fruits, vegetables, and healthy fats, particularly those high in omega-3 fatty acids, have been shown to support prostate function. Some studies suggest that specific nutrients, such as zinc and selenium, may also play a role in reducing the risk of BPH and promoting overall prostate health. Incorporating these nutritional strategies can be a proactive way for aging males to manage their health effectively.

The psychological impact of a prostate diagnosis, whether BPH or cancer, cannot be overlooked. Men may experience feelings of fear, anxiety, and depression, particularly when facing treatment decisions or lifestyle changes. Support groups and patient resources are available to help men cope with these challenges. Engaging with others who share similar experiences can provide valuable emotional support and foster a sense of community, which is essential for mental well-being and resilience during this phase of life.

Prostate Cancer

Prostate cancer is one of the most prevalent cancers affecting men, particularly as they age. Understanding the disease is crucial for adult males and older men, especially given its association with benign prostatic hypertrophy (BPH). Prostate cancer often develops silently, making awareness of symptoms and risk factors essential. The earlier it is detected, the better the treatment outcomes, which is why screening methods such as PSA tests and digital rectal exams are recommended for men over 50 or those with a family history of prostate disease.

Lifestyle modifications play a significant role in managing benign prostatic hypertrophy, which can coexist with or precede prostate cancer. Regular physical activity, a balanced diet rich in fruits and vegetables, and maintaining a healthy weight are all important factors. Additionally, reducing alcohol consumption and quitting smoking can help improve overall prostate health. These changes not only alleviate symptoms of BPH but may also lower the risk of developing prostate cancer.

Nutritional interventions specifically targeting prostate health have gained attention in recent years. Diets high in omega-3 fatty acids, antioxidants, and certain vitamins are believed to provide protective effects against prostate diseases. Foods like tomatoes, broccoli, and green tea have been studied for their potential benefits in reducing prostate cancer risk and progression. Men should consider incorporating these foods into their diet as part of a proactive approach to their prostate health.

The psychological impact of a prostate cancer diagnosis can be profound and often leads to feelings of anxiety, depression, and isolation. It is essential for patients to seek support from family, friends, and support groups. Resources are available that provide emotional support and education about the disease, treatment options, and coping strategies. Engaging with others who share similar experiences can be beneficial in navigating the challenges that come with a prostate cancer diagnosis.

Advances in prostate cancer treatments and therapies have significantly improved patient outcomes. Options range from active surveillance to surgery, radiation therapy, and hormone therapy. As research continues to evolve, genetic testing is becoming an increasingly important tool in personalizing treatment plans. Understanding the role genetics play in prostate disease can empower patients and their families to make informed decisions about their health and treatment options. Regular medical check-ups remain vital for early detection and effective management of prostate conditions, ensuring that men can maintain their quality of life as they age.

Early Detection and Screening Methods for Prostate Conditions

PSA Testing

Prostate-specific antigen (PSA) testing has become a cornerstone in the early detection of prostate diseases, particularly prostate cancer. For adult males and older men, understanding the benefits and limitations of this test is crucial. PSA is a protein produced by both normal and malignant cells of the prostate gland, and elevated levels can indicate the presence of prostate conditions. Regular PSA testing can help in identifying issues at an early stage, which is essential for effective management and treatment.

The relationship between PSA levels and benign prostatic hypertrophy (BPH) is significant, as both conditions can affect men as they age. While BPH is a non-cancerous enlargement of the prostate, it can still result in elevated PSA levels, leading to potential confusion in diagnosis. It is vital for men to discuss their PSA results with healthcare providers to understand what these levels mean for their health and to distinguish between benign and malignant conditions.

Lifestyle modifications can also play a role in managing prostate health alongside regular PSA testing. Men are encouraged to adopt a balanced diet, maintain a healthy weight, and engage in regular physical activity. These lifestyle changes can help lower the risk of developing prostate issues and may positively influence PSA levels. Additionally, incorporating specific nutritional interventions, such as increased intake of fruits, vegetables, and omega-3 fatty acids, can support overall prostate health.

The psychological impact of a prostate cancer diagnosis can be profound. Many men experience anxiety and fear about their health, treatment options, and the future. Support from patient groups and resources can be invaluable in helping men navigate this challenging time. Open discussions about sexual health and function post-diagnosis are also critical, as they can affect relationships and self-esteem. Men should feel empowered to seek help and communicate openly with their partners and healthcare providers.

Advances in prostate cancer treatments and therapies continue to evolve, providing hope for better outcomes. Genetic research plays a key role in understanding individual risks and tailoring treatment options. Regular medical check-ups, including PSA testing, are vital for aging males to monitor prostate health effectively. By staying informed and proactive, men can take charge of their health and make educated decisions about their prostate care.

Digital Rectal Examination

Digital Rectal Examination (DRE) is an essential screening tool for assessing prostate health, particularly for adult males and older men. This simple yet effective procedure allows healthcare providers to evaluate the prostate for abnormalities that may indicate conditions such as benign prostatic hypertrophy (BPH) or prostate cancer. During a DRE, the physician uses a gloved finger to examine the prostate gland through the rectal wall, checking for any irregularities in size, shape, or texture. Early detection of these conditions can significantly enhance treatment outcomes and improve the quality of life for patients.

For men experiencing symptoms such as difficulty urinating, frequent urination, or pelvic discomfort, a DRE can be a critical step in understanding their prostate health. While the thought of a DRE may cause anxiety, it is a quick procedure that typically lasts only a few minutes. The benefits of early detection through DRE cannot be overstated, as they play a crucial role in identifying potential prostate issues before they escalate into more serious health concerns.

In addition to DRE, patients should maintain open communication with their healthcare providers about their family history and any genetic factors that may increase their risk for prostate diseases. Men with a family history of prostate cancer should consider discussing a more proactive screening approach, which may include regular DREs coupled with other diagnostic tests such as PSA blood tests. Combining these methods can lead to a more comprehensive understanding of prostate health and facilitate timely interventions.

Lifestyle modifications also play a significant role in managing benign prostatic hypertrophy. Regular exercise, a balanced diet rich in fruits and vegetables, and stress management techniques can help alleviate symptoms associated with BPH. Nutritional interventions, including increased intake of omega-3 fatty acids and antioxidants, are beneficial for prostate health and can complement the results of regular medical check-ups, including DREs.

The psychological impact of a prostate cancer diagnosis can be profound, affecting not only the individual but also their loved ones. Support groups and resources are available to help men navigate these challenges. Understanding the importance of regular medical check-ups, including DREs, can empower men to take control of their prostate health, ensuring early detection and better management of potential issues. Advances in prostate cancer treatments and therapies continue to evolve, underscoring the significance of proactive health measures in improving outcomes for aging males.

Advanced Imaging Techniques

Advanced imaging techniques have significantly transformed the landscape of prostate disease diagnosis and management. These methods, which include MRI, CT scans, and ultrasound, allow for a non-invasive look into the prostate without the need for surgical intervention. This is particularly beneficial for older men, as it reduces the risks associated with invasive procedures while providing critical information for the diagnosis of benign prostatic hypertrophy and prostate cancer.

Lifestyle Modifications to Manage Benign Prostatic Hypertrophy

Dietary Changes

Dietary changes play a crucial role in managing prostate health, particularly for older men facing conditions such as benign prostatic hypertrophy and prostate cancer. As we age, the body undergoes various changes that can affect prostate function. A diet rich in fruits, vegetables, and whole grains can provide essential nutrients that support overall health and may help in reducing the risk of prostate diseases. Incorporating specific foods known for their beneficial properties can be a proactive approach to maintaining prostate health.

Research indicates that certain dietary components can have a direct impact on prostate health. For instance, tomatoes are rich in lycopene, an antioxidant that has been associated with a lower risk of prostate cancer. Additionally, fatty fish, which are high in omega-3 fatty acids, can also contribute to better prostate health by reducing inflammation. By making informed dietary choices, men can take steps to protect their prostate and overall health as they age.

Furthermore, it is important for men to monitor their intake of red and processed meats, as studies have shown a correlation between these foods and an increased risk of prostate issues. Instead, opting for lean protein sources such as chicken, turkey, and plant-based proteins can be beneficial. In conjunction with a balanced diet, maintaining a healthy weight is essential, as obesity has been linked to a higher incidence of prostate disease.

Hydration also plays a significant role in prostate health. Drinking adequate water throughout the day helps in maintaining optimal urinary function, which is particularly important for those experiencing symptoms of benign prostatic hypertrophy. Additionally, reducing caffeine and alcohol consumption may alleviate urinary discomfort and enhance overall well-being.

In conclusion, dietary changes can significantly impact prostate health for adult males and older men. By focusing on nutrient-rich foods, reducing harmful substances, and ensuring proper hydration, individuals can improve their quality of life and potentially lower the risk of prostate diseases. These dietary interventions, combined with regular medical check-ups and lifestyle modifications, can provide a comprehensive approach to managing prostate health effectively.

Exercise Recommendations

Exercise is a crucial component of maintaining prostate health, especially for adult males and older men who may be at higher risk for conditions like benign prostatic hypertrophy (BPH) and prostate cancer. Regular physical activity can help manage symptoms associated with these conditions, improve overall health, and contribute to a better quality of life. Engaging in moderate to vigorous aerobic exercises, such as brisk walking, swimming, or cycling, can enhance cardiovascular health and promote healthy body weight, which is essential for prostate health.

Strength training is another important aspect of an exercise regimen for aging males. Incorporating resistance exercises at least two days a week can help build muscle mass, improve metabolism, and support hormonal balance, all of which can play a role in prostate health. Simple activities such as weight lifting or using resistance bands can be beneficial, and they can be easily adapted to suit individual fitness levels and capabilities.

Flexibility and balance exercises should also be included in an exercise program. Activities like yoga or tai chi can help improve flexibility, reduce stress, and enhance overall well-being. These exercises not only promote physical health but also address the psychological aspects of living with prostate conditions by encouraging mindfulness and relaxation.

It's important for older men to consult with healthcare professionals before starting any new exercise program, especially if they have existing health issues or concerns related to prostate conditions. A tailored exercise plan that takes into account individual health status, fitness level, and personal preferences can help maximize benefits while minimizing risks. Regular check-ins with a physician can ensure that the exercise routine remains safe and effective.

In conclusion, incorporating a balanced exercise routine that includes aerobic, strength, and flexibility training can significantly contribute to the health and well-being of adult males, particularly those facing prostate-related issues. By prioritizing physical activity, men can take proactive steps toward managing their prostate health and improving their overall quality of life. Regular exercise, combined with lifestyle modifications and medical check-ups, can be a powerful approach to navigating the challenges of aging and prostate disease.

Stress Management

Stress management is crucial for adult males, especially those dealing with prostate conditions such as benign prostatic hypertrophy (BPH) and prostate cancer. The physical and emotional toll of these diagnoses can exacerbate stress levels, which may, in turn, affect overall health and quality of life. Understanding how to manage stress effectively can help men maintain a sense of control and improve their well-being during challenging times.

There are various strategies that men can adopt for effective stress management. Mindfulness practices, such as meditation and deep breathing exercises, allow individuals to focus on the present moment, reducing anxiety and promoting relaxation. Regular physical activity can also serve as a powerful stress reliever, as it releases endorphins that foster a positive mood and alleviate feelings of tension. Engaging in hobbies and social activities can further provide a necessary distraction and foster connections with others, which is vital for emotional health.

Nutrition plays a significant role in managing stress and supporting prostate health. A balanced diet rich in fruits, vegetables, whole grains, and lean proteins can improve mood and energy levels. Specific nutrients, such as omega-3 fatty acids found in fish, and antioxidants can help combat stress and inflammation. Additionally, staying hydrated and limiting caffeine and alcohol can further enhance mental clarity and emotional stability, which is particularly important for men facing the challenges of prostate conditions.

The psychological impact of a prostate cancer diagnosis can lead to increased stress and anxiety, making it essential for men to seek support from peers and professionals. Joining patient support groups can provide a safe space to share experiences and coping strategies. These groups not only help in managing stress but also foster a sense of community and understanding among individuals facing similar challenges. Professional counselling may also be beneficial for those struggling to cope with their diagnosis, providing them with tools to navigate their emotional landscape.

In conclusion, effective stress management is vital for adult males, especially those dealing with prostate-related health issues. By adopting healthy lifestyle modifications, seeking support, and prioritizing mental well-being, men can better navigate their health journeys. Regular medical check-ups and open discussions with healthcare providers about stress and emotional health should also be part of a comprehensive approach to managing prostate conditions.

Nutritional Interventions for Prostate Health

Key Nutrients for Prostate Health

Prostate health is crucial for men, particularly as they age. Key nutrients play a significant role in maintaining prostate function and reducing the risk of diseases such as benign prostatic hypertrophy (BPH) and prostate cancer. Nutrients like zinc, selenium, and omega-3 fatty acids have been studied for their potential benefits in promoting prostate health. Understanding their functions can help men make informed dietary choices that support their well-being.

Zinc is an essential mineral that supports immune function and plays a vital role in hormone regulation. Studies suggest that adequate zinc levels may help reduce the risk of prostate enlargement and cancer. Foods rich in zinc, such as oysters, beef, and pumpkin seeds, should be included in the diet of men aiming to maintain optimal prostate health. Additionally, supplementation may be considered, particularly for those with dietary restrictions.

Selenium is another critical nutrient that has garnered attention for its antioxidant properties. Research indicates that selenium may protect prostate cells from oxidative stress, potentially lowering cancer risk. Sources of selenium include Brazil nuts, fish, and whole grains. Men should aim to incorporate these foods into their diets to ensure they meet their selenium needs and support their prostate health effectively.

Omega-3 fatty acids, commonly found in fatty fish like salmon and flaxseeds, are known for their anti-inflammatory properties. Chronic inflammation is a risk factor for various prostate conditions, including BPH and prostate cancer. By including omega-3 rich foods in their diets, men can help mitigate inflammation and promote overall prostate health. Supplements are also available for those who do not consume sufficient dietary sources.

In conclusion, focusing on key nutrients such as zinc, selenium, and omega-3 fatty acids is essential for maintaining prostate health in aging men. A balanced diet rich in these nutrients can help reduce the risk of prostate diseases and support overall well-being. As part of a comprehensive approach to prostate health, men should consider their nutritional intake alongside regular medical check-ups and lifestyle modifications to manage prostate conditions effectively.

Foods to Include

Maintaining prostate health is crucial for older men, particularly in the face of common issues such as benign prostatic hypertrophy (BPH) and prostate cancer. A well-balanced diet can play a significant role in managing these conditions. Foods rich in antioxidants, such as tomatoes, which contain lycopene, have been shown to provide protective effects against prostate cancer. Additionally, incorporating cruciferous vegetables like broccoli and cauliflower can help in regulating hormones that may contribute to prostate issues.

Omega-3 fatty acids are another essential component of a prostate-friendly diet. Found in fatty fish such as salmon and mackerel, these healthy fats have anti-inflammatory properties that can aid in reducing the risk of prostate disease. Furthermore, walnuts and flaxseeds are excellent plant sources of omega-3s, making them beneficial for men who may not consume fish regularly. Including these foods in the diet can promote overall prostate health and support bodily functions.

Fibre-rich foods, including whole grains, beans, and lentils, should also be emphasized in the diets of aging males. These foods not only improve digestive health but may also play a role in hormone regulation. A diet high in fibre can help maintain healthy weight levels, which is vital as obesity can increase the risk of developing prostate conditions. Regular consumption of these foods can contribute to better hormonal balance and overall well-being.

Additionally, reducing the intake of red and processed meats can be beneficial. Some studies suggest a link between high consumption of these meats and increased prostate cancer risk. Instead, men should consider lean protein sources such as poultry and plant-based proteins. This dietary shift can help mitigate potential risks while promoting better health outcomes as men age.

Finally, hydration is an often-overlooked aspect of prostate health. Drinking plenty of water not only promotes overall bodily functions but can also help alleviate urinary symptoms associated with BPH. Herbal teas, especially those with anti-inflammatory properties, can also be included in the diet for added benefits. By focusing on these dietary inclusions, older men can take proactive steps in managing their prostate health and reducing the risk of disease.

Foods to Avoid

When it comes to maintaining prostate health, dietary choices play a crucial role. Certain foods have been linked to worsening symptoms associated with benign prostatic hypertrophy (BPH) and prostate cancer. These foods can contribute to inflammation, hormonal imbalances, and other factors that may exacerbate prostate conditions. Therefore, understanding which foods to avoid is essential for men, especially as they age and face these common health issues.

Red and processed meats are among the top contenders for foods to avoid. Studies have shown that high consumption of these meats can lead to increased risk of prostate cancer. The saturated fats found in red meat can promote inflammation and may interfere with hormone levels that are critical for prostate health. Opting for lean meats, poultry, or plant-based protein sources may be a more beneficial choice for maintaining a healthy prostate.

Dairy products also warrant caution. High intake of calcium from dairy has been associated with an elevated risk of prostate cancer in some studies. Full-fat dairy may contain hormones that could affect prostate health negatively. Men should consider reducing their dairy consumption or choosing alternatives such as almond or soy milk, which may offer a healthier option without the associated risks.

Refined carbohydrates and sugars are another group of foods to avoid. These can lead to obesity and insulin resistance, both of which are risk factors for prostate disease. Foods like white bread, pastries, and sugary drinks can spike blood sugar levels and promote inflammation in the body. Instead, men should focus on whole grains and foods that are low in sugar to support overall health and minimize the risk of prostate issues.

Lastly, alcohol consumption should be moderated. While some studies suggest that moderate alcohol may have protective effects, excessive drinking can lead to health complications, including an increased risk of prostate cancer. Men should monitor their alcohol intake and aim for moderation, ensuring they prioritize hydration and nutrient-dense foods that support prostate health.

Psychological Impact of Prostate Cancer Diagnosis

Coping with a Diagnosis

Receiving a diagnosis related to prostate health can be a life-altering moment for many men. Whether it is benign prostatic hypertrophy (BPH) or prostate cancer, the immediate reaction often involves a mix of confusion, fear, and uncertainty. Understanding these conditions is crucial, as knowledge can empower men to make informed decisions about their health. At this stage, it is essential to recognize that they are not alone in this journey; many have walked a similar path and have found ways to cope and thrive despite the diagnosis.

The psychological impact of a prostate cancer diagnosis cannot be understated. Men may experience a range of emotions, including anxiety, depression, and a sense of loss regarding their health and vitality. It's important to acknowledge these feelings rather than suppress them. Seeking support from loved ones, mental health professionals, or support groups can provide a safe space to discuss concerns and fears. Engaging in open conversations about emotions can lead to better coping strategies and an overall improvement in mental well-being.

Lifestyle modifications play a significant role in managing benign prostatic hypertrophy and potentially alleviating symptoms. Integrating regular physical activity, maintaining a healthy diet, and managing stress can significantly impact overall prostate health. Simple changes, such as reducing caffeine and alcohol intake, can help men feel more in control of their symptoms. Additionally, emphasizing a balanced diet rich in fruits, vegetables, and healthy fats can support prostate health and enhance quality of life.

For those diagnosed with prostate cancer, keeping abreast of advances in treatments and therapies is crucial. Continuous research is leading to innovative therapies that can improve outcomes for patients. Men should engage in discussions with their healthcare providers regarding the latest treatment options and clinical trials. This proactive approach can help men feel more empowered, knowing they are exploring the best available options tailored to their individual needs.

Finally, regular medical check-ups are vital for aging males to monitor prostate health effectively. Early detection through screening methods can lead to better management of prostate conditions. Men should prioritize these appointments and engage in open dialogues with their healthcare providers about their risks and symptoms. By prioritizing their health and staying informed, men can navigate their prostate health journey with confidence and resilience.

Impact on Mental Health

The diagnosis of prostate diseases such as benign prostatic hypertrophy (BPH) and prostate cancer can have profound effects on the mental health of adult males. Men often experience feelings of anxiety, depression, and fear following these diagnoses. The uncertainty surrounding the progression of these diseases, alongside concerns about treatment outcomes, can lead to a significant emotional burden. Understanding these mental health impacts is crucial for both patients and healthcare providers to ensure comprehensive care.

Many older men may find themselves grappling with feelings of isolation and loneliness after receiving a prostate diagnosis. They may withdraw from social activities or avoid discussing their health issues with family and friends, leading to a decline in their overall mental well-being. Support groups and resources are vital in helping these individuals connect with others facing similar challenges, thereby alleviating feelings of isolation and fostering a sense of community.

Mental health can also be influenced by the physical symptoms associated with prostate conditions. In cases of BPH, men may face urinary difficulties that affect their daily lives, impacting their self-esteem and confidence. Additionally, the potential side effects of prostate cancer treatments, including changes in sexual health and function, can further exacerbate feelings of inadequacy and distress. Addressing these concerns holistically is essential for improving mental health outcomes in this population.

Lifestyle modifications, including exercise and dietary changes, can play a significant role in managing both prostate health and mental well-being. Engaging in regular physical activity has been shown to reduce anxiety and depression while promoting overall health. Nutritional interventions that support prostate health can also contribute to an improved sense of well-being, making it important for men to consider these aspects as part of their comprehensive care plan.

Ultimately, the intersection of prostate diseases and mental health highlights the importance of early detection and regular medical check-ups. By prioritizing mental well-being alongside physical health, men can better navigate the challenges posed by prostate conditions. A proactive approach that includes psychological support, open communication, and lifestyle interventions can significantly enhance the quality of life for aging males facing these health issues.

Support Systems

Support systems play a crucial role in managing prostate health, particularly as men age. For those diagnosed with benign prostatic hypertrophy (BPH) or prostate cancer, having a solid support network can make a significant difference in coping with these conditions. Family, friends, and healthcare providers form the backbone of this support system, providing emotional encouragement and practical assistance throughout the treatment process.

In addition to personal support, patient support groups offer a unique avenue for connection among men facing similar challenges. These groups create a safe space for sharing experiences, discussing treatment options, and exchanging advice. The camaraderie found in these settings can alleviate feelings of isolation that often accompany a prostate disease diagnosis. Engaging with others who understand the journey can also empower men to advocate for their health more effectively.

Healthcare providers are essential in establishing support systems for patients. Regular medical check-ups are vital for early detection and screening of prostate conditions. Doctors can guide discussions about lifestyle modifications, nutritional interventions, and the psychological impacts of diagnosis. They also play a key role in informing patients about advances in treatments and therapies, ensuring that men are equipped with the latest information to make informed decisions about their health.

Moreover, the psychological impact of a prostate cancer diagnosis can be profound. Mental health support, whether through counselling or group therapy, is vital in helping men navigate their feelings and fears. Addressing emotional well-being is just as important as physical health, as it can influence treatment outcomes and overall quality of life. By incorporating psychological support into their care, men can better manage the stress and anxiety associated with their conditions.

Lastly, alternative and complementary therapies have gained popularity among men looking for holistic approaches to prostate health. Many individuals find solace in practices such as yoga, meditation, or nutritional supplements alongside conventional treatments. This integrative approach reflects the importance of a well-rounded support system that encompasses not only medical care but also emotional and lifestyle considerations for a healthier future.

Advances in Prostate Cancer Treatments and Therapies

Surgical Options

Surgical options for prostate conditions, such as benign prostatic hypertrophy (BPH) and prostate cancer, are critical considerations for aging males facing these health challenges. As men age, the likelihood of developing prostate issues increases, making it essential for them to understand the available surgical interventions. Procedures range from less invasive methods aimed at alleviating symptoms of BPH to more extensive surgeries required for prostate cancer treatment. Each surgical option comes with its own risks and benefits that should be carefully weighed against the individual's health status and personal preferences.

For benign prostatic hypertrophy, minimally invasive techniques like transurethral resection of the prostate (TURP) and laser therapies have become increasingly popular. These procedures aim to relieve urinary obstruction without the need for major surgery, allowing for quicker recovery times. Patients often experience significant improvements in urinary flow and overall quality of life post-surgery. However, it is crucial for men to discuss the potential side effects, such as sexual dysfunction or urinary incontinence, with their healthcare provider to make informed decisions.

When it comes to prostate cancer, surgical options typically include radical prostatectomy, which involves the complete removal of the prostate gland and some surrounding tissue. This procedure can be life-saving but also carries significant risks, including the potential for long-term complications such as erectile dysfunction and incontinence. The decision to proceed with surgery often depends on the cancer's stage, the patient's overall health, and personal preferences regarding treatment outcomes.

Advancements in surgical techniques, including robotic-assisted surgeries, have improved outcomes for many patients undergoing prostate cancer treatment. These modern approaches allow for greater precision, reduced blood loss, and shorter hospital stays. As technology continues to evolve, men should stay informed about the latest developments in surgical options and discuss these with their urologist to determine the best course of action tailored to their specific situation.

In conclusion, understanding the surgical options available for prostate conditions is essential for older men. This knowledge empowers them to engage in meaningful conversations with their healthcare providers, enabling informed decisions that align with their health goals and lifestyle. Regular medical check-ups and discussions about surgical interventions can significantly impact the management of prostate health as men age, ensuring they maintain a good quality of life through informed choices.

Radiation Therapy

Radiation therapy is a pivotal treatment option for prostate cancer, particularly for older men who are often at higher risk for this disease. It involves the use of high-energy rays or particles to target and destroy cancer cells. Patients may undergo external beam radiation therapy, where the radiation is directed at the prostate from outside the body, or brachytherapy, which involves placing radioactive seeds directly into the prostate. Understanding these methods is crucial for navigating prostate cancer treatment options effectively.

One of the significant advantages of radiation therapy is its ability to preserve surrounding healthy tissue while effectively targeting cancerous cells. This precision reduces the likelihood of side effects, making it a viable option for many men who may be concerned about the implications of more invasive treatments. Furthermore, radiation can serve as a standalone treatment or be combined with other therapies, such as hormone therapy, ensuring a comprehensive approach to prostate cancer management.

In addition to treating prostate cancer, radiation therapy may also be utilized in cases of benign prostatic hypertrophy (BPH) when other treatments fail to alleviate symptoms. By reducing the size of the prostate, radiation can help alleviate urinary difficulties associated with BPH, enhancing the quality of life for older men. This dual application exemplifies the versatility of radiation therapy in addressing male prostate health issues.

Men receiving radiation therapy may experience various side effects, including fatigue, changes in urinary habits, and potential impacts on sexual health. It is crucial for patients to have open discussions with their healthcare providers regarding these side effects and to explore supportive care options. Engaging in patient support groups can provide valuable insights and emotional support during this challenging time, helping men navigate the psychological impacts of their diagnosis and treatment.

Advancements in radiation technology continue to improve treatment efficacy and reduce side effects. Techniques such as image-guided radiation therapy (IGRT) and intensity-modulated radiation therapy (IMRT) allow for more precise targeting of tumors. As research progresses, understanding the genetic factors influencing prostate cancer can further tailor radiation therapy, optimizing outcomes for individual patients. For older men, staying informed about these advancements and maintaining regular medical check-ups are essential components of proactive prostate health management.

Hormonal Treatments

Hormonal treatments play a significant role in managing prostate diseases, particularly benign prostatic hypertrophy (BPH) and prostate cancer. For older men, understanding the implications of hormone therapy is crucial as these treatments can alleviate symptoms associated with BPH and may also be a part of therapeutic strategies in prostate cancer management. The primary hormones involved in these treatments are testosterone and dihydrotestosterone (DHT), both of which influence prostate growth and function. By manipulating these hormones, healthcare providers can help improve quality of life for those affected by prostate conditions.

In the case of BPH, hormonal treatments often involve the use of medications such as alpha-blockers and 5-alpha reductase inhibitors. Alpha-blockers work by relaxing the muscles around the prostate and bladder neck, making it easier to urinate. On the other hand, 5-alpha reductase inhibitors reduce the levels of DHT, which can shrink the prostate over time. These treatments are generally well-tolerated, although patients should be aware of potential side effects, including sexual dysfunction and changes in libido, which are critical considerations for older males.

For prostate cancer, hormonal therapy can be a cornerstone of treatment, especially for advanced stages of the disease. Androgen deprivation therapy (ADT) is often used to lower testosterone levels, which can fuel the growth of cancer cells. This therapy can significantly slow disease progression and is sometimes combined with other treatments, such as radiation or chemotherapy. Men undergoing ADT should be monitored closely for side effects, including bone density loss and metabolic changes, as these may impact overall health and well-being.

Regular communication with healthcare providers is essential for men receiving hormonal treatments for prostate conditions. Patients should discuss any side effects or concerns they experience, as adjustments to the treatment plan may be necessary. Furthermore, lifestyle modifications, including diet and exercise, can complement hormonal therapies, enhance their effectiveness and improving overall prostate health. Engaging with support groups can also provide emotional and psychological benefits, fostering a sense of community and shared experience among those facing similar challenges.

In summary, hormonal treatments are vital in the management of benign prostatic hypertrophy and prostate cancer, offering symptom relief and potential disease control. For older men, understanding these therapies' benefits and risks is essential for making informed decisions about their health. With ongoing advances in treatment options and supportive care resources, men can navigate their prostate health more effectively, ultimately improving their quality of life during the aging process.

Emerging Therapies

Emerging therapies for prostate diseases are at the forefront of medical research, offering hope for men facing conditions like benign prostatic hypertrophy (BPH) and prostate cancer. Innovations in treatment methods focus on improving outcomes and minimizing side effects. These therapies often incorporate advancements in genetic understanding, paving the way for tailored approaches that align more closely with individual patient profiles. As the landscape of prostate health evolves, men need to stay informed about the latest options available to them.

One promising area of research includes the development of targeted therapies that specifically attack cancer cells while sparing healthy tissue. These methods aim to enhance the effectiveness of existing treatments, such as hormone therapy and radiation, by delivering drugs directly to the tumour site. Additionally, immunotherapy is gaining traction, harnessing the body's immune system to recognize and destroy cancer cells. This approach not only improves survival rates but also offers a better quality of life for patients undergoing treatment.

For benign prostatic hypertrophy, emerging therapies emphasize minimally invasive procedures that can alleviate symptoms without the need for extensive surgery. Techniques such as laser therapy and microwave therapy provide options that reduce recovery time and improve patient comfort. These advancements reflect a growing understanding of the importance of maintaining a man's quality of life, especially as he ages and faces various health challenges.

Lifestyle modifications continue to be a critical component in managing prostate health. Recent studies highlight the role of diet and exercise in mitigating symptoms associated with BPH and prostate cancer. Nutritional interventions, such as increased intake of antioxidants and healthy fats, are being investigated for their potential to enhance treatment outcomes. Men are encouraged to adopt these lifestyle changes as part of their overall strategy for prostate health, complementing medical treatments with holistic approaches.

Lastly, the psychological impact of a prostate cancer diagnosis cannot be overlooked. Emerging therapies are not just about physical health; they also encompass mental well-being. Support groups and counselling services are increasingly recognized as essential resources for men navigating the emotional challenges of prostate disease. By addressing both the physical and psychological aspects of these conditions, healthcare providers can offer more comprehensive care that truly meets the needs of aging males.

The Role of Genetics in Prostate Diseases

Genetic Risk Factors

Genetic risk factors play a significant role in the development of prostate diseases, particularly benign prostatic hypertrophy (BPH) and prostate cancer. Studies indicate that men with a family history of these conditions are at a higher risk. Understanding these genetic predispositions can empower men to make informed decisions about their health and screening practices.

The heritability of prostate cancer is well-documented, with specific gene mutations linked to an increased risk. For example, mutations in the BRCA1 and BRCA2 genes, commonly associated with breast cancer, have also been implicated in prostate cancer. Men with these genetic markers should discuss their screening options with healthcare providers to facilitate early detection and intervention.

In addition to hereditary factors, lifestyle and environmental interactions with genetic predispositions can influence the onset of prostate conditions. Factors such as diet, exercise, and exposure to certain chemicals may exacerbate genetic risks. Adult males should consider lifestyle modifications that can mitigate these risks, such as maintaining a healthy weight and incorporating a balanced diet rich in fruits and vegetables.

Moreover, understanding the psychological impact of a prostate cancer diagnosis is crucial. Knowing one's genetic risk can lead to anxiety and stress, which may affect overall well-being. Support groups and counselling can provide essential resources for coping with these emotional challenges, helping men navigate their journey with prostate health more effectively.

Advances in genetic testing and therapies are promising for the future of prostate health. Personalized medicine approaches based on genetic profiles are becoming more prevalent, allowing for tailored treatment plans that address the unique needs of each patient. As research continues, it is vital for aging males to stay informed about their genetic risks and engage actively in discussions with their healthcare providers to optimize their prostate health management.

Family History and Prostate Cancer

Family history plays a significant role in understanding the risk factors associated with prostate cancer. Men with close relatives, such as fathers or brothers, who have been diagnosed with prostate cancer are at a heightened risk themselves. This familial connection suggests that genetic predisposition may influence the likelihood of developing this condition. It is crucial for men, especially as they age, to be aware of their family medical history, as it can inform screening and prevention strategies.

In addition to genetic factors, certain lifestyle choices can also be influenced by family history. For instance, dietary habits, exercise routines, and health management strategies often pass down through generations. Men who come from families with a history of prostate issues may benefit from adopting healthier lifestyles, including balanced diets rich in fruits and vegetables, regular physical activity, and maintaining a healthy weight. These modifications not only contribute to overall well-being but also play a role in managing benign prostatic hypertrophy and lowering the risk of prostate cancer.

Early detection is another critical aspect where family history plays a role. Understanding one's genetic background can lead to earlier screening and proactive health measures. Regular check-ups and discussions about prostate health with healthcare providers can help identify any necessary tests, such as PSA screenings. Men with a family history of prostate cancer should particularly consider starting these screenings at an earlier age, as they may be more susceptible to developing the disease.

The psychological impact of having a family history of prostate cancer can be significant. Men may experience anxiety and stress, worrying about their own health outcomes and the potential for hereditary transmission. Support groups and resources specifically tailored for individuals with a family history of prostate issues can provide valuable emotional support and information. Engaging with others who understand these challenges can foster a sense of community and aid in coping with the psychological burden of such a diagnosis.

Advances in treatments and therapies for prostate cancer are continually evolving, and understanding family history can aid in personalizing treatment options. Genetic testing can help determine the most effective therapies based on an individual's unique genetic makeup. Men concerned about their family history should discuss these advancements with their healthcare providers to explore available options, ensuring they receive the most informed and tailored care possible. By being proactive and informed, men can navigate their prostate health with greater confidence and support.

Genetic Testing

Genetic testing has emerged as a vital tool in understanding prostate diseases, particularly benign prostatic hypertrophy (BPH) and prostate cancer. For adult males, especially those at higher risk due to family history, genetic testing can provide crucial insights into their susceptibility to these conditions. By examining specific genes associated with prostate health, men can better understand their risk profile and make informed decisions regarding screening and preventive measures.

The role of genetics in prostate diseases is becoming increasingly clear. Studies have shown that men with a familial history of prostate cancer are more likely to carry genetic mutations that elevate their risk. This understanding underscores the importance of discussing family medical history with healthcare providers and considering genetic counselling, which can guide men on whether genetic testing is appropriate for them.

In addition to risk assessment, genetic testing can influence treatment decisions for those diagnosed with prostate cancer. Knowing the genetic makeup of the cancer can help healthcare professionals tailor therapies that are more effective for the individual's specific type of cancer. This personalized approach can lead to better outcomes and fewer side effects, making genetic testing a significant advancement in prostate cancer management.

While the benefits of genetic testing are clear, it can also have psychological impacts on men. Receiving information about genetic risks may cause anxiety or distress, particularly if the results indicate a higher likelihood of developing prostate conditions. Therefore, it is essential for healthcare providers to offer support and resources, including patient support groups, to help men navigate these emotional challenges effectively.

Ultimately, regular medical check-ups and discussions about genetic testing should be part of every aging male's health routine. As advancements in genetic science continue to evolve, men have more tools at their disposal to manage their prostate health proactively. By integrating genetic testing into their healthcare strategy, they can enhance early detection efforts and improve their overall quality of life.

Patient Support Groups and Resources for Prostate Health

Importance of Support Groups

Support groups play a crucial role in the lives of men dealing with prostate diseases, such as benign prostatic hypertrophy and prostate cancer. These groups provide a safe space where individuals can share their experiences, fears, and coping strategies. The emotional support gained from fellow members who understand the challenges faced can significantly alleviate feelings of isolation and anxiety. This sense of community fosters a supportive environment where men can discuss their health, treatments, and lifestyle modifications without judgment.

The importance of support groups extends beyond mere emotional solace; they serve as a vital resource for information and education. Members often share valuable insights about early detection and screening methods that they have learned through personal experiences or research. This exchange of knowledge can empower individuals to make informed decisions about their health and treatment options. Furthermore, support groups often host guest speakers, including healthcare professionals, who can provide expert advice on managing prostate conditions effectively.

Engagement in support groups can also positively impact lifestyle modifications and nutritional interventions for prostate health. Members often discuss dietary changes and exercise routines that have benefited their health. This shared information can inspire individuals to adopt healthier habits and improve their overall well-being. By learning from others' successes and challenges, men can make more informed choices that contribute to better management of benign prostatic hypertrophy and prostate cancer.

The psychological impact of a prostate cancer diagnosis can be profound, making support groups particularly valuable. Men often grapple with feelings of fear, depression, and uncertainty about their future. By connecting with others who have faced similar diagnoses, they can find hope and resilience. Support groups offer a platform for members to express their feelings openly, which can be a significant step in the healing process. This emotional support can lead to improved mental health and a greater sense of control over their situation.

Finally, the role of genetics in prostate diseases is an essential topic that can be explored within these support groups. Discussions around genetic predispositions can help members understand their risks and the importance of regular medical check-ups. By sharing experiences related to family history and genetic testing, men can become more proactive in addressing their health concerns. The camaraderie and shared wisdom found in support groups not only enhance individual coping strategies but also promote collective awareness and action towards prostate health.

Online Resources

In today's digital age, online resources play a vital role in providing information about prostate health, especially for adult males facing conditions like benign prostatic hypertrophy and prostate cancer. Websites dedicated to men's health offer comprehensive insights into these diseases, detailing symptoms, risk factors, and the latest research findings. Through reputable sources, men can educate themselves about early detection methods and screening processes, which are crucial for effective management of prostate conditions. The accessibility of this information online empowers men to take charge of their health proactively.

Lifestyle modifications are essential for managing benign prostatic hypertrophy, and numerous online platforms provide guidance on practical changes men can implement. These resources often include exercise routines, dietary recommendations, and stress management techniques that promote overall well-being. By incorporating these modifications, men can not only alleviate symptoms but also improve their quality of life. Online forums and blogs featuring personal success stories can also inspire and motivate others to make similar changes.

Nutrition plays a significant role in prostate health, and many online resources focus on dietary interventions that may benefit men diagnosed with prostate conditions. Articles and videos discuss the importance of specific nutrients, such as lycopene and omega-3 fatty acids, and how they may influence prostate health. Men can find recipes and meal plans that incorporate these beneficial foods, making it easier to adopt a prostate-friendly diet. Additionally, expert opinions and research articles can provide insights into the ongoing studies related to nutrition and prostate health.

The psychological impact of a prostate cancer diagnosis can be profound, and online support groups are invaluable for those navigating this challenging experience. Websites dedicated to cancer support often feature forums where men can share their feelings, seek advice, and connect with others facing similar struggles. These communities offer a sense of belonging and understanding, which can significantly aid in coping with the emotional toll of a prostate disease diagnosis. Access to mental health resources and counselling services through online platforms can further support men in managing their mental well-being.

Advances in treatments and therapies for prostate cancer are rapidly evolving, and staying informed through online resources is essential. Various medical websites provide updates on the latest research, clinical trials, and innovative therapies available. Men can learn about treatment options tailored to their specific condition, including traditional and alternative therapies. By accessing this wealth of information, men can engage in informed discussions with their healthcare providers, making better choices regarding their treatment plans. Regularly checking these resources can help men stay ahead in their health journey.

Community Programs

Community programs play a vital role in supporting men as they navigate the complexities of prostate health. These initiatives often provide resources and information related to benign prostatic hypertrophy and prostate cancer, helping men understand their conditions better. Such programs can offer educational seminars, workshops, and support groups that foster open discussions about symptoms, treatments, and lifestyle adjustments that may alleviate discomfort and improve quality of life.

Additionally, community programs frequently emphasize the importance of early detection and regular screenings for prostate conditions. By promoting awareness of screening methods, these initiatives encourage men to take proactive steps in monitoring their prostate health. This early intervention can lead to better outcomes, especially in cases of prostate cancer, where early diagnosis significantly impacts treatment effectiveness and survivorship.

Lifestyle modifications are another focus of community programs, aiming to educate men about practical changes they can make to manage benign prostatic hypertrophy. This may include guidance on physical activity, dietary recommendations, and stress reduction techniques. Programs often collaborate with health professionals who can provide personalized advice tailored to individual health needs, ultimately empowering men to take control of their prostate health through informed choices.

Moreover, community initiatives recognize the psychological impact of a prostate cancer diagnosis on men and their families. Support groups and counselling services offer a safe space for men to express their fears, share experiences, and receive emotional support. These resources are crucial for mental well-being, helping men cope with the challenges that accompany prostate disease and treatment.

Lastly, community programs can facilitate access to the latest advancements in prostate cancer treatments and therapies. By partnering with healthcare providers and researchers, these initiatives can keep men informed about new clinical trials, medications, and alternative therapies. This connection to cutting-edge information ensures that men have the resources they need to make educated decisions regarding their health, ultimately leading to improved outcomes and a heightened sense of agency in their healthcare journey.

The Importance of Regular Medical Check-ups for Aging Males

Recommended Screening Intervals

When it comes to screening for prostate diseases, understanding the recommended intervals can significantly influence early detection and treatment outcomes. For adult males, particularly those over the age of 50, the consensus among healthcare professionals is to begin regular screenings for prostate cancer, which may involve a prostate-specific antigen (PSA) test and a digital rectal exam (DRE). Men with a family history of prostate cancer or genetic predispositions, such as BRCA mutations, may need to start screening even earlier, around the age of 40 or 45, to catch any potential issues as early as possible.

Benign prostatic hypertrophy (BPH), while not cancerous, is another condition that commonly affects aging males. Regular screenings for BPH are equally important, as the symptoms can significantly impact quality of life. Men experiencing urinary difficulties should consult with their healthcare provider, who may recommend annual evaluations after the age of 50. Recognizing the symptoms and understanding the need for routine checks can help manage BPH effectively and improve overall prostate health.

The intervals for screening can also be influenced by individual risk factors and overall health status. For men with normal PSA levels and no family history, a screening every two years may be sufficient. However, men with elevated PSA levels or other concerning symptoms might be advised to return for more frequent assessments, possibly annually. This tailored approach ensures that each individual receives the most appropriate level of care based on their unique situation.

In addition to regular screenings, lifestyle modifications can play a crucial role in managing prostate health. A diet rich in fruits, vegetables, and healthy fats, alongside regular exercise, can have a positive impact on both BPH and prostate cancer risk. Men should also consider discussing nutritional interventions with their healthcare provider, as certain supplements and dietary changes can support prostate health and potentially delay the onset of disease.

Finally, the psychological impact of a prostate disease diagnosis cannot be overlooked. Many men experience anxiety and uncertainty following screenings, particularly if they receive abnormal results. Access to support groups and patient resources can provide valuable assistance during these challenging times. Regular medical check-ups not only facilitate early detection but also offer an opportunity for men to discuss their concerns, receive guidance on managing their conditions, and maintain a proactive approach towards their health.

Building a Relationship with Healthcare Providers

Building a relationship with healthcare providers is crucial for men dealing with prostate diseases, such as benign prostatic hypertrophy and prostate cancer. Open communication fosters trust and ensure that patients feel comfortable discussing their symptoms and concerns. Regular check-ups and screenings are essential for early detection, making it vital for men to establish a rapport with their healthcare team. By doing so, they can receive personalized care tailored to their specific needs and medical history.

Understanding the importance of lifestyle modifications is another key aspect of this relationship. Healthcare providers can offer valuable insights into managing benign prostatic hypertrophy through diet, exercise, and other lifestyle changes. Men should actively engage with their providers about their daily habits and be open to suggestions that might improve their condition. This partnership can lead to more effective management of symptoms and a better quality of life.

Nutrition plays a significant role in prostate health, and discussing dietary choices with healthcare providers can enhance treatment outcomes. Men should feel encouraged to seek advice on nutritional interventions that can support prostate health, such as foods rich in antioxidants and omega-3 fatty acids. By collaborating with their healthcare team, patients can make informed dietary decisions that complement their medical treatments and overall wellness strategies.

The psychological impact of a prostate cancer diagnosis is profound, and healthcare providers can offer essential support. Building a strong relationship with providers allows men to voice their emotional struggles and seek guidance on coping strategies. Mental health is an integral part of overall health, and having a supportive healthcare team can significantly alleviate feelings of anxiety and depression associated with prostate diseases.

Finally, as advancements in prostate cancer treatments continue to evolve, maintaining an open dialogue with healthcare providers ensures that patients are informed about the latest options available. By establishing a solid relationship, men can confidently discuss new therapies and express their preferences for treatment. This collaborative approach not only empowers patients but also fosters a proactive attitude towards managing their health and navigating the complexities of prostate disease.

Understanding Medical Advice

Understanding medical advice is crucial for adult males, especially as they navigate the complexities of prostate health. Two common diseases that frequently affect aging men are benign prostatic hypertrophy (BPH) and prostate cancer. BPH can lead to uncomfortable urinary symptoms, while prostate cancer poses a significant threat, making early detection and screening vital. Men should be aware of the various screening methods available, including PSA tests and digital rectal exams, which can help in identifying potential issues before they escalate.

Lifestyle modifications can play a pivotal role in managing benign prostatic hypertrophy. Regular exercise, maintaining a healthy weight, and avoiding irritants like caffeine and alcohol can alleviate symptoms and improve quality of life. Additionally, incorporating specific nutritional interventions may support prostate health. Diets rich in fruits, vegetables, and healthy fats, particularly omega-3 fatty acids, have shown promise in promoting overall well-being and potentially reducing the risk of prostate diseases.

The psychological impact of a prostate cancer diagnosis cannot be underestimated. Many men experience anxiety, depression, and fear regarding their health and future. Understanding these emotional responses is important for both patients and their families. Engaging with support groups can provide a sense of community and shared experience, helping individuals cope with their diagnosis. Furthermore, mental health resources should be readily accessible to support men through their treatment journeys.

Advances in prostate cancer treatments and therapies have significantly improved patient outcomes. Options such as hormone therapy, radiation, and newer immunotherapies offer hope and can be tailored to individual needs. The role of genetics in prostate diseases is also an emerging area of study, with genetic testing becoming more prevalent. Understanding one's genetic predisposition can guide proactive measures and personalized treatment plans, empowering men in their health management.

Regular medical check-ups are essential for aging males to catch any potential health issues early, including prostate conditions. Men must prioritize their sexual health and function, especially when dealing with prostate-related issues. Alternative and complementary therapies can also be explored, providing additional avenues for managing symptoms and enhancing quality of life. Overall, informed medical advice is the cornerstone of effective prostate health management, enabling men to make empowered decisions about their health.

Sexual Health and Function in Men with Prostate Conditions

Effects of Prostate Conditions on Sexual Health

Prostate conditions, particularly benign prostatic hypertrophy (BPH) and prostate cancer, significantly impact sexual health in aging males. BPH, a non-cancerous enlargement of the prostate, can cause urinary symptoms that indirectly affect sexual function. Men with BPH often experience difficulties such as decreased libido and erectile dysfunction, which can lead to frustration and a decline in overall quality of life. Understanding the relationship between these conditions and sexual health is crucial for older men navigating these challenges.

Prostate cancer poses both physical and psychological challenges that can also influence sexual health. The diagnosis of prostate cancer often leads to anxiety and depression, which can further diminish sexual desire and performance. Treatments for prostate cancer, such as surgery and radiation, may result in side effects like erectile dysfunction or altered orgasm, affecting a man's sexual identity and relationships. Addressing these issues openly can help men cope better and seek appropriate support.

Early detection and screening methods for prostate conditions are essential in managing sexual health outcomes. Regular check-ups and discussions with healthcare providers about prostate health can lead to timely interventions that may preserve sexual function. Screening methods, including PSA tests and biopsies, allow for the early identification of potential issues, enabling men to make informed decisions about their health and treatment options.

Lifestyle modifications play a vital role in managing benign prostatic hypertrophy and improving sexual health. Engaging in regular physical activity, maintaining a healthy weight, and avoiding excessive alcohol consumption can alleviate symptoms of BPH. Additionally, adopting a nutritious diet rich in fruits, vegetables, and healthy fats can support prostate health. These changes not only enhance physical well-being but can also boost self-esteem and confidence, positively impacting sexual relationships.

The psychological impact of prostate conditions cannot be overstated. Men diagnosed with prostate cancer may benefit from patient support groups and counselling services, which provide a platform to share experiences and strategies for coping. Understanding the emotional aspects of these diseases is crucial for fostering resilience and encouraging men to seek help. As advancements in treatments and therapies continue, it becomes increasingly vital for men to stay informed and proactive about their prostate health and its effects on their sexual well-being.

Treatment Options for Sexual Dysfunction

Sexual dysfunction is a common concern among aging males, particularly those who are dealing with prostate conditions such as benign prostatic hypertrophy (BPH) and prostate cancer. These conditions not only affect urinary function but can also significantly impact sexual health. Understanding the treatment options available is crucial for managing these issues effectively. This subchapter will explore various approaches to treating sexual dysfunction, helping men navigate their options and make informed decisions about their health.

One of the primary treatment options for sexual dysfunction is pharmacotherapy. Medications such as phosphodiesterase type 5 inhibitors, including Viagra and Cialis, are often prescribed to enhance erectile function. These medications work by increasing blood flow to the penis, making it easier to achieve and maintain an erection. However, it is essential for men to consult with their healthcare providers to determine the most suitable medication, taking into consideration any underlying health conditions or concurrent treatments for prostate diseases.

In addition to medication, lifestyle modifications can play a significant role in improving sexual function. Regular exercise, a balanced diet, and maintaining a healthy weight can enhance overall well-being and may alleviate some symptoms of sexual dysfunction. For men with BPH, managing urinary symptoms through lifestyle changes can also positively affect sexual health. Reducing alcohol consumption and quitting smoking are particularly beneficial, as these factors can contribute to erectile difficulties.

Another option for treating sexual dysfunction is therapy or counselling. Psychological factors, such as anxiety and depression, can profoundly affect sexual performance. Engaging with a therapist can help address these emotional aspects, providing coping strategies and improving the overall quality of life. Support groups for men facing prostate conditions can also offer valuable insights and shared experiences, fostering a sense of community and understanding.

Finally, alternative and complementary therapies, such as acupuncture and herbal supplements, are being explored for their potential benefits in treating sexual dysfunction. While some men may find these therapies helpful, it is crucial to approach them with caution and under the guidance of a healthcare professional. By combining medical treatments, lifestyle changes, psychological support, and alternative therapies, men can adopt a comprehensive approach to managing sexual dysfunction and enhancing their quality of life.

Open Communication with Partners

Open communication with partners is essential for men facing prostate diseases such as benign prostatic hypertrophy and prostate cancer. Discussing symptoms, treatment options, and emotional responses can create a supportive environment that fosters understanding and reduces anxiety. Partners play a crucial role in the journey of managing these conditions, and sharing concerns can lead to better coping strategies and improved overall health outcomes.

When men are open about their prostate health, it not only benefits themselves but also helps their partners understand what they are going through. This transparency can address fears and misconceptions about the diseases and their implications. Encouraging partners to ask questions and express their feelings can strengthen the relationship and create a sense of teamwork in tackling the challenges posed by prostate conditions.

Moreover, many lifestyle modifications can be implemented when both partners are involved. For instance, dietary changes and exercise routines can be more effective when shared. Cooking healthy meals together or participating in physical activities can enhance emotional bonds while simultaneously promoting prostate health. This collaborative approach can make lifestyle changes feel less daunting and more achievable.

Additionally, the psychological impact of a prostate cancer diagnosis can be overwhelming for both the patient and their partner. Open discussions about fears, treatment side effects, and emotional struggles can help alleviate stress and foster a supportive atmosphere. It is essential for partners to recognize that they, too, may experience feelings of anxiety and uncertainty, and sharing these feelings can lead to mutual support and understanding.

Finally, seeking external support through patient support groups can be beneficial for both partners. These groups provide a platform for sharing experiences and gaining insights from others in similar situations. By communicating openly and seeking resources together, couples can navigate the complexities of prostate diseases more effectively, ensuring that both partners feel heard, supported, and empowered in their journey toward health and wellness.

Alternative and Complementary Therapies for Prostate Health

Herbal Remedies

Herbal remedies have gained significant attention in recent years, especially among aging males seeking alternative ways to manage prostate health. Many men are increasingly turning to natural solutions like saw palmetto, Pygeum, and stinging nettle to alleviate symptoms associated with benign prostatic hypertrophy (BPH). These herbs are believed to help reduce urinary frequency and improve overall prostate function, offering a holistic approach to care that resonates with those wary of traditional medications.

In addition to addressing BPH, some herbal remedies are being explored for their potential benefits in the realm of prostate cancer. Research suggests that certain plant compounds, such as lycopene found in tomatoes and turmeric's active ingredient curcumin, may possess anti-cancer properties. These substances are thought to contribute to cellular health and may even play a role in preventing the progression of prostate malignancies, making them appealing options for men looking to enhance their nutritional interventions.

The psychological impact of a prostate cancer diagnosis can be profound, and many men search for supportive therapies to cope with the emotional strain. Herbal remedies can serve as a complementary approach, with adaptogens like ashwagandha and rhodiola known for their stress-reducing properties. By incorporating these herbs into daily routines, older men may find not only physical relief but also emotional balance, which is critical during their treatment journey.

As advancements in prostate cancer treatments continue to evolve, the integration of herbal remedies into standard care practices offers an exciting avenue for research. Understanding the role of genetics in prostate diseases highlights the importance of personalized approaches, including the potential benefits of combining genetic insights with herbal therapies. This integration may empower patients to make informed decisions about their health, blending traditional and alternative methods for a more comprehensive treatment plan.

Regular medical check-ups remain essential for aging males, and discussing herbal remedies with healthcare providers can lead to a more tailored approach to prostate health. As more evidence emerges regarding the efficacy of these natural treatments, the conversation around alternative and complementary therapies will expand. Engaging with patient support groups can further enhance men's understanding of herbal remedies, fostering a community of shared experiences and knowledge that benefits all men facing prostate-related challenges.

Acupuncture and Other Therapies

Acupuncture is an ancient practice that has gained recognition in modern medicine for its potential benefits in managing various health conditions, including those affecting prostate health. For adult males, particularly older men dealing with benign prostatic hypertrophy (BPH) or prostate cancer, acupuncture may provide relief from symptoms and improve overall quality of life. The therapy involves inserting thin needles into specific points on the body to stimulate energy flow and alleviate discomfort, making it a valuable complementary approach alongside traditional medical treatments.

In addition to acupuncture, other alternative therapies have emerged as options for managing prostate conditions. Herbal remedies, for instance, are frequently explored by men seeking natural interventions for BPH and prostate cancer. Certain herbs, such as saw palmetto and Pygeum, have been shown to support prostate health by reducing inflammation and improving urinary function. However, it is crucial for patients to discuss these therapies with their healthcare providers to avoid potential interactions with prescribed medications.

Lifestyle modifications play a significant role in enhancing the effectiveness of acupuncture and other therapies. Regular physical activity, a balanced diet rich in antioxidants, and stress management techniques can strengthen the body's response to treatment. For older men, incorporating these changes can lead to better outcomes not only for prostate health but also for overall wellness. Engaging in activities like yoga or tai chi may complement acupuncture by promoting relaxation and improving circulation.

The psychological impact of a prostate cancer diagnosis can be profound, and integrating alternative therapies like acupuncture may help alleviate anxiety and depression. Many patients report feeling more empowered and in control of their health when they explore various treatment options. Support from patient groups that focus on alternative therapies can also provide valuable resources and emotional support, fostering a sense of community among those facing similar challenges.

As advances in prostate cancer treatments continue to evolve, the inclusion of alternative therapies represents a holistic approach to care. Men are encouraged to stay informed about their options and engage in regular medical check-ups. By combining traditional medical interventions with acupuncture and other complementary therapies, adult males can address prostate conditions effectively while improving their overall health and well-being.

Evaluating Effectiveness and Safety

Evaluating the effectiveness and safety of treatments for prostate diseases is essential for informed decision-making among adult males. As men age, conditions like benign prostatic hypertrophy (BPH) and prostate cancer become increasingly common. Understanding the potential benefits and risks associated with various treatment options can empower patients to engage actively in their healthcare. This process often involves a detailed discussion with healthcare professionals about the anticipated outcomes of different therapies, including surgical interventions, medications, and lifestyle modifications.

In the context of benign prostatic hypertrophy, evaluating treatment effectiveness encompasses monitoring symptom relief and quality of life improvements. Medications such as alpha-blockers and 5-alpha-reductase inhibitors are commonly prescribed to alleviate urinary symptoms. However, it's crucial to assess not only the immediate relief of symptoms but also the long-term effects of these drugs on overall prostate health. Patients should regularly review their treatment progress with their doctors to make necessary adjustments based on how well the therapy is working.

For prostate cancer, the evaluation of treatment effectiveness and safety is more complex due to the disease's varying aggressiveness and the diversity of treatment options available. Surgical treatments, radiation therapy, and hormonal therapies each carry distinct risks and benefits, which must be carefully weighed. Patients are encouraged to participate in shared decision-making, where they can discuss their values and preferences with their healthcare providers, ensuring that the chosen treatment aligns with their personal goals and lifestyle.

Lifestyle modifications play a pivotal role in managing prostate health, particularly for men with benign prostatic hypertrophy. Dietary changes, regular exercise, and stress reduction techniques have shown promise in improving symptoms and enhancing overall wellbeing. Evaluating the effectiveness of these lifestyle interventions involves not only subjective symptom reporting but also objective measures such as urinary flow rates and quality of life assessments, creating a comprehensive view of the impact of these changes.

Lastly, the psychological impact of a prostate cancer diagnosis cannot be overlooked in evaluating treatment effectiveness. Men may experience anxiety, depression, or changes in sexual health and function as a result of their diagnosis and treatment journey. Incorporating mental health support and community resources into the evaluation process can significantly improve patient outcomes. Being aware of the psychological dimensions of prostate disease ensures a holistic approach to treatment, ultimately contributing to better health and quality of life for aging males.

Conclusion

Summary of Key Points

Understanding the key points regarding prostate health is essential for adult males, particularly as they age. Two prevalent conditions affecting older men are benign prostatic hypertrophy (BPH) and prostate cancer. BPH can lead to uncomfortable urinary symptoms, while prostate cancer is a serious disease that requires early detection for better treatment outcomes. Recognizing these conditions and seeking timely medical advice can significantly impact a man's health and quality of life.

Early detection and screening methods play a crucial role in managing prostate conditions. Regular check-ups and tests, such as the PSA (Prostate-Specific Antigen) test, can help identify potential issues before they escalate. For aging males, understanding the importance of these screenings is vital, as early intervention can lead to more effective treatments and better prognoses for conditions like prostate cancer.

Lifestyle modifications are also key in managing benign prostatic hypertrophy. Engaging in regular physical activity, maintaining a healthy weight, and avoiding certain foods can alleviate symptoms associated with BPH. Additionally, nutritional interventions focusing on a diet rich in fruits, vegetables, and healthy fats can support prostate health and may reduce the risk of developing prostate diseases.

The psychological impact of a prostate cancer diagnosis cannot be overlooked. Men may experience anxiety, depression, and a sense of loss of control over their health. Support from patient groups and resources can provide essential emotional backing, helping individuals navigate their feelings and connect with others facing similar challenges. Furthermore, advances in treatment options, including surgery, radiation, and hormone therapies, have improved the outlook for many diagnosed with prostate cancer.

Lastly, sexual health and function are important considerations for men dealing with prostate conditions. Open discussions with healthcare providers can help address concerns and explore alternative and complementary therapies that may support prostate health. Regular medical check-ups, combined with a proactive approach to lifestyle and nutrition, empower men to take charge of their health and well-being as they age, ensuring a better quality of life despite any prostate-related challenges.

Encouragement for Proactive Health Management

Proactive health management is crucial for adult males, especially as they age and face conditions like benign prostatic hypertrophy (BPH) and prostate cancer. Being informed about these diseases empowers men to take charge of their health. Understanding the symptoms and risks associated with prostate conditions encourages timely medical visits and screenings, leading to early detection. Men should recognize that their health is in their hands and that regular check-ups are vital for maintaining prostate health and overall well-being.

Lifestyle modifications play a significant role in managing benign prostatic hypertrophy. Engaging in regular physical activity, maintaining a healthy weight, and avoiding excessive alcohol and caffeine can alleviate symptoms. Additionally, dietary choices, such as increasing the intake of fruits, vegetables, and healthy fats, can contribute positively to prostate health. Men are encouraged to think of these changes not just as remedies, but as integral parts of a healthy lifestyle that can enhance their quality of life.

Nutritional interventions are equally important for prostate health. A diet rich in omega-3 fatty acids, antioxidants, and specific vitamins can help mitigate the risks associated with prostate diseases. Foods such as fatty fish, tomatoes, and cruciferous vegetables have been linked to better prostate health outcomes. Men should be proactive about their diet, understanding how what they eat can influence their risk of developing prostate conditions and how it can aid in their management.

The psychological impact of a prostate cancer diagnosis cannot be overlooked. Many men experience anxiety, depression, or fear when faced with such a diagnosis. It is essential for men to seek support, whether through patient support groups or talking to mental health professionals. Acknowledging these feelings and discussing them openly can foster resilience and improve coping strategies, which are crucial for navigating the challenges that come with prostate conditions.

Advances in treatments and therapies for prostate cancer offer hope for many men. Staying updated on new medical interventions, such as immunotherapy and targeted therapies, can empower men to make informed decisions about their health. Proactive health management involves not only understanding one's condition but also being aware of the available resources and support systems.

With the right mindset and lifestyle choices, men can significantly influence their health outcomes and live fulfilling lives despite the challenges posed by prostate diseases.

Pause for Thought

- As men age prostate health becomes a critical concern, the two most common conditions affecting this demographic are benign prostate hypertrophy (BPH) and prostate cancer. BPH involves enlargement of the prostate gland which can lead to uncomfortable urinary symptoms which can significantly affect the quality of life.
- Prostate cancer remains one of the most prevalent form of cancer among men thus making understanding its risk and management essential for older men and their partners. To this end early detection and screening methods play a vital role in managing prostate health.
- It is felt that screening practices such as the blood test assessing the value of the prostate specific antigen (PSA) coupled with the digital rectal examination are crucial for early diagnosis. These methods can facilitate timely interventions that may improve outcomes and reduce the risk of complications associated with prostate diseases.
- Encouraging lifestyle modifications can greatly assist men in managing BPH. This can be achieved by engaging in regular physical activity, maintaining a healthy weight and avoiding irritants such as caffeine and alcohol can help alleviate symptoms associated with BPH. This can be

facilitated by incorporating specific exercises targeting pelvic floor muscles which can enhance urinary control and improve overall prostate health.

- Nutritional interventions also play a significant role in promoting prostate health. A diet rich in fruits, vegetables, and healthy fats, particularly omega-3 fatty acids, has been linked to a lower risk of prostate issues. Foods high in antioxidants, such as tomatoes and broccoli, may also provide protective benefits against prostate cancer. By focusing on nutrition, aging men can take proactive steps towards better prostate health and overall wellbeing.
- The diagnosis of prostate cancer can be far reaching affecting not only the patient but their families and carers. Support groups and resources are essential in providing emotional support and guidance through treatment and recovery. Advancements in prostate cancer treatments, including targeted therapies and immunotherapy, offer hope for improved outcomes.
- The relationship between BPH and prostate cancer is an important consideration for aging men. BPH is not cancerous, but its symptoms can mimic those of prostate cancer, leading to confusion and anxiety. Hence the need for regular screening and early detection.
- The psychological impact of a prostate diagnosis, whether BPH or cancer cannot be ignored as men may experience feelings of fear, anxiety and

depression, particularly when facing treatment decisions on lifestyle changes.

- Engaging with others who share similar experiences can provide valuable emotional support and foster a sense of community, which is essential for mental well-being and resilience during this phase of life.
- Prostate cancer often develops silently, making awareness of symptoms and risk factors essential. The earlier the condition is detected, the better the treatment outcomes. Hence the recommendation for PSA test and digital rectal examinations for men from 50 years of age or those with a family history of prostate disease.

Take Home Nuggets

- In maintaining prostate health, dietary choices play a crucial role. Foods rich in antioxidants such as tomatoes because of their lycopene content, offer protection against prostate cancer, so too are cruciferous vegetables like broccoli, and cauliflower which functions through hormonal regulation which may contribute to prostate issues. Omega-3 fatty acids are particularly friendly to the prostate and is found in fatty fish such as salmon and mackerel. This has anti-inflammatory properties. Other foods like walnut and flaxseeds are excellent sources of omega-3 fatty acids. These are therefore useful additions to the diet of adult and aging men. They are believed to be involved in hormone regulation. Adequate water intake will further promote prostate health. On the other hand foods like red meat and processed meats are best avoided , so too are diary products. High calcium intake has been associated with increased risk of prostate cancer. Almond and soya milk are better options to cow's milk. Carbohydrates and sugars because of their association with obesity and insulin resistance are best avoided, they can also lead to a spike in blood sugar, thus promoting inflammation in the body.

- Advances in prostate cancer treatments and therapies have significantly improved patient outcomes. Management options range from active surveillance to surgery, radiation therapy and hormone therapy. Genetic testing is becoming an increasingly important tool in personalising treatment plans. Understanding the role of genetics in prostate disease can empower patients and their families in making decisions about their health and treatment options.
- PSA testing has become a cornerstone in the early detection and follow up of prostate diseases, understanding the benefits and limitations of this test is crucial. PSA is a protein produced by both normal and malignant cells of the prostate gland; an elevated level can indicate the presence of prostate disease. Regular testing can help in identifying issues at an early stage, which is essential for effective management.
- Digital rectal examination (DRE) is an essential screening tool for assessing prostate health, particularly for adult males as well as older

men. This simple procedure allows health care providers to evaluate the prostate for abnormalities that may indicate BPH or prostate cancer.

- During a DRE, a health care provider uses a gloved finger to examine the prostate gland through the rectal wall, checking for any irregularities in size , shape or texture. Early detection of these abnormalities can significantly enhance treatment outcomes and improve the quality of life for patients.
- For men experiencing symptoms such as difficulty urinating, frequent urination, or pelvic discomfort a DRE can be a critical step in understanding their prostate health. Though thoughts of a DRE may cause anxiety, it is a quick procedure that typically last only a few minutes. The benefits of this simple quick examination play a crucial role in identifying potential prostate issues before they escalate into more serious health concerns.
- Men with a family history of prostate cancer should consider discussing a more proactive screening approach which may include regular DRE coupled PSA diagnostic test. Combining these assessments can lead to a more comprehensive understanding of prostate health and allow for more timely interventions.
- Genetic risk factors play a significant role in the development of prostate diseases; particularly BPH and prostate cancer. Men with a family history of these conditions are at higher risks. Specific gene mutations are linked to increased risks, for example, mutations in the BRCA1 and BRCA2

genes commonly associated with breast cancer have also been implicated in prostate cancer. It is important that men with these mutations discuss their screening options with their health care providers.

- Advances in prostate cancer treatments and therapies have significantly improved patient outcomes. Options such as hormone therapy, radiation and newer immunotherapies offer hope and can be tailored to individual needs. Simultaneously, genetic testing is becoming more prevalent, thus by understanding one's genetic predisposition, personalized treatment plans can be developed, thus empowering men in their health care. We emphasise the need for regular medical check ups for aging males to identify any potential issues early.
- Both BPH and prostate cancer significantly impact sexual health in aging males. Men with BPH often experience decreased libido and erectile dysfunction, which can be frustrating and lead to a decline in overall quality of life. Prostate cancer poses both physical and psychological challenges that can also influence sexual health. The diagnosis of cancer often leads to anxiety and depression which can further diminish sexual desire and performance. Treatments for prostate cancer such as surgery and radiation may lead to erectile dysfunction or altered orgasm; affecting a man's sexual identity and relationships.

Chapter 13: The Return to Self: A New Era of Men's Health

The Quiet Turning Point

There comes a moment in every man's life when the noise fades. The expectations, the bravado, the pressure to endure without question — all of it falls silent. What remains is the truth he has avoided, postponed, or simply never been taught to see.

That moment is now.

You have travelled through the pages of this book not as a passive reader, but as a man reclaiming something that was always yours: ownership of your body, your choices, and your future. This final chapter is not an ending. It is a return — a return to yourself.

The Weight of Unspoken Battles

Men carry battles that rarely make it into conversation. The pelvic discomfort dismissed as "normal." The fatigue explained away as "just stress." The sexual changes hidden behind humour. The emotional strain buried under responsibility.

For generations, men have been conditioned to push through pain, to minimise symptoms, to treat vulnerability as a threat rather than a tool. But silence has a cost. It steals years. It erodes confidence. It fractures relationships. It dims the spark that makes a man feel alive.

Understanding your health is not weakness. It is mastery. It is strategy. It is leadership of the highest order — leadership of yourself.

A New Model of Male Health

Throughout this book, you've been introduced to a different way of thinking about your body — one rooted in clarity, autonomy, and function. This new model of male health is built on five pillars:

Autonomy

You are the primary decision-maker in your health journey. No one knows your body better than you.

Knowledge

Understanding your anatomy, your pelvic floor, your hormones, your stress responses — this is power.

Prevention

Health is not something to rescue at the brink of collapse. It is something to cultivate daily.

Functionality

Strength, mobility, sexual health, continence, energy — these are not luxuries. They are the foundations of a life well lived.

Integration

Your mind, your relationships, your purpose, your biology — they are not separate chapters. They are one story.

The Man Who Leads Himself Picture the man you are becoming.

He knows his numbers — blood pressure, weight trends, prostate health markers. He understands his pelvic floor — how it supports him, how to protect it, how to restore it. He recognises stress patterns — and interrupts them before they take root. He invests in sleep, hydration, movement, and recovery — not as chores, but as acts of self-respect. He builds a life that supports his biology — not one that constantly fights against it.

This man is not defined by age, circumstance, or past choices. He is defined by awareness, intention, and courage.

Tools for the Next Decade

As you step forward, carry these practical commitments with you:

- Conduct an annual self-audit of your physical, mental, and sexual health.
- Maintain pelvic health as a lifelong practice, not a crisis response.
- Manage stress and inflammation with deliberate daily habits.
- Stay literate in your sexual health — understand changes, seek help early, and protect your confidence.

- Build a supportive ecosystem: clinicians you trust, partners who understand you, mentors who challenge you.

These tools are not complicated. They are consistent. And consistency is what transforms men.

Your Legacy of Strength

Every man leaves a legacy — not just in what he builds, but in how he lives. Your health is not a private matter. It shapes your relationships, your work, your presence, your longevity, and the example you set for the next generation.

Strength is not the absence of struggle. Strength is the willingness to face yourself honestly and act with intention.

You are not a passenger in your health journey.

You are the architect.

You are the protector of your future self.

You are the author of the next chapter of your life.

A Closing Reflection

Your health is not a chapter in your story — it is the ink.

Every choice you make writes the next line.

Choose boldly.

Choose wisely.

Choose yourself.

And as you close this book, remember this is not the end.

This is the beginning of the man you were always meant to be.

Pause for thought

- There comes a moment in every man's life when the noise fades. The expectations, the bravado, the pressure to endure without question – all of it falls silent. What remains is the truth he has avoided, postponed or simply never been taught to see! That moment is now!
- I hope this book helped you reclaim something that was always yours. Ownership of your body, your choices and your future. This is not meant to be an end, it is a return- a return to yourself.
- Men carry battles that he rarely talks about. The pelvic discomfort, he dismisses as normal, the fatigue he explains as just stress, the sexual changes that he hides behind humour, the emotional strain that he buries under responsibility.
- From our world, men have been conditioned to push through pain, minimize symptoms and to threat vulnerability as a threat rather than a tool. But silence has a cost. It steals years. It erodes confidence. It fractures relationships. It dims the spark that makes a man feel alive.

- Understanding your health is not weakness, it is mastery. It is strategy. It is leadership of the highest order – leadership of yourself.
- There is a different way of thinking about your body, one routed in clarity, autonomy, and function.
- Men have come to realize that they are the primary decision maker on their health journey. No one knows your body better than you.
- Understanding your anatomy, your pelvic floor, your hormones, your stress responses – gives you power.
- Health is not something to rescue at the brink of collapse. It is something to cultivate daily.
- Foundations of a life well lived requires strength, mobility, sexual health, continence, and energy, these are necessities not luxuries.

Take Home Nuggets

- Your mind, your relationship, your purpose, your biology – they are not separate chapters, they are one story.
- The man who leads himself can picture the man he is becoming. He invests in sleep, hydration, movement and recovery not as chores but as acts of self-respect.

- He ought to build a life that supports his biology, not one that constantly fights against it. Man is not defined by age, circumstance or past choices. He is defined by awareness, intention and courage.

- As you step forward, carry these practical commitments with you – conduct an annual audit of your physical, mental and sexual health. Maintain pelvic health as a lifelong practice not as a crisis response. Manage stress and inflammation with deliberate daily habits. Stay literate in your sexual health – understand changes, seek help early and protect your confidence. Build a supportive ecosystem. This may include clinicians you trust, partners who understand you, mentors who challenge you. Consistency is what transforms men.

- Your legacy of strength: every man leaves a legacy , not just what he builds but in how he lives. Your health is not a private matter, it shapes your relationships, your work, your presence, your longevity and the example you set for the next generation.

- Strength is not the absence of struggle. It is the willingness to face yourself honestly and act with intention.

- You are not the passenger in your health journey. You are the architect, the protection of your future self, you are the author of the next chapter of your life.

- Your health is not a chapter in your story – it is the ink; every choice you make writes the next line.
- Chose boldly, choose wisely, choose yourself.
- Remember, this is not the end, it is the beginning of the man you were always meant to be.

www.ingramcontent.com/pod-product-compliance
Ingram Content Group UK Ltd.
Pitfield, Milton Keynes, MK11 3LW, UK
UKHW061701190726
13853UKWH00008B/2343